An Introduction to Epidemiology

SECOND EDITION

THOMAS C. TIMMRECK, PhD

Professor of Public Health and Health Care Administration
Department of Health Science and Human Ecology
California State University, San Bernardino

JONES AND BARTLETT PUBLISHERS
Sudbury, Massachusetts
BOSTON   TORONTO   LONDON   SINGAPORE

World Headquarters

Jones and Bartlett Publishers
40 Tall Pine Drive
Sudbury, MA 01776
978-443-5000
info@jbpub.com
www.jbpub.com

Jones and Bartlett Publishers Canada
P.O. Box 19020
Toronto, ON M5S 1X1
CANADA

Jones and Bartlett Publishers International
Barb House, Barb Mews
London W6 7PA
UK

Acquisitions Editor	Paul Shepardson
Production Editor	Lianne B. Ames
Manufacturing Buyer	Jane Bromback
Editorial Production Service	Sue Gleason
Design Publishers	Publishers' Design and Production Services, Inc.
Typesetting	Publishers' Design and Production Services, Inc.
Cover Design	Chad Timmreck–45 design
Printing and Binding	Courier-Westford
Cover Printing	Courier-Westford

Library of Congress Cataloging-in-Publication Data

Timmreck, Thomas C.
    An introduction to epidemiology / Thomas C. Timmreck.—2nd ed.
      p.   cm.
    Includes bibliographical references and index.
    ISBN 0-7637-0635-3
    1. Epidemiology.   I. Title.
    [DNLM: 1. Epidemiological Methods.   2. Epidemiology.   WA 950 T5841
1998]
    RA651.T56   1998
    614.4—dc21
    DNLM /DLC
    for Library of Congress   98-15823
                                                      CIP

Printed in the United States of America
98 97 96   10 9 8 7 6 5 4 3

Dedication

To all of my dedicated students who have enjoyed, yet diligently
struggled through their epidemiology learning experiences, the
second edition of this book is dedicated to you.

Acknowledgment

A great deal of appreciation is extended to Ellen for her diligence and
support in the editing of the original manuscript of
An Introduction to Epidemiology

About the Author

Thomas C. Timmreck, Ph.D. has been actively involved in the field of public health, health science, and health services since his professional career began in 1971. His work has brought him to public health departments, community health services, hospitals, nursing homes, environmental health services, and both public and private social and health agencies. Dr. Timmreck has served on the full-time faculty at Texas Tech University, Idaho State University, Northern Arizona University, and is currently a Professor of Public Health and Health Care Administration, Department of Health Science and Human Ecology at California State University San Bernardino. Dr. Timmreck has also served on the adjunct faculty of the University of Redlands, University of Southern California, Chapman University, California State University Long Beach, Loretto Heights College, University of Colorado at Denver, University of Denver and Western International University in Phoenix, teaching both graduate and undergraduate courses. He has over 50 professional publications in a variety of subject areas including public health, health services, long-term care and gerontology, health education and health promotion, and behavioral health, and is the author of four nationally published books. Dr. Timmreck received his Ph.D. in health science from the University of Utah. In addition, he holds two master's degrees, one in community health and community health education from Oregon State University and one in counseling psychology and human relations and behavior from Northern Arizona University, and a Bachelor of Science degree in Health Science from the Brigham Young University. He also received a graduate certificate in gerontology from the Rocky Mountain Gerontology Center at the University of Utah. Dr. Timmreck has been a Registered Sanitarian and has taught public health and epidemiology courses for over 23 years.

Contents

Contents

Contents

Preface

The field of epidemiology has come a long way since the exciting days of infectious disease investigations by famous scientists such as Louis Pasteur, Dr. Robert Koch, and Dr. John Snow. The knowledge explosion in the fields of biology and medical science have advanced at such a rapid rate that it is difficult to keep up with. Epidemiology has benefited greatly from these advances, as it has from the knowledge gains made in the social and behavioral sciences. Advances in the field of statistics have aided biomedical and behavioral science research efforts by providing effective and sound analysis of research findings. However, these advances also have affected the perception of some biomedical science and epidemiology professionals as to what constitutes the field of epidemiology. Such perceptions have tended to cloud the importance of the basics of epidemiology which seem to be becoming lost to the processes of analyzing the findings of biomedical research.

Many recent books bearing the title of *epidemiology* are in fact biostatistics books, with limited information on the basics of epidemiological investigations or the study of epidemics. Biostatistics, an important branch of traditional statistics, is essential in completing the last phases of an epidemiological investigation, the analysis of the data. However, biostatistics is not epidemiology. Some epidemiology books seem to be written by biostatisticians for biostatisticians, with many of the basics left out, or at the most, quickly glossed over, in order to get to the biostatistics. Other epidemiology books are written by physicians with many advanced public health degrees and other outstanding credentials, who assume the student also has advanced levels of biomedical knowledge and background. Such books, written by advanced scientists for the other biomedical scientists, leave introductory students lost and bewildered.

This book was written and developed as an introductory epidemiology text for the student who has minimal training in the biomedical sciences and statistics. *Introduction to Epidemiology* is based on the premise of filling the role of a very basic text and that the advanced analysis of empirical research studies, using advanced statistical methods, are more akin to biostatistics than epidemiology and, therefore, are not included in this book and are left to biostatistics courses and books.

Many fine books are already available on statistics, empirical research design, and biostatistics and need not be included in an introductory epidemiology textbook. This book takes the introductory student of epidemiology up to and through descriptive statistics and stops at the threshold of inferential statistics. Thus, if the student wishes to know how to conduct advanced experimental studies and then analyze the results with T-tests, multivariate analysis, or ANOVAs, additional biostatistics and related statistical books and research resources should be sought.

Preface to the Second Edition

In this era of increased communicable diseases, new and unknown infections, and mutating pathogens, epidemiology has become more important than ever before. Interest in disease investigation is heightened by the regular reporting of disease outbreaks and unusual infections by newspapers, radio and television—including tabloid TV programs. More and more health science, health education and promotion, nursing and health care academic degree programs are seeing the importance of studying epidemiology, and now include the course in their programs of study. Epidemiology is now studied at both the undergraduate and graduate level, if for no other reason than to heighten disease awareness and promote disease prevention in students who are soon to be health care practitioners.

This book, *An Introduction to Epidemiology*, has been known for its ease of use, readability, and for being student-friendly. The second edition has become even more user-friendly with added pictures provided by the Centers for Disease Control and Prevention, "case files," and "news files," and has undergone some reorganization. The new edition also includes an extensive new case on the "History and Epidemiology of Polio." Additions to the Appendix include some Internet epidemiology-related addresses, epidemiology-related professional associations, and *Epi Info*. Several assignments are now set up to encourage the use of computers, and the concept of relative risk is presented in a simple straightforward fashion.

This book was written as a comprehensive basic introductory textbook for graduate and undergraduate courses in epidemiology or for entry level practitioners new to the practical work of epidemiology. The original premise behind the development of the book was that enough information and material are available at the introductory level of epidemiology that it need not be a biostatistics course. Colleagues, professors who teach the course, and students alike have firmly supported the necessity of a solid separate course and book on the fundamentals, keeping it basic epidemiology without turning to inferential statistics and biostatistics. Thus, *An Introduction to Epidemiology* remains unchanged in its fundamental approach, retaining student and reader friendliness and what made the book a unique introductory text in the first edition.

Foreword

Epidemiology is a fun and challenging subject to study as well as an interesting field to pursue as a career. Most solid undergraduate degree programs and graduate programs in community health and public health, environmental health, occupational health and industrial hygiene, health education and health promotion, health services administration and other health-related degree programs areas require a basic introductory course in epidemiology and that is one reason this book was written. *Introduction to Epidemiology* also can be valuable as a handbook for practicing epidemiologists. Thus, it is hoped that this book will be a useful and practical handbook for introductory epidemiology courses, as well as epidemiologists working in the field. They may be specialists in international projects in developing countries, or industrial hygienists within major industrial plants, or infectious disease nurses in hospitals and medical centers, chronic disease epidemiologists in government agencies, behavioral scientists conducting behavioral health epidemiological investigations, or staff epidemiologists in local public health departments.

C H A P T E R

1

Foundations of Epidemiology

CHAPTER OBJECTIVES

This chapter on foundations and basic concepts of epidemiology

- presents basic concepts, constructs, and principles foundational to epidemiology;
- defines *epidemiology, epidemiologist,* and related terms;
- presents the purposes, goals, scope, and uses of epidemiology;
- presents some basic concepts, constructs, and principles foundational to the role of the epidemiologist;
- presents the epidemiology triangle;
- reviews types and classifications of epidemics;
- presents an advanced epidemiology triangle for chronic diseases and behavioral disorders;
- presents the concepts and principles of *case* as used in epidemiology;
- presents the three levels of prevention used in public health and epidemiology;
- presents key terms and study questions for review of chapter concepts.

INTRODUCTION

What is epidemiology? What does epidemiology mean, and how is it defined? By turning to basic medical terminology to learn the meaning of this term, first we discover that the prefix

> **epi-** means "on, upon, befall,"

as in the medical term *epidermis*, which means "upon the body (skin)." The root

> **demo** means "people, population, man,"

as in the word *demographics*, which is the study of the statistics of populations. The suffix

> **-ology** means "the study of."

In true medical terminology fashion, one reads the suffix first, then the prefix and the root. Thus, the term epidemiology, if taken literally, means "that which befalls man."[1]

EPIDEMIOLOGY DEFINED

Some public health professionals view epidemiology as a science. Others view epidemiology as a method rather than a pure science, as it is not a clearly defined field. This book assumes that epidemiology is a scientific methodology. Epidemiology is an investigative method used to detect the cause or source of diseases, disorders, syndromes, conditions, or perils that cause pain, injury, illness, disability, or death in human populations or groups. An epidemiologist is often considered a "detective of diseases and epidemics."

Epidemiology has been defined in several ways. One definition is the study of the nature, cause, control, and determinants of the frequency and distribution of disease, disability, and death in human populations. Epidemiology also involves characterizing the distribution of health status, diseases, or other health problems in terms of age, sex, race, geography, religion, education, occupation, behaviors, time, place, person, etc. This characterization is done in order to explain the distribution of a disease or health-related problems in terms of the causal factors. Epidemiology is useful in assessing and explaining the impact of public health control measures, prevention programs, clinical intervention, and health services on diseases or other factors that impact the health status of a population. The epidemiology of a disease can include the description of its presence in a population and the factors controlling the particular disease's presence or absence.[2,3]

Concerned with the types and extent of injuries, conditions, or illnesses that beset groups or populations, epidemiology also deals with risk factors that impact, influence, provoke, and affect the distribution of diseases, defects, disabilities, and death.[3,4] As a scientific method, epidemiology is used to study patterns of occurrence influencing the factors listed above. The epidemiologist has the task of determining if there has been an increase, or a decrease in these factors over various time periods—days, weeks, months, years. The task also includes determining if one certain location or geographical area has an increase or decrease more than other locations or areas. A third concern is the characteristics of the people involved and if they differ or are alike in some way. In other words, the epidemiologist is highly interested in the *time, place,* and *person* aspects of disease, defect, disability, or death occurrences. The distribution of pathological conditions in human populations or those factors which influence this distribution are all the focus of epidemiology.[5,6]

EPIDEMIOLOGIST DEFINED

An **epidemiologist** (*-ist*, a suffix meaning "specialist") is a public health scientist who is responsible for carrying out all useful and effective activities needed for successful epidemiology practice. The epidemiologist uses **inductive** and **deductive reasoning**, is concerned with describing the distribution of disease, and fitting observations about disease occurrence into known scientific and medical knowledge. The epidemiologist uses sequences of reasoning and makes inferences from observations about occurrences of disease, defect, disability, injury, or death in groups or populations. The epidemiologist in his or her professional work activities draws upon the medical, biological, and behavioral sciences (anthropology, psychology, sociology, education), as well as statistics, demographics, health and medical care services, and computer sciences.[1,4,5]

The training of an epidemiologist can range from physicians with cross-training in public health and epidemiology, to doctorates in health science and public health to master's degrees and some bachelor's degrees in public health and health science. Some professionals pursue a bachelor's and master's degree with concentrations in epidemiology and become highly trained specialists in the field. Some preventive medicine physicians specialize in epidemiology. Epidemiologists are employed at all levels of federal, state, and local governments within the appropriate health agencies. They also find careers in health care organizations, private and voluntary health organizations, hospitals, the military, and private industry. Epidemiologists are also employed by universities and medical schools to teach the subject or do epidemiological research.

PURPOSES OF EPIDEMIOLOGY

According to Lilienfeld and Lilienfeld three general purposes of epidemiological studies exist.[5] The following three items are the updated purposes of epidemiology:

1. to explain the **etiology** (study of the cause of disease) of a single disease or group of diseases, conditions, disorders, defects, disabilities, syndromes, or death by analyzing medical and epidemiologic data using information management combined with information from any appropriate field or discipline including the social/behavioral sciences;

2. to determine if epidemiological data are consistent with the proposed hypotheses and with current scientific, behavioral, and biomedical knowledge;

3. to provide a basis for developing control measures and prevention procedures for groups and populations at risk, and for developing needed public health measures and practices; all of which are used for evaluation of the success of the measures, practices and intervention programs.

SCOPE AND APPLICATION OF EPIDEMIOLOGY

Historically, epidemiology was developed using infectious disease epidemics as a study model. The foundation of epidemiology still relies on disease models, methods, and approaches. Many epidemiological methods and approaches were developed historically while searching for the causes of the many devastating communicable diseases and epidemics that existed at the time. The knowledge and approaches used in early developments in the field are still found useful to modern day epidemiologists.

Even in ancient times, some epidemics were traced to noninfectious causes. In the 1700s James Lind traced scurvy to the lack of citrus in the diet (Chapter 3). Other nutritional deficiency diseases were linked to the lack of vitamins A and D. Several studies have associated lead poisoning to various ailments, colic, gout, mental retardation, and nervous disorders in children, artists, and potters. For example, it was observed in ancient times that artists using lead paints, who constantly put a point on their paint brushes with their lips and tongue later developed lead poisoning symptoms, mental diseases, and related chronic diseases. Similar observations were made about potters who used lead-based glazes to coat pots. In recent times, epidemiology has been found effective in developing cause-effect associations in noninfectious conditions such as drug abuse, suicide, automobile accidents, chemical poisoning, cancer, and heart disease. The areas of chronic disease and behavioral epidemiology are the fastest growing branches of the field.[3,7,8]

As an investigative method, epidemiology is the foundation of public health and preventive medicine. Epidemiology is used to determine the needs of disease control programs, to develop preventive programs and health services planning activities, and to establish patterns of endemic diseases, epidemics, and pandemics.

Endemic (**en-** is the prefix for "in or within") is the ongoing, usual level of, or constant presence of a disease within a given population or geographic area—the usual prevalence of a specific disease within a given area or group.

Hyperendemic (**hyper-** is the prefix for "above") is a term associated with endemic but not commonly used. It denotes a persistent level of activity beyond or above the expected prevalence, often associated with select, small, or distinct populations such as might be found in a hospital, nursing home or other institution. It also signifies a communicable disease that persists at a high yet continuous incidence level above the normal prevalence rate in a population and is found equally distributed in all ages and groups. A related but distinctly different type of endemic occurrence of disease in populations is holoendemic.

Holoendemic (**holo-** the prefix meaning "whole or all") describes a disease that is highly prevalent in a population and is commonly acquired early in life in most all of the children of the population. The prevalence of the disease decreases as the age of the group increases, so that the disease is less evident in adults than in children. Diseases fitting this category include chickenpox and in tropical climates, malaria.

Epidemic is an outbreak or occurrence of one specific disease from a single source, in a group, population, community, or geographical area, in excess of the usual level of expectancy. An epidemic exists when new cases exceed the prevalence of a disease. An acute outbreak—sharp increase of new cases that affect a significant group—is usually thought of as an epidemic. The seriousness and severity of the disease also influences the definition of an epidemic. If the disease is life threatening only a few cases need occur (such as in rabies) to constitute an epidemic.

Pandemic (**pan-** is a prefix for "all or across") is an epidemic that is widespread across a country, continent, or a large populace, possibly worldwide. AIDS is a pandemic disease.

INCIDENCE AND PREVALENCE DESCRIBED

How a disease outbreak affects a population and whether the disease is endemic or an epidemic in a population is described and determined in a specific manner. **Incidence** is one way a disease outbreak is determined. Incidence describes the extent that people, within a population who do not have a disease, develop the disease during a specific time period. The key to determining incidence is to look at the number of *new* cases of a disease in specific populations over a *specific period of time*. The focus is on new cases within a specific time within a specific group of people. High levels of incidence can indicate that an epidemic is at hand. Incidence can be observed by plotting an epidemic curve.

 Prevalence is the number of people within a population who have a certain disease, disorder, or condition at a given point in time. Prevalence is the counterpart of incidence, and without the incidence of disease there is no prevalence of disease. The key to prevalence is to look at the population from a cross-section view, at a specific point in time. It is like stopping the clock for a moment and asking how many cases of a disease exist in a group of people at that moment. This is called **point prevalence**. Incidence tells us about the occurrence of *new* cases. Prevalence tells us about the ongoing level of a disease in a population at a given point in time. Prevalence relies on two factors: (1) how many people have had the disease in the past (based on the previous incidence) and (2) the duration of the disease in the population. Incidence rates, prevalence rates, point prevalence, and the interrelationships of these variables are presented in Chapter 5.[2,3,5,10]

USES OF EPIDEMIOLOGY

Public health has found epidemiology most useful in assisting its mission, aims, and operations of protecting the health of populations and groups. Table 1.1 gives seven possible uses of epidemiology, and even though not a complete nor exhaustive list, it presents the basics.

TABLE 1.1 Seven uses of epidemiology

1. **To study the history of disease**
   - Epidemiology studies the trends of a disease for the prediction of trends.
   - The results of epidemiological studies are useful in planning for health services and public health.
2. **Community diagnosis**
   - What are the diseases, conditions, injuries, disorders, disabilities, defects causing illness, health problems, or death in a community or region?
3. **Look at risks of individuals as they affect groups or populations**
   - What are the risk factors, problems, behaviors that affect groups?
   - Groups are studied by doing risk factor assessments and health appraisal approaches, e.g., health risk, appraisal, health screening, medical exams, disease assessments, etc.
4. **Assessment, evaluation, and research**
   - How well do public health and health services meet the problems and needs of the population or group?
   - Effectiveness; efficiency; quality; quantity; access; availability of services to treat, control, or prevent disease; injury; disability; or death are studied.

(continued)

TABLE 1.1   (Continued)

---

5. **Completing the clinical picture**
   - Identification and diagnostic processes to establish that a condition exists or that a person has a specific disease.
   - Cause-effect relationships are determined, e.g., strep throat can cause rheumatic fever.

6. **Identification of syndromes**
   - Help to establish and set criteria to define syndromes, some examples are: Down, fetal alcohol, sudden death in infants, etc.

7. **Determine the causes and sources of disease**
   - Epidemiological findings allow for control, prevention, and elimination of the causes of disease, conditions, injury, disability, or death.

It is important to note that a diagnosis or verification of a condition must be completed prior to starting an epidemiological study. This is much like the situation facing a police detective investigating a murder. He or she must determine that a crime has been committed before investigating it.

THE EPIDEMIOLOGY TRIANGLE

An outbreak of a disease in a population often involves several factors and entities. Many people, objects, avenues of transmission, and organisms can be involved in the spread of disease. To better understand and study this multifaceted phenomenon, an epidemiological model is helpful.

A single factor must be present for an infectious disease to occur, and that single factor is referred to as an *agent*. In communicable diseases, for example, the spirochete is the agent of syphilis; a bacteria is the agent of cholera. In occupationally related diseases, lead is the agent of lead poisoning; asbestos is the agent of asbestosis.

Epidemiology uses an ecological view to assess the interaction of various elements and factors in the environment and disease-related implications. Ecology is the relationship of organisms, one to another. Organisms share a similar environment and contribute to that environment. All diseases or conditions cannot always be attributed to a single cause or factor. When more than a single cause must be present for a disease to occur, this is called **multiple causation**. A single bacterium living in isolation is not sufficient to cause an outbreak of a disease and cannot by itself be responsible for the outbreak nor be labeled as the cause. The mode of transmission has to be considered, the level of sanitation within the community, the ability of the organism to grow and propagate, an environment or medium conducive to propagation, the communicability of the organism, the level of immunity within the population, the density of the population or the proximity of the cases to one another also contribute to the level or intensity of an outbreak.

When the colonists settled America, they introduced smallpox to the Native Americans. Epidemics became rampant and entire tribes died as a result. In the 1500s the entire native population of the island of Jamaica died when smallpox was introduced. The lack of exposure, levels of immunity in these people, various modes of transmission, lack of sanitation, lack of knowledge, and environmental conditions all allowed such epidemics to run wild and wipe out entire populations. A multitude of epidemiological circumstances allowed such epidemics to happen. The interrelatedness of four epidemiological factors often contribute to an outbreak of a disease. The four factors include (1) the role of the host, (2) an agent or disease-causing organism, (3) the environmental circumstances needed for a disease to thrive, survive, and spread, and (4) time-related issues.

Interrelatedness of the various factors that can contribute to a disease outbreak are presented best in a model. Figure 1.1 illustrates the traditional triangle of epidemiology. This model is useful in showing the interaction and interdependence of *environment, host, agent,* and *time* as used in the investigation of diseases and epidemics. This traditional triangle is based on the communicable disease model. The epidemiology triangle is used to analyze the role and interrelatedness of each of the four factors in the epidemiology of infectious diseases, that is, the *influence, reactivity,* and *effect* each factor has on the other three.

To understand the triangle of epidemiology one must have an understanding of the terms used in the triangle. The **agent** is the cause of the disease. Bacteria, virus, parasite, fungus, or mold are various agents found in the cause of infectious diseases. In other disease, conditions, disability, injury, or death situations, the agent may be a chemical such as a solvent, a physical factor such as radiation or heat, a nutritional deficiency, or some other substance, such as rattlesnake poison. One or several agents may contribute to an illness.

The **host** is an organism, usually a human or an animal, that harbors a disease. The host may or may not get the disease. A host offers subsistence and lodging for a pathogen. (A **pathogen** is a disease-causing microorganism or related substance.) The level of immunity, genetic makeup, levels of exposure, state of health, and overall fitness within the host can determine the effect a disease organism can have upon it. The makeup of the host and the organism's ability to accept the new environment can also be a determining factor, as some organisms thrive only under limited, ideal conditions. For example, many infectious disease organisms can exist only in a limited temperature range.

The **environment** is those favorable surroundings and conditions external to the human or animal that cause or allow disease transmission. Environmental factors can include the biological aspects as well as the social, cultural, and physical aspects of the environment. The surroundings in which an organism lives and the effect the surroundings

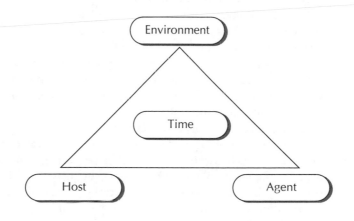

FIGURE 1.1 The triangle of epidemiology.

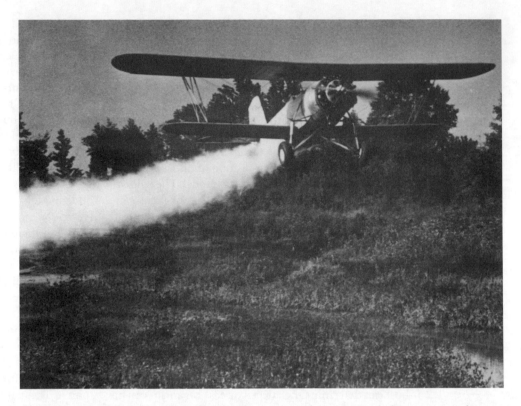

FIGURE 1.2   Public health officials often attack the *reservoir* of an *agent* at the *environment* leg of the triangle of epidemiology. The *chain of infection* can be broken by destroying the *vector* in the environment in which it lives. Airplanes are often used to spray the watery breeding places (environment) of mosquitoes in order to kill this *vector* of malaria, St. Louis encephalitis, and yellow fever. (Picture courtesy of Centers for Disease Control and Prevention, Atlanta, Georgia)

have on it are a part of the environment. Environment can be within a host or external to it in the community.

Time accounts for incubation periods, life expectancy of the host or the pathogen (agent), duration of the course of the illness or condition. Additional time issues include severity of illness in relation to how long a person is infected or until the condition causes death or passes the threshold of danger toward recovery. Delays in time from infection to symptoms, duration and threshold of an epidemic in a population (epidemic curve) are time elements the epidemiologist is concerned with. (See Chapters 2 and 9 for further information on disease-related issues and epidemic curves.)

The mission of the epidemiologist is to break one of the legs of the triangle of epidemiology, which disrupts the connection between environment, host, and agent, stopping the continuation of an outbreak. Similarly, the goals of public health are the control and prevention of disease (see Figure 1.2). By breaking one of the legs of the triangle, public health intervention can partially realize these goals and stop epidemics. An epidemic can be stopped when one of the elements of the triangle is interfered with, altered, changed, or removed from existence, so that the disease no longer continues along its mode of transmission and routes of infection.

SOME DISEASE TRANSMISSION CONCEPTS

Several disease transmission epidemiological concepts that relate to or influence the epidemiology triangle are fomite, vector, reservoir, and carrier.

Fomites (*fomes* = singular) are inanimate objects that serve a role in disease transmission. Fomites can be pencils, pens, drinking glasses, doorknobs, faucets, clothing, or any inanimate object that conveys infection by being contaminated with disease-causing organisms and then touched by another person (see Figure 1.3).

A **vector** is an insect, such as a fly, flea, mosquito, or small animal, such as a mouse, rat, or other rodent. A vector is any living nonhuman carrier of disease that transports and serves the process of disease transmission. The vector spreads an infectious agent from an infected human or animal to other susceptible humans or animals through its waste products, bite, body fluids, or indirectly through food contamination.

Reservoirs are humans, animals, plants, soil, or inanimate organic matter (feces or food) in which infectious organisms live and multiply. As infectious organisms reproduce in the reservoir, they do so in a manner that allows disease to be transmitted to a susceptible host. Humans often serve as both reservoir and host. When an animal transmits a disease to a human this is referred to as **zoonosis**. The World Health Organization states that **zoonoses** are those diseases and infections which are transmitted between vertebrate animals and man (W.H.O. Technical Report #378 of the Expert Committee on Zoonoses, 1967).

Another related term which describes a process that can contribute to the spread of disease is *carrier*. A **carrier** contains, spreads, or harbors an infectious organism (see Figure 1.4). The infected person harboring the disease-producing organism is often absent of discernible clinical manifestation of the disease. Yet, the person or animal serves as a potential source of infection and disease transmission for other humans (or animals). The carrier condition can occur throughout the entire course of a disease or the course of the person's life if not treated and can be inapparent because the carrier may not be sick (healthy carriers). Some carriers of certain diseases may be infected and can be carriers for their entire lives, such as Typhoid Mary (Chapter 3). Tuberculosis is another disease commonly

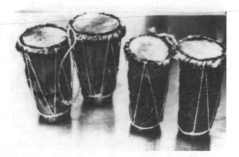

FIGURE 1.3 Diseases can be transmitted in many ways. The epidemiologist must consider every possible means of transmission when investigating an outbreak of disease. These drums, purchased in Haiti, served as a *fomite* and were responsible for transmitting cutaneous anthrax to the 22-year-old female who had purchased them. (Picture courtesy of Centers for Disease Control and Prevention, Atlanta, Georgia)

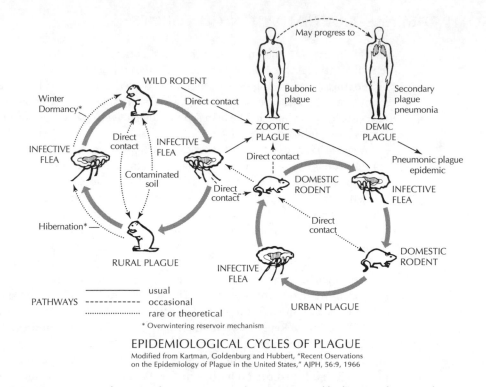

EPIDEMIOLOGICAL CYCLES OF PLAGUE

Modified from Kartman, Goldenburg and Hubbert, "Recent Oservations on the Epidemiology of Plague in the United States," AJPH, 56:9, 1966

FIGURE 1.4   Rodents and coyotes are often *carriers* of bubonic plague. Fleas serve as *vectors* in transmitting this disease to humans as shown in these epidemiological cycles of the bubonic plague. (Courtesy of Centers for Disease Control and Prevention, Atlanta, Georgia)

known to have carriers. Some carriers can be cured of this condition. Typhoid Mary could have been cured by surgery (removal of the gall bladder was the treatment at the time). If she had lived in modern times, antibiotics would have been used effectively.[2,3,4]

Carriers have been found to have several different conditions or states. Six types of carriers have been identified by the public health and medical fields.

Active carrier   An individual who has been exposed to and harbors a disease-causing organism and has done so for some time, even though they may have recovered from the disease is a carrier.

Convalescent carrier   An individual who has been exposed to and harbors a disease-causing organism (pathogen) and is in the recovery phase of the course of the disease but is still infectious is a convalescent carrier.

Healthy carrier   An individual who has been exposed to and harbors a disease-causing organism (pathogen) but has not become ill or has not shown any of the symptoms of the disease is a healthy carrier. This could be referred to as a subclinical case.

Incubatory carrier   An individual who has been exposed to and harbors a disease-causing organism (pathogen), is in the beginning stages of the disease, is showing symptoms, and has the ability to transmit the disease is an incubatory carrier.

Intermittent carrier   An individual who has been exposed to and harbors a disease-causing organism (pathogen) and who can intermittently spread the disease is an intermittent carrier and can spread the disease at different places or intervals.

Passive carrier   An individual who has been exposed to and harbors a disease-causing organism (pathogen) but has no signs or symptoms of the disease is a passive carrier, which is the same as a healthy carrier.[11,12]

MODES OF DISEASE TRANSMISSION

Several **modes of disease transmission** have been identified. There are various methods by which an agent can be passed from one host to the next, or can exit the host to infect another susceptible host—either a person or an animal. There are two general modes of disease transmission: direct transmission and indirect transmission.

    Direct transmission, also referred to as **person-to-person transmission**, is the direct and immediate transfer of the pathogen or agent from a host/reservoir to a susceptible host. Direct transmission can occur through direct physical contact or direct person-to-person contact, such as touching with contaminated hands, skin-to-skin contact, kissing, or sexual intercourse.

    Indirect transmission occurs when pathogens or agents are transferred or carried by some intermediate item, organism, means, or process to a susceptible host, resulting in disease. Fomites, vectors, air currents, dust particles, water droplets, water, food, oral-fecal contact, and other mechanisms that effectively transfer disease-causing organisms are means of indirect disease transmission. Indirect transmission is done in one or more of the following ways: **airborne** (via droplets or dust particles), **waterborne, vehicleborne**, or **vectorborne transmission**. *Airborne transmission* occurs when droplets or dust particles carry the pathogen to the host and infect it. *Waterborne transmission* occurs when a pathogen such as cholera or shigellosis, is carried in drinking water, swimming pools, streams, or lakes used for swimming. *Vehicleborne transmission* is related to fomites, such as eating utensils, clothing, washing items, combs, shared drinking bottles, and so on.

    Airborne transmission occurs when a person sneezes, coughs, or talks, spraying microscopic pathogen-carrying droplets into the air which can be breathed in by nearby susceptible hosts. It also occurs when droplets are carried through a building's heating or air conditioning ducts, or are spread by fans throughout a building or complex of buildings.

    Some epidemiologists classify droplet spread as direct transmission, because it usually takes place within a few feet of the susceptible host and because it is direct. Logically, however, the droplets from a sneeze or cough use the intermediary mechanism of the droplet to carry the pathogen. Thus, it is an indirect transmission. This is also a form of person-to-person transmission and is a common way for influenza and the common cold to be spread. Droplet spread can also be done by air-moving equipment and air-circulation processes (heating and air conditioning) within buildings, which carry dropletborne disease great distances, often to remote locations, causing illness. Tuberculosis and Legionnaire's disease have been spread this way (see case example, pages 302–305).

Some *vectorborne* disease *transmission* processes are simple mechanical processes, as when the pathogen uses a host (for example, a fly, flea, louse, or rat) as a mechanism for a ride, for nourishment, or as a physical transfer process in order to spread. This is called **mechanical transmission**. When the pathogen undergoes changes as part of its life cycle, while within the host/vector and before being transmitted to the new host, it is called **biologic transmission**. Biologic transmission is easily seen in malaria, in which the female *Anopheles* mosquito's blood meal is required for the *Plasmodium* protozoan to complete its sexual development cycle. This can occur only with the ingested blood nutrients found in the intestine of the *Anopheles* mosquito.

THE CHAIN OF INFECTION

There is a close association between the triangle of epidemiology and the **chain of infection** (Figure 1.5). Disease transmission occurs when the **pathogen** or agent leaves the **reservoir** through a **portal of exit** and is spread by one of several **modes of transmission**. The pathogen or disease-causing agent enters the body through a **portal of entry** and infects the host if the host is susceptible.

The *etiological agent/pathogen link* can include bacteria, viruses, worms, chemicals, or any other plant or animal substance or factor that can cause disease, disability, illness, syndrome, or death. The *source/reservoir* is the medium or habitat in which pathogens or infectious agents thrive, propagate, and multiply rapidly. Reservoirs are humans, animals, or certain environmental conditions or substances, such as food, feces, or decaying organic matter, that are conducive to the growth of pathogens. Many communicable or infectious diseases have human reservoirs and some animal reservoirs. Two types of human or animal reservoirs are generally recognized: symptomatic ill persons who have a disease, and carriers, or those who harbor a pathogen, who are asymptomatic and yet can transmit the disease.

Once a pathogen or agent leaves its reservoir, it goes by *mode of transmission* to a susceptible host, either by direct transmission (person-to-person contact) or by indirect transmission (airborne droplets or dust particles, vectors, fomites, foodborne substances). The final link in the chain of infection is thus the susceptible individual or *host*—usually a human or an animal. The host is generally protected from invasion of pathogens by the skin, mucous membranes, and physiological responses (mucous membranes' weeping to cleanse themselves, acidity in the stomach, cilia in the respiratory tract, coughing, and the natural response of the body's immune system). If the pathogen is able to enter the host, the result will most likely be illness if the host has no immunity to the pathogen. Susceptibility is based on levels of immunity. Natural immunity can come from genetic makeup; that is, some people seem better able to resist disease than others. Active, natural immunity

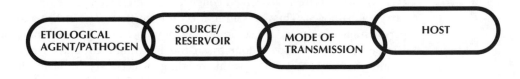

FIGURE 1.5   The chain of infection.

also occurs when the body develops antibodies and antigens in response to a pathogen invading the body. Active immunity is developed from vaccines; from a case of the disease, whether mild or serious; or from bacterial toxins. Passive immunity comes from antibodies entering a baby from its mother's placenta or from antitoxin or immune globulin injections.[13]

NEWS FILE

Pediculosis (Person-to-Person Transmission)

Head Lice: The Epidemic Continues

Some people think of head lice as a nuisance that bothers only the lower class and those with bad personal hygiene. Yet a nationwide epidemic of pediculosis continues to run rampant in both public and private schools.

The bloodsucking lice (Anoplura order) prefer mammal hosts and rarely infest even closely related species, including pets. Head lice limit themselves to the hair of the head near the nape of the neck and the ears. The life cycle of head lice is spent on the host, usually on the same person. The three-stage growth cycle of egg, nymph, and adult takes about three weeks. When head lice are not on the host, they die in a day or two. The head louse is very small, about 2 to 3 mm and can be found grasping the hair shaft near the scalp with its special claws. The adult female louse lives about a month, laying 150 or more eggs called nits, about 10 a day. Nits are not to be confused with solidified glubules of hair spray or dandruff. The yellowish-white, oval-shaped nit found glued to the bottom of the hair shaft, takes about a week to hatch.

Little disease is transmitted through lice, but they are a problem themselves. They suck blood and inject saliva during the infestation, causing itching and secondary infections from excreta, bites, and scratching.

Transmission occurs either directly, from contact with an infested person, or indirectly through fomites such as shared scarves, hats, coats, brushes, combs, sweaters, and bedding. The louse cannot jump or fly, so fomite transmission is used, mostly in schools, where children may try on and wear each other's clothing. Because lice like a frequent blood meal and a warm and fuzzy environment, person-to-person transmission is most common. Control comes largely from not sharing combs, brushes, and head clothing or sleeping with infested persons.

The only way to get rid of nits and lice is to use pesticide treatment which comes in the form of special shampoos, cream rinses, and topical lotions, with shampoos containing permethrin being most common and effective if used according to directions. Clothing and bedding must be washed in hot soapy water and dried in a hot dryer to destroy lice and nits. Nits must also be removed from the hair with fine-toothed combs. Children should be kept out of school until treatment is complete and successful.

(Source: California Morbidity, *March 1996, Division of Communicable Disease Control, California Department of Health Services)*

CLASSES OF EPIDEMICS/OUTBREAKS

Epidemics are classified differently depending on how they spread through a community or population. The three most common classifications are common source, propagated, and mixed epidemic.

A **common source epidemic** occurs when a group of persons is exposed to a common infection or source of germs (pathogenic agents), as when unvaccinated schoolchildren are exposed to other children with measles. Common source epidemics usually fall into three subcategories: point source, intermittent, and continuous epidemic. When the agent or pathogen comes from a single source, such as food, this is called a **point source epidemic**. For example, a group of people attend a church potluck picnic, where most of them share potato salad from a large common bowl. The majority of those who have eaten the potato salad fall ill because it was contaminated by staphylococcus bacteria. In a point source epidemic, **persons** exposed in one **place** at one **time** become ill within the incubation period of the agent (pathogen) obtained from a single source.

In some disease outbreaks, however, susceptible persons are exposed to the disease off and on over a period of time—days, weeks, or longer. Tuberculosis is often spread this way, through airborne transmission from coughing. Because tuberculosis is spread by direct person-to-person contact and because people move around and interact with many other people, the spread of the disease is irregular and somewhat unpredictable, with an irregular pattern—resulting in an **intermittent epidemic**.

When an epidemic spreads through a community or population at a high level, affecting a large number of people within the population without diminishing, it is considered continuous. As exposure grows and spreads, with people becoming ill on a regular basis, and even increasing for a time, this outbreak is considered a **continuous epidemic**.

When a single common source cannot easily be identified, yet the epidemic or disease outbreak continues to spread from person to person, growing in numbers and usually in an exponential growth pattern, it is considered a **propagated epidemic**. In this type of epidemic, cases occur over and over, exceeding one incubation period. The epidemic curve usually has a series of successive peaks, reflecting the increase in numbers of cases in each generation if the epidemic is not controlled or stopped. The epidemic can wane after a few generations. In some diseases, natural immunity or death can cause susceptibles to diminish. Resistance to the disease can occur along with treatment or immunization of all which reduce susceptibles. Disease transmission is usually by direct, person-to-person contact, or by fomiteborne, vehicleborne, or vectorborne transmission. Syphilis and other sexually transmitted diseases (STDs) are examples of such direct transmission. Hepatitis B and AIDS/HIV in needle-sharing drug users are examples of vehicleborne transmission. Malaria spread by mosquitoes is an example of vectorborne transmission.

Some disease outbreaks may have both common source and propagated epidemic features. A **mixed epidemic** occurs when a common source epidemic is followed by person-to-person contact and the disease is spread as a propagated outbreak. In some cases it is difficult to determine which came first. During the mid-1980s, at the beginning of the AIDS epidemic in San Francisco, HIV spread rapidly in bathhouses. Homosexual men had sexual contact before entering the bathhouses. Yet the bathhouses would be considered the common source aspect of the epidemic, and the person-to-person spread through sexual intercourse would be the source of direct transmission. Direct disease transmission from person-to-person contact occurred in some individuals before and after entering a bath-house. The common source of the bathhouses was clearly a point for public health inter-vention and control, so the bathhouses were closed in an attempt to slow the epidemic.

THE ADVANCED TRIANGLE OF EPIDEMIOLOGY

The epidemiology triangle as used in communicable disease is basic and foundational to all epidemiology. However, infectious diseases are no longer the leading cause of death in industrialized nations. Thus, a more advanced model of the triangle of epidemiology is needed. This new model includes all facets of the communicable disease model, and to be useful with the current causes of diseases, conditions, disorders, defects, injury, and death it must reflect current causes of illness and conditions. Thus, behavior, lifestyle factors, environmental causes, ecological elements, physical factors, and chronic diseases must be taken into account. Figure 1.6 presents an adapted and advanced model of the triangle of epidemiology, better reflecting the behavior, lifestyle, and chronic disease issues found in modern times.

The advanced model of the triangle of epidemiology, like the traditional epidemiology triangle, is not comprehensive or complete. However, the advanced model recognizes that disease states and conditions affecting a population are complex and that causative factors are many. It gives recognition to the fact that many factors and elements contribute to disease and maladies in populations. The concept of *agent* is replaced with *causative factors*, which implies the need to identify multiple causes or etiologic factors of disease, disability, injury, and death. In Chapter 10, the web of causation is presented and developed as an effective model of investigation into chronic disease and behaviorally founded causes of disease, disability, injury, and death. The web of causation shows the importance of looking for many causes or an array of contributing factors to various maladies. (One example is the web of causation for lead poisoning found in Chapter 10.)

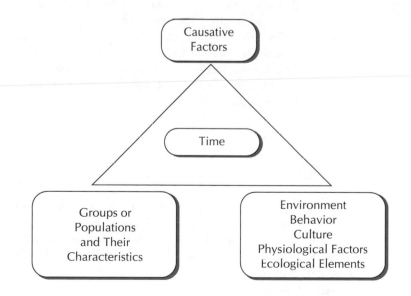

FIGURE 1.6   Advanced model of the triangle of epidemiology.

TABLE 1.2   Some broad aims and goals of epidemiology

Some aims of epidemiology are to

- determine the primary agent or ascertain causative factors;
- understand the causation of disease, disorders, or conditions;
- determine the characteristics of the agent or causative factors;
- define the mode of transmission;
- define and determine contributing factors;
- identify and explain geographic disease patterns;
- determine, describe, and report the natural course of disease, disability, injury, and death;
- determine control methods;
- determine preventive measures;
- aid in the planning and development of health services;
- provide administrative and planning data.

GOALS OF EPIDEMIOLOGY

Once both epidemiological triangles are understood, then a clearer understanding of the goals of epidemiology can be reached. In addition to the three purposes of epidemiology as suggested by Lilienfeld and Lilienfeld, several goals of epidemiology must be considered and reviewed (Table 1.2).[6,9]

One other aim of epidemiology is the development of a foundation for, and justification of preventive and control measures against diseases, conditions, disabilities, injuries, and death which affect groups of people but have not yet been developed or discovered.[11] Epidemiology also has the goal of developing hypotheses to demonstrate disease distribution patterns based on human characteristics. Specially designed studies are used to verify or disprove the hypotheses. Another goal is to test the validity and reliability of the constructs and assumptions on which preventive and control approaches are established. And yet another aim of epidemiology is to assist in the classification of conditions, illnesses, and diseases into groups that have common etiological characteristics, factors, and clinical pictures.[11]

CASE CONCEPTS IN EPIDEMIOLOGY

Epidemiology is based on examining, studying, and assessing the effects of disease, illness, and injury in groups and populations. However, the epidemiologist must not lose sight of the fact that populations or groups are made up of individuals. The diseased states of individuals are what make up cases. Each case or person with a disease becomes significant to the epidemiological investigation, as each is a part of the puzzle and is needed to complete the epidemiological picture.

Several case-related epidemiological concepts are important to the study of and investigation into a disease outbreak. When an epidemic is confirmed and the epidemiology investigation begins, one activity of the epidemiologist is to look for and examine cases of the disease. A **case** is a person who has been diagnosed with having a disease. Any individual in a population group, identified as having a particular disease, disorder, injury, or condition is also considered a case. A clinical record of an individual, someone identified in a screening process, a person identified from a survey of the population, or a general data registry can also be an epidemiologic case. Thus, the epidemiological definition of a case is not the same as the clinical definition, as a variety of criteria may be used to identify cases in epidemiology.

When establishing the existence of an epidemic, the epidemiologist looks for the first case of the disease that has been introduced into the population group, and that person is referred to as the **primary case**. The first case of the disease brought to the attention of the epidemiologist is the **index case**. The index case is not always the primary case but may be. Those persons who become infected and ill once a disease has been introduced into a population and who became infected from contact with the primary case are **secondary cases**. (See *herd immunity* in Chapter 2.)

In Chapter 5 you will be reviewing the concept of period prevalence, which is used to determine the usual, ongoing level of certain diseases in a select population over a specific time period. When assessing period prevalence, a **recurring case** is treated as if the person never had the disease or as if the person was never ill, and thus is viewed as a new case. Certain communicable diseases, injuries, or conditions can have several recurrences. An example of a disease that is prone to recurring is gonorrhea. Certain types of poisonings and occupational or behaviorally related conditions can recur over and over, if no intervention is taken.

A **new case** is a part of incidence and treated as such. A new case can be a first occurrence or can be a new case of the same disease. See the definition of *incidence* and *incidence rate* for a clearer understanding of the importance of new cases in incidence rates.

A **suspect case** is an individual or group of individuals who have all of the signs and symptoms of a disease or condition, yet have not been diagnosed as having the disease, nor has the cause of the symptoms been connected to a suspected pathogen. For example, a cholera outbreak could be in progress and a person could have vomiting and diarrhea, symptoms consistent with cholera. However, the cholera bacteria has not been identified as being in the person, nor has the disease been definitely confirmed as cholera, as it could be one of the other gastrointestinal diseases such as salmonella food poisoning.

As epidemics occur across time and in different places, each case must be described exactly the same way each time in order to standardize disease investigations. As cases occur in each separate epidemic, they must be described and diagnosed consistently from case to case, using the same diagnostic criteria. This is called **case definition**, or use of a standard set of criteria to determine whether a person exposed to a certain disease has that disease or condition. When standard disease diagnosis criteria are used by all physicians assisting in outbreak investigations, the epidemiologist can compare the numbers of cases of a disease that occur in one outbreak (numbers of new cases in a certain place and time) with those in different outbreaks of the same disease (cases from different epidemics in different places and times). Computerized laboratory analysis that is now available, even in remote communities, has increased the capability of arriving at a case-specific definition. With advanced computer-assisted support directly and quickly available from the Centers for Disease Control and Prevention (CDC), case definition of almost all diseases has become extremely accurate and specific. Different levels of diagnosis (suspect, probable, or confirmed) are generally used by the physician who is assisting in epidemic investigations.

As more information (such as laboratory results) becomes available to the physician, he or she generally upgrades the diagnosis. When all criteria are met and they meet the case definition, the case is classified as a confirmed case. If the case definition is not matched, then the exposed person is labeled not a case, and other possible diseases are considered until the case definition fits. Elaborate diagnoses are not always needed in some epidemics, in which obvious symptoms can be quickly seen, as in measles and chickenpox.[13]

As cases begin to die from disease or injury, the number of deaths from a specific disease or cause in a certain period per 100 episodes of the disease that occurred in that period are calculated. This is called the **case fatality ratio**. A ratio is used rather than a rate, as some deaths could be the results of episodes that began at an earlier time. Case fatality ratio is presented in greater detail in Chapter 4. As cases die, epidemics decline.

If people become ill enough to require hospitalization, the severity of the illness is of concern. **Case severity** is found by looking at several variables that are effective measures of it. One such measure is the average length of stay in a hospital (ALOS). The longer the ALOS the greater the severity of the illness. Subjectively, severity is also measured by how disabling or debilitating the illness is, the chances of recovery, how long the person is ill, and how much care is needed to attend to the person/case.[2,3,4,5]

LEVELS OF PREVENTION

In describing and characterizing the different levels of health care services, three levels have been established. **Primary care** is the first level of care and is the level of entry into the health care system such as a visit to the family physician, emergency room, or clinic. **Secondary care** is usually given in the hospital environment, extended care in a nursing home, or the usual care provided by a home health agency. Secondary levels of care can include minor or general surgery and routine and advanced nursing care. **Tertiary care** is the third and highest level of care. This level of care is found in larger, advanced-care hospitals which use the highest levels of technology such as open heart surgery, brain surgery, and specialty intensive care units such as a neonatal intensive care.

From the clinical model which uses three classes of medical care, three levels of prevention have emerged. The three levels are: primary, secondary, and tertiary prevention.

The notion behind three levels of prevention is that of detection and intervention into the cause, risk factors, and precursors of disease. Basic to all epidemiologic thought is that of prevention and control of disease in populations. Epidemiology is more interested in the prevention and control of disease than secondary and tertiary curative approaches found in traditional clinical medicine. Detection of and intervention into any and all maladies that plague mankind is of key importance. Prevention, though hard to measure and demonstrate empirically is less costly both in terms of human suffering and economic savings than crisis intervention and treating disease and conditions after they have occurred. The least productive and most costly attempts at improving the health status of populations is to treat diseases once they are in their advanced stages with limited hopes of full recovery.

Prevention aims to inhibit the development of diseases and maladies prior to their ever developing. Prevention concepts have expanded to include interrupting or slowing the progression of diseases or disorders. It is from these expanded notions that the three levels of prevention were developed.

Primary Prevention

Primary prevention involves halting any occurrence of a disease or disorder before it happens. Health promotion, health education, and health protection are three main facets of primary prevention. Lifestyle changes; community health education; health screening; school health education; health activation; good prenatal care; good behavioral choices; proper nutrition; safety and healthy conditions at home, school or the work place are all primary prevention activities. Fundamental public health measures and activities such as sanitation; infection control; immunizations; protection of food, milk, and water supplies; environmental protection; and protection against occupational hazards and accidents are all basic to primary prevention. Basic personal hygiene and public health measures have had a major impact on halting communicable disease epidemics. Immunizations, infection control (e.g., hand washing), refrigeration of foods, garbage collection, solid and liquid waste management, water supply protection and treatment, and general sanitation have reduced infectious disease threats to populations. Thus, the main causes of disease in industrialized nations no longer are the communicable diseases. Instead chronic disease, lifestyle, and human behavior are now the main contributing factors in the causes of death in the United States and industrialized nations (see Figure 1.7). The leading factors contributing to the causes of death are smoking and tobacco use, alcohol and substance abuse, accidents, diet, lack of physical fitness, emotional and mental health problems, and environmental health concerns. Prevention at its basic levels now has to be behaviorally directed and lifestyle oriented. Basic health promotion and protection activities of public health must never be ignored, discounted, or diminished. If these activities are not kept at a high level, communicable diseases can return to being the main cause of suffering, disease, and death. With public health activities being maintained, efforts at the primary prevention level have to focus on influencing individual behavior and protecting the environment. In the future less focus should be given to treatment and health care by physicians, and should be replaced with a major effort in primary prevention including adequate economic support for prevention programs and activities.[2,3,4,15]

Secondary Prevention

Secondary prevention is aimed at health screening and detection activities used to discover **pathogenic** states in individuals within a population. (*Pathogenic* means disease producing states; the term *pathological*, meaning due to disease, is also commonly used.) If pathogenic states are discovered early, diagnosis and early treatment can prevent conditions from progressing, from spreading within the population, and can stop or at least slow the progress of disease, disability, disorders, or death. Secondary prevention has the aim of blocking the progression of disease or an injury from developing into an impairment or disability.[2,3,11,15]

One area of health promotion that has been interesting to the public and effective in prevention has been health screening programs, often found in health fairs. Whether such programs are conducted through health fairs or as specialized programs within industry or at senior citizen housing complexes, the results are the same—early detection, referral, and prompt treatment to either cure the disease or halt it at the earliest stages of development as possible. At the very least, early detection can slow the progress of a disease, prevent

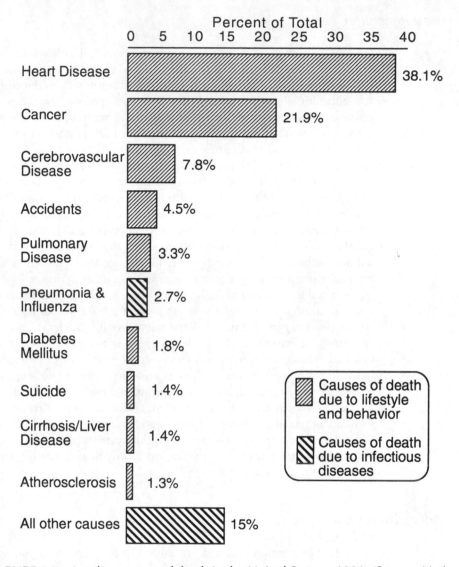

FIGURE 1.7   Leading causes of death in the United States—1991. (Source: National Center for Health Statistics, U.S. Public Health Service)

complications, limit disability, and halt or reverse the communicability of an infectious disease. Early intervention and treatment of a disease in single cases can prevent groups or major populations from acquiring communicable diseases. Such interventions provide primary prevention for persons not exposed and secondary prevention for those already infected. Additionally, secondary prevention can maintain already healthy behaviors and reverse unhealthy lifestyles through health education and behavior change programs, such as smoking cessation, weight loss, stress reduction, health counseling, or early admission into a drug treatment program.[2,3,15]

Tertiary Prevention

The aim of the third level of prevention is to retard or block the progression of a disability, condition, or disorder in order to keep it from becoming advanced and in need of excessive care. **Tertiary prevention** consists of limiting any disability by providing rehabilitation where disease, injury, or a disorder has already occurred and has caused damage. At this level the goal is to help those diseased, disabled, or injured individuals to avoid wasteful use of health care services and avoid becoming dependent upon health care practitioners and health care institutions. Prompt diagnosis and treatment followed by proper rehabilitation and post treatment recovery, along with proper patient education, behavior change, and lifestyle changes are all necessary so that diseases or disorders will not recur. At the very minimum, the progression of the disease or disorder or injury needs to be slowed and checked.[14,15]

Rehabilitation is any attempt to restore an afflicted person to a useful, productive, and satisfying lifestyle and to provide the highest quality of life possible, given the extent of the disease and disability. Rehabilitation is one component of tertiary prevention. Patient education, after care as well as health counseling and some aspects of health promotion can be important components of tertiary prevention.

CONCLUSION

Overall, the main function of epidemiology is to ascertain, in a population, those groups with high rates of disease, disability, injury or death and those with low rates. The epidemiologist asks questions that will help discover what the well group is doing that the ill group is not doing or what the sick population is doing that is different from the well population. This is done so that the causes of illness can be determined. The effectiveness of the modern epidemiological method lies in relating chronic diseases to the lifestyle and behaviors of different groups. By doing so, epidemiology unravels the multitude of causes of disease for which prevention and control programs can be developed.[16]

Concerned with control and a preventive approach to studying the cause and spread of disease, epidemiology has been found effective, not only in the behavior and lifestyle areas, but also is useful in the early stages of understanding uncontrolled diseases. Prevention activities include the disruption of the patterns of causation. Even before all aspects of the disease are known or understood, epidemiology can help establish whether there is one cause or a combination of causes. Epidemiology has been a solid contributor to preventive medicine and in reducing morbidity and mortality. With the cost of health care escalating, epidemiology has a definite role in contributing to the control and prevention of not only uncontrolled communicable diseases, but chronic as well as lifestyle and behaviorally related diseases and conditions.[17]

EXERCISES

Key Terms

Define and explain the following terms.

agent	new case
airborne transmission	pandemic
biologic transmission	pathogen
carrier	pathogenic
case	persons
case definition	person-to-person transmission
case fatality ratio	place
case severity	point prevalence
chain of infection	point source epidemic
common source epidemic	portal of entry
continuous epidemic	portal of exit
deductive reasoning	prevalence
direct transmission	primary care
endemic	primary case
environment	primary prevention
epidemic	propagated epidemic
epidemiologist	recurring case
epidemiology	rehabilitation
etiology	reservoir
fomite	secondary care
holoendemic	secondary case
host	secondary prevention
hyperendemic	suspect case
incidence	tertiary care
index case	tertiary prevention
indirect transmission	time
inductive reasoning	vector
intermittent epidemic	vectorborne transmission
mechanical transmission	vehicleborne transmission
mixed epidemic	waterborne transmission
modes of disease transmission	zoonoses
multiple causation	zoonosis

Study Questions

1.1 Define and explain the role of the epidemiologist, including academic degrees and training common to the field.

1.2 **Injuries Due to Falls.** Falls are the greatest cause of injury-related deaths in the United States. Between 16,000 and 17,000 persons die from injuries due to falls each year. For example, in Washington state the annual number of deaths from falls is approximately 300.

TABLE 1.3   Case 1. Children's activities that produce injuries

Activity	Frequency	Percent
Unknown	642	30.8
Playing	349	16.8
Bicycle-tricycle	197	9.5
Walking	189	9.1
Stairs	118	5.7
Running	79	3.8
Sleep-related	76	3.7
Gymnastics	64	3.1
Sitting	59	2.8
Climbing	51	2.5
Roller skating	43	2.1
Jumping	30	1.4
Bathing	29	1.4
Tree climbing	25	1.2
Horseback riding	23	1.1
Being carried	23	1.1
Sports	21	1.0
Skiing	20	1.0
Other (includes skateboarding)	41	1.9
TOTAL	2,079	100.0%

In an attempt to examine fatalities and patterns among nonfatal falls a retrospective study of the nature and causes of injuries attributed to falls was conducted. The main cause of death of children is accidents.[16] See Table 1.3.

Case 1.1 Children's Hospital   A study of 4,963 injury-related emergency room (ER) visits at Children's Hospital showed that 2,079 injuries (42%) were due to falls. Sixty percent of these occurred in April through September. More males (58%) than females were treated. Saturday and Sunday were the days with the highest frequency of injuries treated and the evening (3–11 PM) was the peak period of treatment of injuries due to falls. Most common types of injuries were lacerations (42%), contusions (18%), and fractures (14%). Of the 2,079 persons seen in the ER with injuries due to falls, 1,470 (71%) were treated and released, and 153 were admitted.[14]

Of all the 2,079 injury-related, emergency room visits, 223 involved repeat visits: 101 children had two injuries due to falls and 7 children were treated for 3 falls. More repeaters were treated in August (18%) than any other month. Sunday and Monday accounted for 43% of repeat injuries, but the time of day did not appear to be a factor in repeated visits to the ER.[14] (See Table 1.3 for children's activities known to produce injuries as reported in the state of Washington.)

1.3   From Case 1.1, present the facts related to *time*, and explain the role time plays in accidents in children.

1.4   Using the advanced model of the epidemiology triangle and Case 1.1, describe and discuss the causative factors (agent) contributing to falls in children. What are the environmental, behavioral, cultural, physiological, ecological factors (environment) which contribute to falls? What are the traits and characteristics of the group and population (host) that contribute to falls?

1.5   Which of the types of falls would best lend themselves to primary prevention activities? What types of secondary prevention activities might one expect to be needed from the list of accidents?

Case 1.2 Emergency Medical Services (EMS)   Emergency responses were made to 1,551 nonindustrial injuries due to falls. Of the total, 869 falls (56%) occurred at home and 682 (44%) occurred elsewhere. The very young (less than 4 years old) and the very old (80+ years) were the most vulnerable to falls. Persons over age 60 accounted for 44% of the total emergency calls due to nonindustrial falls. On weekends most injuries from falls occurred in the home. Time pattern analysis revealed that the greatest number of injuries due to falls at home occurred in the late afternoon and evening, between 3 PM and midnight.

Three socioeconomic strata were identified from census tract information. Age and sex was tabulated for the three strata areas based on falls in the home. The greatest use of the EMS was by those over 60 years of age in all three strata levels. Those 40–59 in the low socioeconomic group and infants through 9 years of age in the low socioeconomic group were next highest users. The highest socioeconomic group had the lowest rates for each age group.[14] The percentages given are out of total emergency responses by the EMS. Table 1.4 represents percentages of falls per total population based on the rates per 100,000 people. In Table 1.4

- Population for the high socioeconomic group was 143,798.
- Population for the medium socioeconomic group was 249,381.
- Population for the low socioeconomic group was 138,413.

TABLE 1.4   Case 2. Home falls and emergency medical service response in the state of Washington

Age Group	High Socio-economic Rate/ 100,000	% Total Popu-lation	Medium Socio-economic Rate/ 100,000	% Total Popu-lation	Low Socio-economic Rate/ 100,000	% Total Popu-lation
0–9	87.95	3.8	199.88	6.4	260.24	2.9
10–19	35.94	4.8	87.43	6.7	104.81	2.9
20–39	29.69	8.2	60.77	14.9	104.76	9.1
40–59	60.66	6.8	168.42	9.7	288.89	5.1
60+	444.05	3.4	355.18	9.3	420.66	5.9
TOTAL	—	27.05	—	46.91	—	26.04

1.6 As learned from the above case on Emergency Medical Services (EMS), what importance does age play in falls? Present statistics and provide a discussion of reasons for the age related statistics and differences.

1.7 Explain the effect of socioeconomic status on falls as responded to by the EMS, as shown in Table 1.4 and from the case on the EMS and falls. What levels of socioeconomic status have falls most often? Which age groups plus socioeconomic groups have highest rate of falls? Why? Explain. Which age groups plus socioeconomic groups have lowest rate of falls? Why? Explain. What role does age play in the assessment? Why? Explain.

1.8 Explain the epidemiology triangle and compare and contrast it to the advanced epidemiology triangle. How are the two triangles alike and how do they differ? Include a discussion of each component and the interrelatedness of the various components of the triangles.

1.9 Review Figure 1.7, then explain the implications of the ten leading causes of death on public health and epidemiology including the three levels of prevention.

1.10 Compare and contrast incidence with prevalence. Explain how these two principles differ and identify which is a subelement of the other.

1.11 Using the three levels of prevention and related epidemiological and public health activities, discuss how these apply to polio.

1.12 Using the three levels of prevention, how would you apply them to a 45-year-old female who had the following risk factors? Smoking for 25 years, heavy alcohol consumption, high fat diet, no exercise as she worked 12 hour days as an administrative assistant in a high-pressure law firm, and is now in physical therapy recovering from a stroke that affected one whole side of her body and her speech.

REFERENCES

1. Chabner, D.E. 1981. *Language of Medicine*, 2nd edition. Philadelphia: W.B. Saunders.
2. Timmreck, T.C. 1997. *Health Services Cyclopedic Dictionary*, 3rd edition. Sudbury, MA: Jones and Bartlett Publishers Inc.
3. Mausner, J. and A.K. Bahn. 1974. *Epidemiology: An Introductory Text*. Philadelphia: W.B. Saunders.
4. Shindell, S., J.C. Salloway, and C.M. Oberembi. 1976. *A Coursebook in Health Care Delivery*. New York: Appleton-Century-Crofts.
5. Lilienfeld, A.M. and D.E. Lilienfeld. 1980. *Foundations of Epidemiology*, 2nd edition. New York: Oxford University Press.
6. Lilienfeld, D.E. 1978. "Definitions of Epidemiology," *American Journal of Epidemiology*, 107, pp. 87–90.
7. Buck, C., A. Llopis, E. Najera, and M. Terris. 1988. *The Challenge of Epidemiology: Issues and Selected Readings*. New York: Pan American Health Organization.
8. Hughes, P.H. and G.A. Crawford. 1974. "The High Drug Use Community: A Natural Laboratory for Epidemiological Experiments in Addiction Control," *American Journal of Public Health (Supplement)*: Vol. 64, December, pp. 11–15.
9. Hennekens, C.H. and J.E. Buring. 1987. *Epidemiology in Medicine*. Boston: Little, Brown and Company.
10. Rothman, K.J. 1986. *Modern Epidemiology*. Boston: Little, Brown and Company.

11. Thomas, C.L. (Editor.) 1981. *Taber's Cyclopedic Medical Dictionary*, 14th edition. Philadelphia: F.A. Davis Company.

12. Nester, E.W., B.J. McCarthy, C.E. Roberts, and N.N. Pearsall. 1973. *Microbiology*. New York: Holt, Rinehart & Winston.

13. Epidemiology Program Office. 1992. *Principles of Epidemiology: An Introduction to Applied Epidemiology and Biostatistics*, 2nd edition. Atlanta: Centers for Disease Control and Prevention (CDC), Public Health Service.

14. MacMahon, B. and T.F. Pugh. 1970. *Epidemiology Principles and Methods*. Boston: Little, Brown and Company.

15. Picket, G. and J.J. Hanlon. 1990. *Public Health: Administration and Practice*. St. Louis: Times Mirror/Mosby.

16. Centers for Disease Control and Prevention. 1978. Injury Due to Falls. *MMWR (Morbidity and Mortality Weekly Report)* Vol. 27, No. 23, pp. 192, 197–198.

17. Lilienfeld, D.E. 1978. Definitions of Epidemiology. *American Journal of Epidemiology*, Vol. 107, No. 2, pp. 87–90.

CHAPTER

2

Practical Disease Concepts in Epidemiology

CHAPTER OBJECTIVES

This chapter on disease concepts in epidemiology

- reviews the essential concepts of infectious diseases;
- compares acute diseases with chronic diseases;
- presents various classifications of communicable and noncommunicable diseases and conditions and their sources, transmission, and cause;
- reviews time and incubation factors in communicable diseases;
- reviews the role of zoonosis in communicable disease in humans;
- presents the notifiable diseases in the United States and the notifiable disease reporting system;
- reviews immunity and immunizations against infectious diseases;
- reviews herd immunity and disease control and prevention in populations;
- presents key terms and study questions for review of chapter concepts.

INTRODUCTION

Historically, epidemiology development was founded on tracking and studying infectious diseases as they affected populations of humans and animals. Thus, the model of epidemiology study is based on communicable and infectious disease outbreaks. The student of epidemiology should have a solid knowledge of the source, cause, spread, course, and control of communicable diseases. However, epidemiology is not limited to infectious diseases alone. In recent times epidemiology has been used to determine the source, cause, course, retardation, and maintenance of chronic diseases and disorders. Behaviorally founded and lifestyle caused diseases are also of great concern to epidemiology and will continue to be a major focus of epidemiology in the future.

Epidemiology has been of key importance in ascertaining the causes and control of human death, disabilities, diseases, defects, disorders, conditions, dysfunctions, syndromes, injuries, and illness throughout the world. In recent times epidemiology has been effective in the investigation of an array of maladies that go beyond communicable diseases and include the areas of human behavior, lifestyle, and chronic disease as they contribute to health and/or life threatening outcomes. Epidemiology has been used in investigating the cause of suicide, drug abuse, automobile accidents, dog bites, gunshot wounds, genetic disorders, obesity, and other behavior related maladies. Historically communicable disease has been the foundation of epidemiology, thus, this chapter presents basic information on infectious diseases. Additionally other basic information on noninfectious sources of disease and conditions including nutritional deficiency, psychiatric, and chronic diseases is provided.

ESSENTIALS OF COMMUNICABLE DISEASE

Disease processes are complex and require an understanding of anatomy, physiology, histology, biochemistry, microbiology, and related medical sciences. This book cannot attempt to provide a comprehensive foundation of all these fields of study. Thus, only the basics of diseases, their classification and processes will be provided in this chapter.

Disease is an elusive and somewhat vague concept and is defined socially and culturally as well as scientifically. Any disruption in the function and structure of the body can be considered a disease. **Disease** is defined as a pattern of responses by a living organism to some form of invasion by a foreign substance or injury, which causes an alteration of the organism's normal functioning. Disease can be further defined as an abnormal state in which the body is not capable of responding to or carrying on its normally required functions. Disease is also a failure of the adaptive mechanisms of an organism to counteract adequately the invasion of the body by a foreign substance, resulting in a disturbance in the function or structure of some part of the organism.[1,2,3,4,5]

Disease is multifactorial and may be prevented or treated by changing any or all of the factors contributing to the diseased state. Infectious diseases are caused by invading microscopic organisms called pathogens. Understanding diseases relies on understanding the etiological factors of a disease. Pathogens are the source of or cause of communicable diseases.

Pathogens are organisms or substances such as bacteria, viruses, or parasites that are capable of producing diseases. **Pathogenesis** is the development, production, or process of generating a disease. Another related concept is that of pathogenicity. **Pathogenic** refers to disease-causing or producing and **pathogenicity** describes the potential ability and strength of a pathogenic substance to cause disease. A nonpathogen is any microorganism, substance, or agent that has little or no ability to cause disease. Acute diseases are often highly communicable, infectious diseases. Diseases that are **infective** are those which the pathogen or agent has the capability to enter, survive, and multiply in the host (body). Another pathogen-related issue is the strength of the disease.

The host plays a major part in the ability of a microorganism to cause disease, that is, pathogenicity depends on the contributions of the host such as nutrients and a life-sustaining environment as well as the innate ability of the pathogen to cause disease. Closely associated to pathogenicity is virulence.

Virulence is the extent of pathogenicity or strength of different organisms. The ability of the pathogen to grow, to thrive, and to develop are factors of virulence and pathogenicity of organisms. The growth of the organism in one place makes the pathogen have strength or virulence. The capacity and strength of the disease to produce severe and fatal cases of illness is virulence.

One other factor that makes an organism pathogenic is its ability to enter the host. Some microorganisms affect plants; others affect only animals; others affect humans. Some can affect all three. Other pathogens are zoonotic microorganisms invading both humans and animals. The ability to get into a susceptible host and cause a disease within the host is termed **invasiveness**, which is the capacity of a microorganism to enter into and grow in or upon tissues of the host; whereas communicability of an organism depends more upon the environment, susceptible hosts, fomites, and vectors. Transmission of a disease is not solely a product of invasiveness but includes a set of factors and conditions which come into play at the time the disease is being spread, such as pathogenicity and virulence.

Those factors contributing to the source of or causation of a disease are referred to as **etiology**. It is fundamental to epidemiology to recognize that a simple casual association of an agent or substance to disease does not mean the same as disease causality. The actual cause of the disease must be directly associated with the onset of the disease. Cause-effect relationships must be based on common sense approaches, proven biomedical and scientific principles.[1,2,3,4,5] *Causality* and *association* both are presented in detail in Chapter 10.

Antibiotics work against pathogens because of their toxicity. That is, the antibiotic substance contains elements that are more toxic to bacteria than to the human body. **Toxins** are poisons and consequently kill bacteria or viruses by poisoning them. The strength of a substance or chemical is measured by how little it takes to work as a poison and how quickly it acts. The shorter the duration and the less of the substance needed to cause the desired organism to die, the more toxic it is and is said to have a high level of **toxicity**. For example, arsenic is a toxin once used to treat syphilis.[2]

Diseases have a range of seriousness, effect, duration, severity, and extent (Table 2.1). Based on these and other variables diseases are classified into three levels.

1. **Acute**—relatively severe, of short duration and often treatable; usually the patient either recovers or dies.

2. **Subacute**—intermediate in severity and duration, having some acute aspects to the disease but of longer duration and with a degree of severity that detracts from a complete state of health and is longer in duration than an acute disease. Expected to eventually heal, the patient may fully recover and does not have a chronic disease.

TABLE 2.1   Comparison of chronic disease with acute disease

	Chronic	*Acute (Infectious)*
Duration of Illness	Long-term, once acquired it lasts until death	Short-term or brief
Agent or Causative Factors	Environmental, lifestyle behavior, chemicals, substances, or unknown	Pathogens (microorganisms)
Treatment	Symptoms and pain are treated; minimal cure rate experienced	Antibiotics or chemicals directed at the pathogens
Course of the Disease and Pathological Changes	Intervention into pathogenesis is minimal and disease is usually not reversible	Intervention is usually effective and the disease is most often reversible
Goal of Care	Retard advancement of the disease; control, maintenance, rehabilitation	Total cure
Duration of Care	Long-term from onset to end of life	Short-term, until cured

3. Chronic—less severe but of long and continuous duration, lasting over long time periods if not a lifetime. The patient may not fully recover and the disease can get worse over time. Life is not immediately threatened, but may be over the long term.[1,2,3,4,5]

THE NATURAL COURSE OF DISEASE

Each disease has a natural course of progression if no medical intervention is taken and the disease is allowed to run its full course. The process of disease begins with an individual being susceptible to the disease and with a pathogenic agent virulent enough to cause illness. The natural course of the disease (also referred to as the natural history of the disease) is well documented for some diseases but not well understood in others. (See Figure 2.3 on page 39 to review the natural course of an upper respiratory disease, and Figure 9.8 to review the natural course of the disease poliomyelitis.) The natural course of the disease begins with the susceptible person's exposure to a pathogen. The pathogen propagates itself and then spreads within the host. Each disease, each pathogen, and each individual host varies in how a disease responds, spreads, and affects the body. The progress of a disease can be halted at any point, either by the strength of the response of the body's natural immune system or through intervention with antibiotics, therapeutics, or other medical interventions (Figure 2.1). The body responds first by undetected and unfelt changes. As the pathogen continues to propagate, changes are experienced by the host, marked by the onset of such symptoms as fever, headache, weakness, muscle aches, malaise, and upset stomach. The disease reacts within the body in the manner peculiar to that disease. The body responds, and generally the person either begins to recover and gets well, or health diminishes. The illness gets worse, eventually the pathogen overpowers the body, and the subject ends up disabled or dies. Figure 2.2 is a generalized presentation of the natural course of disease.

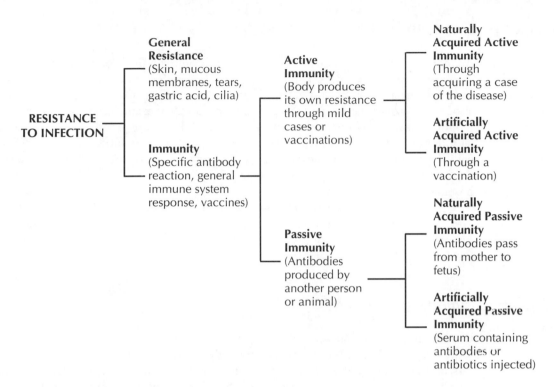

FIGURE 2.1   How the human body resists infections.

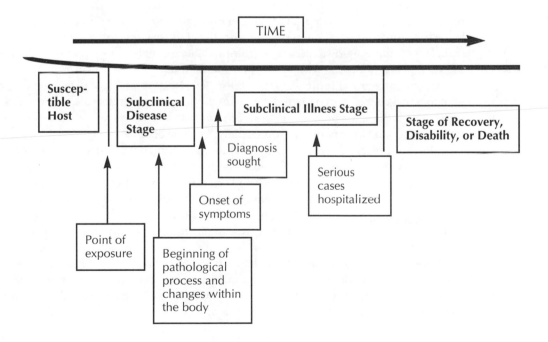

FIGURE 2.2   Natural course of a communicable disease.

GENERAL CLASSIFICATION OF DISEASES

An individual may have more than one acute or chronic condition or disease at one time. Two or more infectious diseases can exist at one time in the human body, a phenomenon sometimes overlooked by the diagnosing health care provider. One infectious disease can also lead to or open the way for other infectious diseases. For example, an open lesion in the mouth (canker sore) caused by a virus can then result in a more serious secondary bacterial infection. Illness, injury, and or invasive treatment often result in a lowered defense within the immune system and can allow secondary infections to occur. For example, it is quite common for an elderly person to enter a hospital with a broken hip and while in the hospital get viral pneumonia.

Chronic and communicable diseases also occur simultaneously within the body. Additionally, some infectious diseases can become chronic. For example, a sinus infection can turn into chronic sinusitis. For ease of understanding and study, diseases and conditions are classified into five broad categories.

Five Major Classifications of Diseases

Congenital and hereditary diseases—are often caused by genetic and familial tendencies toward certain inborn abnormalities, injury to the embryo or fetus by environmental factors, chemicals, or agents such as drugs, alcohol, smoking, innate developmental problems possibly caused by chemicals or agents or can be a fluke of nature. Examples are Down syndrome, hemophilia, and heart disease at an early age.

Allergies and inflammatory diseases—are diseases caused by the body reacting to an invasion of or injury by a foreign object or substance. Allergies, a virus, bacteria, or other microscopic and microbiological agents can cause an inflammatory reaction in the body. Some inflammatory reactions may result from the body forming antibodies against its own tissue, for example ingrown toenails or arthritis. Other examples range from slivers of wood, metal, or plants under the skin, to hay fever and asthma.

Degenerative or chronic diseases—cause deterioration of body systems, tissue, and functions; degeneration of parts and systems of the body. Degenerative diseases are often associated with the aging process, but in some cases may not be age-related. Arteriosclerosis, arthritis, and gout are examples of degenerative chronic diseases.

Metabolic diseases—cause the dysfunction, poor function, or malfunction of certain organs or physiological processes within the body leading to disease states. Glands or organs that fail to secrete certain biochemicals to keep the metabolic process functioning within the body cause metabolic disorders. For example, adrenal glands no longer function properly; the cells may no longer utilize glucose normally causing diabetes; or the thyroid gland no longer functions properly resulting in a goiter, hyperthyroidism, or cretinism (hypothyroidism).

Cancer/neoplastic diseases—are characterized by abnormal growth of cells that form into a variety of tumors both benign and malignant and can occur in persons at all ages. Cancers are malignant tumors that are easily diagnosed and are categorized by the type of tissue that has been affected and/or the location.[2]

TABLE 2.2   Classification of sources of disease or illness

Classification	Examples of Sources
Allergies	Asthma, anaphylactic reactions, lesions
Chemical	Drugs, acids, alkali, heavy metals (lead, mercury), poisons (arsenic), some enzymes
Congenital	Spina bifida, polycystic kidney disease, cerebral aneurysm
Hereditary	Familial tendency diseases such as alcoholism, genetic or chromosome structure that passes disability, disease, or disorders on to offspring, syndromes
Iatrogenic	Nosocomial infections, disease, or injury caused by care or treatment in a health care facility
Idiopathic	Diseases of unknown cause or origin or a morbid state of spontaneous origin
Infectious	Bacteria, viruses, parasites
Inflammatory	Stings, poison ivy, wounds, slivers or impaled objects, arthritis, serum sickness, allergic reactions
Metabolic	Dysfunctional organs within the body producing hypothyroidism, hyperthyroidism, exophthalmic goiter
Nutritional	Vitamin deficiencies such as scurvy or protein deficiencies such as Kwashiorkor
Physical agents	Excessive cold or heat, electrical shock, radiation, injury
Psychological	Biochemical imbalances in the brain as in schizophrenia; loss of or destruction of brain tissue such as in Alzheimer's disease
Traumatic	Wounds, bone fractures, contusions, mechanical injury
Tumors	Environmental or behaviorally stimulated tumors, such as cancer of the lung from smoking
Vascular	Smoking, stress, lack of proper diet, lack of exercise and other behaviorally related implications that contribute to heart and cardiovascular diseases

(Adapted from Green, L.W., and C.L. Anderson. 1982. *Community Health*, 4th edition. St. Louis: C.V. Mosby)

Diseases are classified in many additional ways. Table 2.2 presents another approach to the classification of diseases, this time by source. The classification is alphabetical with no attempt to give importance or priority by classification.

Another way of classifying infectious or communicable diseases is to list the diseases by the means of transmission. The ability of a disease to be transmitted from one person to the next or to spread in a population is referred to as the **communicability of the disease**. Communicability of a disease is determined by the capacity of a pathogen or agent to be transmitted from a diseased or infected person to another person who is not immune and is susceptible. Five different means of transmission can be used to classify certain infectious diseases. The five classifications are: fomiteborne, zoonosis or vectorborne,

TABLE 2.3   Classification of major infectious diseases by mode of transmission

Airborne Respiratory Diseases	Intestinal Discharge Diseases	Open Sores or Lesion Diseases	Zoonosis or Vectorborne Diseases	Fomiteborne Diseases
Chickenpox	Amebic dysentery	AIDS	African sleeping sickness	Anthrax
Common colds	Bacterial dysentery	Anthrax	Encephalitis	Chickenpox
Diphtheria	(shigellosis)	Erysipelas	Lyme disease	Common colds
Influenza	(staphylococcal)	Gonorrhea	Malaria	Diphtheria
Measles	Cholera	Scarlet fever	Rocky Mountain	Influenza
Meningitis	Giardiasis	Smallpox	spotted fever	Meningitis
Pneumonia	Hookworm	Syphilis	Tularemia	Poliomyelitis
Poliomyelitis	Poliomyelitis	Tuberculosis	Typhus fever	Rubella
Rubella	Salmonellosis	Tularemia	Yellow fever	Scarlet fever
Scarlet fever	Typhoid fever			Streptococcal
Smallpox	Hepatitis			throat
Throat infections				infections
Tuberculosis				Tuberculosis
Whooping cough				

TABLE 2.4   Classification of microbe sources of disease/pathogens

Organisms	Disease
Bacteria	
bacilli	Diphtheria (aerobic—*Corynebacterium*)
	Botulism (anaerobic—*Colstridum botulinum*)
	Brucellosis (*Brucella abortus*)
	Legionellosis (*Legionellae*)
	Salmonellosis (*Salmonella*)
	Shigellosis (*Shegella*)
	Cholera (*Vibrio cholerae*)
cocci	Impetigo (staphylococci)
	Toxic shock (staphylococci)
	Streptococcal sore throat (streptococci)
	Scarlet fever (streptococci)
	Erysipelas (streptococci)
	Pneumonia (pneumococci)
	Gonorrhea (gonococci)
	Meningitis (meningococci)
spiral organisms	Syphilis (*Treponema pallidum*)
	Rat bite fever (*Spirillum minus*)
	Lyme disease (*Borrelia burgdorferi-a* spirochete)

TABLE 2.4   (*Continued*)

Organisms	Disease
acid-fast organisms	Tuberculosis (*Mycobacterium tuberculosis*) Leprosy (*Myocobacterium tuberculosis*)
Rickettsia (very small bacteria)	Rocky Mountain spotted fever (*Rickettsia rickettsii*) Typhus (*Rickettsia prowazekii*)
Virus	Chickenpox (herpes virus) Influenza Type A—associated with epidemics and pandemics Type B—associated with local epidemics Type C—associated with sporadic minor localized outbreaks Measles (*Morbillivirus*) Mumps (*Paramyxovirus*) Poliomyelitis (Types 1, most paralytogenic, 2, 3 less common) Rabies Smallpox (*Variola* virus)
Fungus	Mycosis
Mold	Ringworm
Yeast	Biastomycosis Dermatophytosis

airborne/respiratoryborne, intestinal (alvine) discharge (which includes water and food-borne), and open lesions. Table 2.3 presents the five classifications and some of the major, related diseases and mode of transmission.[4,5,6,7,9]

CLASSIFICATION OF DISEASE BY CAUSE

Diseases can also be classified by the source or cause from which they come. The most common cause of infectious diseases are pathogens or disease-causing organisms. There are seven major classifications of pathogens that cause disease in humans (and in some animals). Most of these pathogens are microscopic organisms and are not visible to the naked eye. The different classes of microorganisms are presented with examples in Table 2.4.[1,2,4,5,6,8,10]

In addition, three microscopic animal sources of disease exist. The classification of the three animal sources are presented in Table 2.5. The organism is presented with an example of the disease which it causes.[1,2,4,5,6,8,9,10]

TABLE 2.5   Classification of animal sources of disease/pathogens

Organisms	Disease
Protozoan (one celled)	
ameba	Dysentery
plasmodium	Malaria
Worms (metazoan)	
roundworms	Ascaris (large roundworms)
pinworms	
tapeworms	
flukes	
trichinella	Trichinosis
Arthropods (lice)	Pediculosis
	Scabies (*Sarcoptes scabiei*)

INANIMATE SOURCES OF ILLNESS AND DISABILITY

Microorganisms and microscopic animals are not the only sources of disease, conditions, or death in humans. Many causes of illness, conditions, and injury exist; some are of man's own doing, some are naturally occurring, and others are environmentally related. Still other conditions are self-inflicted at work, in industry, at home, or in the process of getting to and from work. Table 2.6 presents the different inanimate sources of illness and disability. The *source*, an *example of illness or disability* is presented as is the *mode of entry* into the body.[11,12]

TABLE 2.6   Classification of inanimate sources of illness and disability

Source	Illness/Disability	Mode of Entry
Dusts		
silica	Silicosis (fibrosis of lung tissue)	Inhalation
asbestos	Asbestosis (fibrosis of lung tissue)	
	Lung cancer	
Fumes		
lead	Lead poisoning	Inhalation
		Skin
Smoke	Asphyxia due to oxygen deficiency	Inhalation
	Smoke poisoning	
	Asphyxia due to carbon monoxide	
Gases, mists,	Asphyxia or chemical poisoning	Inhalation
aerosols,	(Depending upon the source)	
and vapors		
Electrical	Burns, neurological damage, death	Skin

TABLE 2.6   *(Continued)*

Source	Illness/Disability	Mode of Entry
Noise	Hearing loss, deafness	Nervous system
Ionizing radiation	Cancer, dermatitis	Skin/tissue
Nonionizing radiation	Burns, cancer	Skin/tissue
Thermal	Burns, cancer	Skin/tissue
Ergonomics	Muscle, skeletal, tissue problems	Skin/tissue
Stress	Mental, emotional, physiological, behavioral	Nervous system
Bites	Snakebite poisoning, lacerations, tissue damage	Skin/tissue
Stings	Poisoning, death	Skin/tissue
Chemical ingestion	Arsenic, malathion poisoning, death	Respiratory, digestive, skin/tissue

PORTALS OF ENTRY OF INFECTIOUS DISEASE AGENTS INTO THE HUMAN BODY

Ten different modes of entry into the body of infectious disease agents have been identified. Listed below are the ten different modes of entry with the more common entries listed in order.

- Respiratory
- Oral
- Reproductive
- Intravenous
- Urinary
- Skin
- Gastrointestinal
- Cardiovascular
- Conjunctival
- Transplacental

TIME: INCUBATION PERIODS IN COMMUNICABLE DISEASES

To become ill, an individual has to acquire a pathogen that is infectious in nature. In other words, a person has to be inoculated with a disease. This brings to mind a picture of an *Anopheles* mosquito biting (inoculation by injection) an unsuspecting, susceptible individual on a warm spring evening, infecting the person with a disease such as malaria. The incubation period is the time that elapses between inoculation and the appearance of the first signs or symptoms of the disease. In the case of the victim with the mosquito bite, the incubation for malaria would be about 15 days (10 to 35 days) from the time of the bite until the victim started to have shaking chills, fever, sweats, malaise, and a headache for about one day and then on and off every 48 hours. The interval between exposure to malaria and the appearance of the first detectable signs or symptoms of the illness is malaria's incubation period. Difficulty in determining exposure to the inoculation of or exposure to an illness makes ascertaining the starting point of the incubation period difficult. Vague prodromal signs of illness make it difficult to determine the end point of the illness and the signs and symptoms of different diseases are often alike, i.e., malaria could initially be mistaken for flu. The **prodromal period** is the second stage of illness and the period in which signs and symptoms of a disease first appear (see Table 2.7). The easiest diagnosis is often arrived at when a disease comes from a single exposure of short duration. Identification of the sources of infection and a person developing the first classical signs of a disease greatly helps in disease diagnosis.[1,2,4,5,8]

To better understand the role incubation periods play in the course of a disease, see Figure 2.3. The course of a respiratory disease with the incubation period is shown. The disease starts

TABLE 2.7   Incubation periods for major communicable diseases (list is incomplete)

Disease	Incubation Period	Period of Communicability
Botulism	12 to 36 hours	When exposed
Chickenpox	2 to 3 weeks	From 5 days before vesicles appear to 6 days after
Common cold	12 to 72 hours (usually 24 hrs)	From 1 day before onset to 5 days after
Conjunctivitis	1 to 3 days	Always while infection active and present
Diphtheria	2 to 5 days	2 weeks or less and not more than 4 weeks
Dysentery (amebic)	2 to 4 weeks (wide variation)	During intestinal infection; untreated, for years
Epstein-Barr virus	4 to 7 weeks	While symptoms are present
Gonorrhea	2 to 5 days (may be longer)	Indefinite unless treated
Hepatitis (serum)	45 to 160 days (usually 80 to 100)	Many weeks before onset of symptoms
Herpes simplex virus	Up to 2 weeks	As long as 7 weeks after symptoms disappear
Impetigo (contagious)	4 to 10 days or longer	Until lesions heal
Influenza	1 to 3 days	Often 3 days from clinical onset
Measles (rubeola)	10 days to onset, rash at 14 days	From prodromal period to 4 days after rash onset
Meningitis	2 to 10 days	1 day after beginning of medication
Mumps	12 to 26 days (usually 18 days)	From 6 days before symptoms to 9 days after
Pediculosis	Approximately 2 weeks	While lice remain alive
Pneumonia, bacterial	1 to 3 days	Unknown
Pneumonia, viral	1 to 3 days	Unknown
Poliomyelitis	3 to 21 days (usually 7 to 12 days)	7 to 10 days before and after symptoms
Pinworm (enterobiasis)	2 to 6 weeks	Continual as exposed

TABLE 2.7   *(Continued)*

Disease	*Incubation Period*	*Period of Communicability*
Rabies	2 to 8 weeks or longer	From animals, 3 to 5 days before symptoms and during the course of the disease
Respiratory viral infection	A few days to a week or more	Duration of the active disease
Ringworm	4 to 10 days	As long as lesions are present
Rubella (German measles)	8 to 10 days (usually 14 days)	1 week before and to 4 days after onset of rash
Salmonella food poisoning	6 to 72 hours (usually 36 hrs)	3 days to 3 weeks (wide variation)
Scarlet fever	1 to 3 days	Treated cases 10 to 21 days, untreated—months
Staphylococcus food poisoning	2 to 4 hours	Continual as exposed
Streptococcal sore throat	1 to 3 days	Treated cases 10 to 21 days, untreated—months
Smallpox	7 to 17 days (usually 10 to 12)	First 7 days
Syphilis	10 days to 10 weeks (usually 3 weeks)	Variable and indefinite if not treated
Tetanus	4 days to 3 weeks	When exposed
Trichinosis	2 to 128 days (usually 9 days) after ingestion of infected meat	When exposed
Tuberculosis	4 to 12 weeks (primary phase)	As long as tubercle bacilli are discharged by patient or carrier
Typhoid fever	1 to 3 weeks (usually 2 weeks)	As long as typhoid bacilli appear in feces
Whooping cough	7 to 21 days (usually by 10 days)	From 7 days after exposure to 3 weeks after onset of typical paroxysms

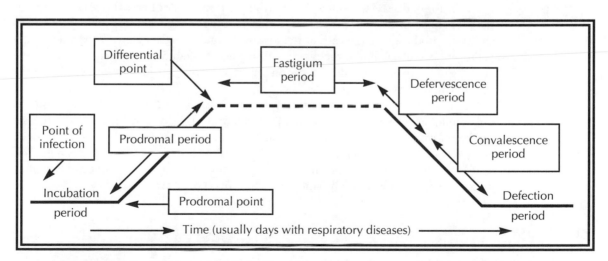

FIGURE 2.3   Course of an infectious respiratory disease. Prodromal symptoms: Nasal discharge, headache, mild fever, general aching, irritability, restlessness, digestive disturbances, cough, sore throat. (Adapted from Green, L., and C.L. Anderson. 1982. *Community Health*, 4th ed. St. Louis: C.V. Mosby)

with the pathogen invading or inoculating the host. The pathogen multiplies in the host during the incubation period. A respiratory disease may or may not be transmissible during this period. Some diseases are transmissible in the last 2 or 3 days of the incubation period, for example, measles and chickenpox. As can be seen in Table 2.7, incubation periods vary from disease to disease. Incubation periods can vary in individuals who have more active immune systems to retard the pathogen's growth within the body, lengthening the incubation period. It has been observed that diseases with short incubation periods generally produce a more acute and severe illness, while long incubation diseases are less severe. The prodromal period begins with the first signs and symptoms of the disease. In most respiratory diseases this is usually one day. Disease transmission is greatest during the prodromal period due to the high communicability of the disease at this stage and the symptoms not being well-pronounced.

The **fastigium period** is the period when the disease is at its peak. Diagnosis is easiest at or directly after the differential point. Many respiratory illnesses produce the same symptoms in the prodromal stage making diagnosis difficult. In the fastigium period, even though highly communicable, patients do not spread the disease much. Usually in this phase of the disease a person is home in bed or in the hospital.

Defervescence is the period when the symptoms of the illness are declining. As patients feel they are recovering from a disease in this period, they may not take care of themselves and can have a relapse as the disease has not yet run its course and the immune system is not as strong as it should be. If the body's defenses are weakened and cannot effectively fight off the pathogens, at this stage a relapse may occur. This is also a period when transmission of the disease is quite high as the patient may be up and about yet not recovered and is still infectious.

Convalescence is the recovery period. The person may still be infectious at this point, but is feeling much better, is out and about, and spreading the disease.

Defection is the period during which the pathogen is killed off or brought into remission by the body's immune system. In some diseases, defection and convalescence may be the same stage. If isolation is required, it is in the defection stage when isolation is lifted.[6]

A factor of disease that affects not only upper respiratory diseases but many others, is the strength or virulence of the disease. Virulence is the strength of the disease agent and its ability to produce a severe case of the disease or cause death. Related to virulence of a pathogen, is the viability of the disease causing agent. **Viability**, a related concept, is the capacity of the pathogen or disease-causing agent to survive outside of the host and to exist or thrive in the environment.

When a disease such as a respiratory disease has not yet manifested itself or produces only a mild case of a disease or condition, it is referred to as being **subclinical**. Some diseases can be shown to be present by clinical tests such as blood analysis, and the presence of an antigen reaction can be identified. However, clinical symptoms may not be apparent. This state is also referred to as a subclinical infection or subclinical case, as such a condition must be confirmed immunologically while failing to show clinical symptoms.

ZOONOSIS

It has been long understood that animals can be the host, vector, or source of certain infections and diseases (see Figure 2.4). Historically it was recognized that certain diseases can be transmitted from animals to humans. **Zoonosis** is defined as any infection or infectious disease transmissible from animals to humans. The diseases may be endemic or epidemic. Thus, another way some diseases are classified and studied is based on the ability of the disease to be transmitted to humans from animals. More than 185 diseases have been known to be transmitted to humans from animals.[10] Some common zoonotic diseases include

AIDS	dermatophilosis	Rocky Mountain spotted fever
amebiasis	leprosy	salmonellosis
anthrax	Lyme disease	shigellosis
bovine papular stomatitis	pasteurollosis	streptococcosus infections
brucellosis	plague	tetanus
California encephalitis	Q-fever	trichinosis
cat-scratch fever	rabies	tularemia
Colorado tick fever	rat-bite fever	yellow fever
cowpox	rickettsialpox	zoonotic scabies
dengue fever		

Life cycle of *Taenia solium*

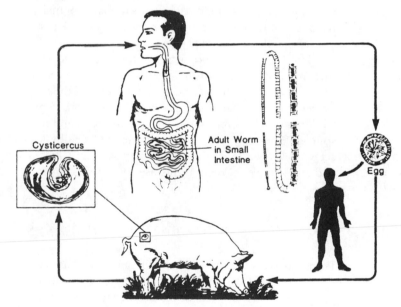

FIGURE 2.4   Example of zoonosis and the disease transmission cycle. The two-host life cycle of *T. solium* involves humans as definitive hosts for the intestinal stage adult tapeworm that is acquired by eating undercooked pork contaminated with cysticerci. Swine, the intermediate host, become infected with the larval stage by ingesting eggs shed in the feces of a human tapeworm carrier. Humans may inadvertently acquire larval-stage infection through the fecal-oral route. (Source: Centers for Disease Control and Prevention, "Locally acquired neurocysticercosis—North Carolina, Massachusetts, and South Carolina, 1989–1991." *Morbidity and Mortality Weekly Report*, Public Health Services, U.S. Department of Health and Human Services, Vol. 21, No. 1, Jan. 10, 1992, pp. 1–4)

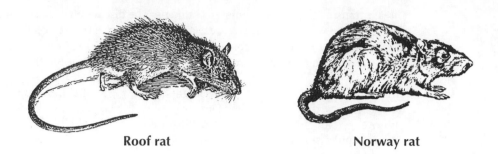

Roof rat   **Norway rat**

Both are vectors of disease

Some animals can be carriers of a disease without showing any signs or symptoms. For example, coyotes can carry plague, never becoming sick from the disease, yet spreading it to rodents and humans via a flea vector. Humans may get bitten by a flea while in the woods or at home, get ill a few days later, and make no connection of the disease to the inoculation by the insect. Historically the animal to flea to human set of events was a connection not easily made. For hundreds of years humans got malaria from mosquito bites and never realized that the disease came from the mosquito. The same was also true for the sequence of events in flea bites and plague.

Humans are most protective of their domestic animals and any implication that an owner may get a disease from a pet is not well received. Yet the possibility exists and must not be overlooked by the epidemiologist. One of the most common disorders overlooked by pet owners is that of allergies in the family caused by the furry animals in their home. Children or adults may suffer allergies for years and never consider the family pet as the source of the allergic condition, until tested by a physician. Tularemia (rabbit fever), cat-scratch fever, worms from dogs, and parrot fever (psittacosis) have long been known to exist and are examples of zoonotic diseases.

INTERNATIONAL CLASSIFICATION OF DISEASES

For many years the World Health Organization has been responsible for the classification of diseases. The current set of classifications is in its ninth edition and is referred to as ICD-9. ICD-9 is designed for the classification of morbidity and mortality information for statistical purposes, for indexing hospital records by disease and treatment procedures, and for data storage and retrieval. The ICD-9 was found to be of limited use in hospital settings so a clinical modification was done and is referred to ICD-9-CM (CM stands for clinical modification). The process of adapting ICD-9 for clinical settings was taken up by the U.S. National Committee on Vital Health Statistics through its subcommittee on hospital statistics. A study done by the American Hospital Association and the American Medical Record Association found the ICD suitable for indexing hospital records. After various editions, revisions, and adaptations the current ICD-9-CM was put into use in 1979 with some updates periodically made. ICD-9-CM is published as a three-volume set: Volume 1 Diseases: Tabular List, Volume 2 Diseases: Alphabetic Index, Volume 3 Procedures: Tabular List and Alphabetic Index.

Four and five digit numbers are used to give a numerical code to the various diseases and associated conditions. Thus, each condition, subcondition, or a modification of a disease or condition has been assigned a number. The ICD-9-CM also includes injuries and conditions not necessarily considered diseases. When a person is seen by a health care provider for a routine checkup, health screening, or some non-treatment encounter and is not currently sick, yet has a problem or condition which influences the person's health status, a special "V" code is added. Injury, poisoning, and accidents are indicated by "E" codes.

The ICD-9-CM contains lists of hundreds of diseases and disorders in a general overall classification system. In part, the classification system uses a body systems approach to classifying the various diseases that invade each body system. Listed below is the general overall ICD-9-CM classification structure:

- Infectious and parasitic diseases
- Neoplasms (cancer)
- Endocrine, nutritional, and metabolic diseases and immunity disorders
- Diseases of the blood and blood-forming organs
- Diseases of the nervous system and sense organs
- Diseases of the circulatory system
- Diseases of the respiratory system
- Diseases of the digestive system
- Diseases of the genitourinary system
- Complications of pregnancy, childbirth, and the puerperium
- Diseases of the skin and subcutaneous tissue
- Diseases of the musculoskeletal system and connective tissue
- Congenital anomalies
- Certain conditions originating in the perinatal period
- Injury and Poisoning
- V-codes = Classification of factors influencing health status and contact with health services
- E-codes = Classification of external causes of injury and poisoning

ICD-10-CM as of 1996 is in use in 28 countries and has been translated into 37 languages. ICD-10 is to be used for mortality reporting in the United States in 1999 and death certificates are to be coded with ICD-10 codes.

ICD-10-CM has numerous changes from the ICD-9-CM including the addition of a "z" code for outpatient encounters, a code format change to an alpha-numeric system, an increase in a number of codes (sixth digit added, left-right body designations) and will present more specific coding. It uses a sequencing prioritizing process that pertains to diseases or conditions affecting more than one body system. Chapter structures are changed to include body system chapters, and body site classification is commonly used. Language is modified to be consistent with current clinical practice.

Final versions of ICD-10-CM and ICD-10-PCS (Procedural Coding System) are due out in late spring of 1998 and are due to be fully implemented by October, 2000.

NOTIFIABLE DISEASES IN THE UNITED STATES (CENTERS FOR DISEASE CONTROL AND PREVENTION)

In the United States there are currently 49 notifiable diseases. Statutes have been passed and regulations developed at the federal level making the reporting of notifiable diseases a legal requirement. Similar legal requirements are also found at the state level in all states. Physicians, hospitals, labs, clinics, and other health care providers which may come in contact with patients, who have certain serious diseases are required by law to report all cases of notifiable diseases. Reporting of certain diseases such as AIDS and sexually transmitted diseases (STDs) has not always been accurate nor efficiently done. Some health care providers choose to

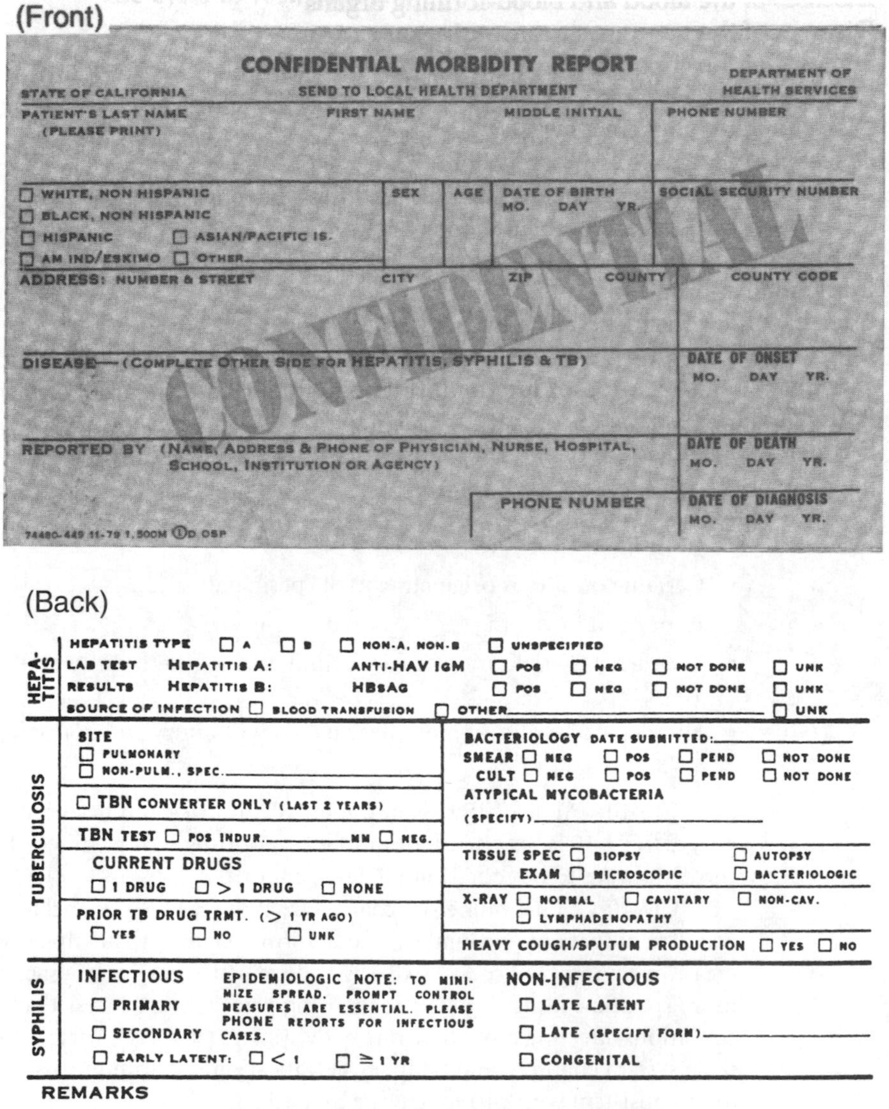

(Front)

CONFIDENTIAL MORBIDITY REPORT

STATE OF CALIFORNIA — SEND TO LOCAL HEALTH DEPARTMENT — DEPARTMENT OF HEALTH SERVICES

PATIENT'S LAST NAME (PLEASE PRINT) | FIRST NAME | MIDDLE INITIAL | PHONE NUMBER

☐ WHITE, NON HISPANIC
☐ BLACK, NON HISPANIC
☐ HISPANIC ☐ ASIAN/PACIFIC IS.
☐ AM IND/ESKIMO ☐ OTHER

SEX | AGE | DATE OF BIRTH MO. DAY YR. | SOCIAL SECURITY NUMBER

ADDRESS: NUMBER & STREET | CITY | ZIP | COUNTY | COUNTY CODE

DISEASE—(COMPLETE OTHER SIDE FOR HEPATITIS, SYPHILIS & TB) | DATE OF ONSET MO. DAY YR.

REPORTED BY (NAME, ADDRESS & PHONE OF PHYSICIAN, NURSE, HOSPITAL, SCHOOL, INSTITUTION OR AGENCY) | DATE OF DEATH MO. DAY YR.

PHONE NUMBER | DATE OF DIAGNOSIS MO. DAY YR.

CONFIDENTIAL

74480-449 11-79 1,500M OSP

(Back)

HEPATITIS

HEPATITIS TYPE ☐ A ☐ B ☐ NON-A, NON-B ☐ UNSPECIFIED
LAB TEST RESULTS HEPATITIS A: ANTI-HAV IGM ☐ POS ☐ NEG ☐ NOT DONE ☐ UNK
HEPATITIS B: HBsAG ☐ POS ☐ NEG ☐ NOT DONE ☐ UNK
SOURCE OF INFECTION ☐ BLOOD TRANSFUSION ☐ OTHER ☐ UNK

TUBERCULOSIS

SITE ☐ PULMONARY ☐ NON-PULM., SPEC.
☐ TBN CONVERTER ONLY (LAST 2 YEARS)
TBN TEST ☐ POS INDUR. ___ MM ☐ NEG.
CURRENT DRUGS ☐ 1 DRUG ☐ > 1 DRUG ☐ NONE
PRIOR TB DRUG TRMT. (> 1 YR AGO) ☐ YES ☐ NO ☐ UNK
BACTERIOLOGY DATE SUBMITTED:
SMEAR ☐ NEG ☐ POS ☐ PEND ☐ NOT DONE
CULT ☐ NEG ☐ POS ☐ PEND ☐ NOT DONE
ATYPICAL MYCOBACTERIA (SPECIFY)
TISSUE SPEC EXAM ☐ BIOPSY ☐ AUTOPSY ☐ MICROSCOPIC ☐ BACTERIOLOGIC
X-RAY ☐ NORMAL ☐ CAVITARY ☐ NON-CAV. ☐ LYMPHADENOPATHY
HEAVY COUGH/SPUTUM PRODUCTION ☐ YES ☐ NO

SYPHILIS

INFECTIOUS ☐ PRIMARY ☐ SECONDARY ☐ EARLY LATENT: ☐ < 1 ☐ ≥ 1 YR
EPIDEMIOLOGIC NOTE: TO MINIMIZE SPREAD, PROMPT CONTROL MEASURES ARE ESSENTIAL. PLEASE PHONE REPORTS FOR INFECTIOUS CASES.
NON-INFECTIOUS ☐ LATE LATENT ☐ LATE (SPECIFY FORM) ☐ CONGENITAL

REMARKS

FIGURE 2.5 Example of card used for notifiable disease reporting, state of California.

protect the patients with AIDS or STDs by not reporting the cases, thus distorting the reported statistics. Telephone as well as preprinted card reporting systems (see sample below in Figure 2.5) have been established to make reporting easy for the health care provider.

Some professionals refer to notifiable diseases as reportable diseases. What makes a disease of such seriousness or concern that it has to be reported? Two major factors which make a disease notifiable are the ability of the disease to cause death and the communicability of the disease. Increased chances of dying from a disease or increased chances of a disease spreading through populations are of great concern to public health officials, therefore, such diseases must have extensive control. Notification to public health officials of diseases posing a threat to large populations provides a starting point for local epidemiological investigations. If preventive measures have failed, such as immunizations not being acquired, then the reporting process alerts public health and political officials that measures need to be taken to intervene in the event of an outbreak of life and health threatening diseases. Notifiable disease reporting allows for the tracing of sources of infection, modes of transmission, routes of spread, identification of the vehicles (vectors and fomites) of the infection and allows for the identification of time, person and place (geographical location and clustering) issues of concern about these specific diseases.[14,15]

The *Morbidity and Mortality Weekly Report* lists on a regular basis a graphic presentation of the trends of occurrence (decrease and increase) of the top 12 to 14 notifiable diseases (see Figure 2.6). Table 2.8 lists the year's cumulative occurrence of the notifiable diseases. Figure 2.7 illustrates the notifiable disease reporting system as used in the United States.

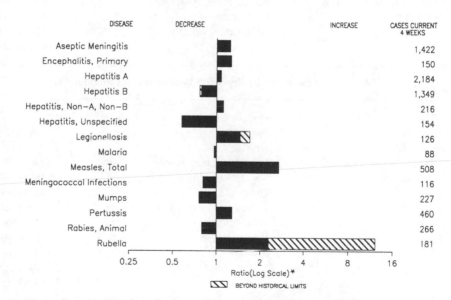

*Ratio of current 4-week total to mean of 15 4-week totals (from comparable, previous, and subsequent 4-week periods for past 5 years).

FIGURE 2.6 Example of notifiable disease increase and decrease comparison over a 4-week period. (Source: The Centers for Disease Control and Prevention, "Notifiable diseases reports, comparison of 4-week totals ending October 27, 1990," *Morbidity and Mortality Weekly Report*, Public Health Services, U.S. Department of Health and Human Services, Vol. 39, No. 43, Nov. 2, 1990, p. 780)

TABLE 2.8   Notifiable and reportable diseases (disease reporting requirements)

Disease to Be Reported Immediately by Telephone

Anthrax	Domoic acid poisoning (shellfish)	Rabies
Botulism	*Escherichia coli (E. coli)*	Scombroid fish poisoning
Cholera	Hantavirus	Viral hemorrhagic fever
Ciguatra fish poisoning	Hemolytic uremic syndrome	Yellow fever
Dengue fever	Meningococcal infections	Outbreaks of any disease
Diarrhea of the newborn	Paralytic shellfish poisoning	
Diphtheria	Plague	

Disease or Suspected, to Be Reported Within One Day of Identification

Amebiasis	*Haemophilus influenzae*	Salmonellosis
Anisakiasis	Hepatitis A	Shigellosis
Habesiosis	Listeriosis	Streptococcal infections
Campylobacteriosis	Lymphocytic choiomeningitis	Swimmer's itch (schistosomal
Colorado tick fever	Malaria	dermatitis)
Conjunctivitis	Measles (rubeola)	Syphilis
Encephalitis	Meningitis	Trichinosis
Food-borne diseases	Pertussis (whooping cough)	Tuberculosis
(2 or more cases—any	Poliomyelitis (paralytic)	Typhoid fever
outbreak)	Psittacosis	Vibrio infections
	Relapsing fever	Water-associated diseases
		Yersiniosis

Disease to Be Reported Within Seven Calendar Days

AIDS	Hepatitis B	PID
Brucellosis	Hepatitis C	Reyes syndrome
Chancroid	Hepatitis D	Rheumatic fever, acute
Chlamydial infections	Hepatitis, other acute	Rocky Mountain spotted fever
Coccidioidomycosis	Kawaski syndrome	Rubella (German measles)
Cysticercosis	Legionellosis	Rubella syndrome, congenital
Echinococcosis (hydatid)	Leprosy (Hansen's disease)	Tetanus
Ehrlichiosis	Leptospirosis	Toxic shock syndrome
Giardiasis	Lyme disease	Toxoplasmosis
Gonococcal infections	Mumps	Tularemia
	Nongonococcal urethritis	Occurrence of any unusual
		diseases

Reportable Noncommunicable Diseases and Conditions

Alzheimer's disease	Cancer	Pesticide exposure
Animal bites	Disorders characterized by	
	lapses of consciousness	

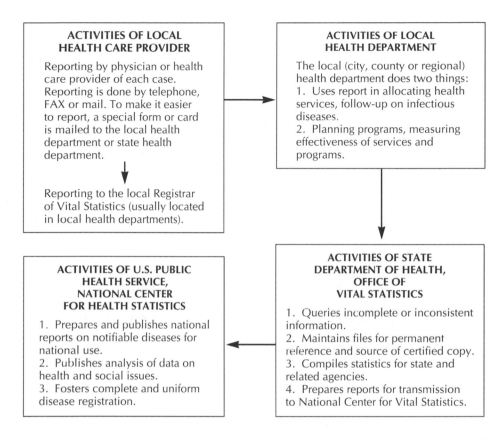

ACTIVITIES OF LOCAL HEALTH CARE PROVIDER

Reporting by physician or health care provider of each case. Reporting is done by telephone, FAX or mail. To make it easier to report, a special form or card is mailed to the local health department or state health department.

Reporting to the local Registrar of Vital Statistics (usually located in local health departments).

ACTIVITIES OF LOCAL HEALTH DEPARTMENT

The local (city, county or regional) health department does two things:
1. Uses report in allocating health services, follow-up on infectious diseases.
2. Planning programs, measuring effectiveness of services and programs.

ACTIVITIES OF U.S. PUBLIC HEALTH SERVICE, NATIONAL CENTER FOR HEALTH STATISTICS

1. Prepares and publishes national reports on notifiable diseases for national use.
2. Publishes analysis of data on health and social issues.
3. Fosters complete and uniform disease registration.

ACTIVITIES OF STATE DEPARTMENT OF HEALTH, OFFICE OF VITAL STATISTICS

1. Queries incomplete or inconsistent information.
2. Maintains files for permanent reference and source of certified copy.
3. Compiles statistics for state and related agencies.
4. Prepares reports for transmission to National Center for Vital Statistics.

FIGURE 2.7   The notifiable disease reporting system as used in the United States.[6,7,9,14]

IMMUNIZATIONS: PROTECTING THE PUBLIC FROM DISEASE

Before the polio vaccine became available in 1955, a peak of 58,000 cases of polio occurred in one year (1952). One out of every 2 cases resulted in permanently crippling the victim. Prior to the first live virus vaccine for measles being licensed in 1963, the United States had 4 million cases every year. Additionally there were 4,000 cases of encephalitis, which resulted in 400 deaths and 800 cases with irreparable brain damage. The immunization of 60 million children from 1963 to 1972 cost $180 million but saved $1.3 billion by averting 24 million cases of measles; 2,400 lives were saved, 7,900 cases of retardation prevented, and 1,352,000 hospital days saved.[1,2,4,5,13]

The rubella epidemic of 1964–65 caused 30,000 babies to be born with rubella syndrome, 20,000 of whom lived more than one year. Before the rubella vaccine was licensed in 1969, 58,000 cases per year were reported.[1,2,4,5,13]

Mumps was the leading cause of childhood deafness and juvenile diabetes. One out of 300 cases of mumps can result in impaired hearing. In diphtheria one out of every 10 victims dies.[1,2,4,5,13]

The importance of the immunization process is very important to all individuals of the United States. According to the Centers for Disease Control and Prevention, if fewer than 80% of the children in a given area have been inoculated for one of the contagious diseases, the danger of serious outbreaks or localized epidemics remains; every unvaccinated child is at risk.[1,2,4,5,13]

Three types of **immunity** are possible in humans: *acquired, active,* and *passive* immunity. **Acquired immunity** is obtained by having had a dose of a disease that stimulates the natural immune system, or by artificially stimulating the immune system by a vaccination. In **active immunity** the body produces its own antibodies. This can occur through a **vaccine** or in response to having a specific disease pathogen invade the body. Acquired and active immunity are similar. **Passive immunity**, which is sometimes called natural passive immunity, is acquired through transplacental transfer of a mother's immunity from diseases to the unborn child. Passive immunity can also come from the introduction of already produced antibodies into a susceptible case.[1,2,4,5,13]

In Table 2.9 is a list of the diseases for which vaccines have been developed. Many well-known diseases still lack vaccines, many are under study, and others are close to being developed. One vaccine that is hoped for is an AIDS vaccine, yet the possibilities of an AIDS vaccine are still limited at this time. Some vaccines are only partially effective and require booster shots, and others, like the smallpox vaccine, work very well.

Vaccinia, the smallpox vaccine, is a highly effective immunizing agent. Vaccinia vaccine brought about the supposed global eradication of smallpox. The last naturally occurring case of smallpox was reported in Somalia in 1977. In May 1980, the World Health Assembly certified that the world was free of naturally occurring smallpox. Even though this report was made worldwide, many public health professionals are skeptical of a true eradication and the belief that another epidemic of smallpox is not possible. Nonetheless, the vaccinia vaccine is a fine example of the effectiveness of wide uses of immunizations in the eradication of disease.[16]

TABLE 2.9   Diseases for which vaccines are used

Anthrax	Pneumonia
Cholera	Polio
Diphtheria	Rabies
German measles (rubella)	Smallpox
Hepatitis A	Spotted fever
Hepatitis B	Tetanus
Influenza	Tuberculosis
Measles	Typhoid fever
Meningitis	Typhus
Mumps	Whooping cough
Pertussis	Yellow fever
Plague	

A chickenpox vaccine is being experimentally used.
A malaria vaccine is being tested (Jan. 1997).

(Source: "Summary of notifiable diseases in the U.S., 1990," *Morbidity and Mortality Weekly Reports*, Centers for Disease Control and Prevention, Vol. 39, 53, Oct. 4, 1991)

The introduction of a substance that can cause the immune system to respond by developing antibodies against a disease is what the immunization process is all about. Some substances are given orally (polio for example). Most are given by injection or skin pricks. Specific antigens from inactivated bacteria, viruses, or microbe toxins are introduced into the body in the form of a vaccine. An **antigen** is any substance that is capable of stimulating the formation of **antibodies** within the body. The ability of the antigen system to have the strength, activity, and effectiveness to respond to disease is referred to as **antigenicity**. The goal of the vaccine is to have the antibodies react in a specific manner and in a detectable way within the body's immune system. The antigens stimulate the immune system to make the body think it has had the disease. The body's immune system responds by developing antibodies and a natural immunity against the disease. If the pathogen later enters the body, the immune system recognizes it and the body is protected from the disease by the immune system's rapid response to it. Some vaccines last a lifetime and others may not. Recent reports indicate that revaccination may be required for some diseases as one gets older. Booster shots keep the immune process active within the body. If antigens and antibodies disappear over time, then a booster shot is needed to strengthen or reactivate the immune response. Booster shots are also given at the outset of an immunization program to help build the body's immune defense systems to the fullest extent possible.[1,2,4,5,13]

When the body cannot respond quickly enough or with enough strength, then help is needed. **Antibiotics** are used to assist the immune system in its fight against pathogens. Common antibiotics are substances such as penicillin, tetracycline, streptomycin, or any other substance that destroys or inhibits the growth of pathogenic microorganisms.[2,5,13]

Table 2.9 lists diseases for which vaccines have been developed and which are in current use in the United States.

HERD IMMUNITY

Herd immunity is based on the notion that if the herd (a population or group) is mostly protected from a disease by immunizations, then the chance of a major epidemic occurring is highly limited. Jonas Salk, one of the developers of the polio vaccine, has suggested that if a herd immunity level of 85% were available within a population, a polio epidemic would not occur. **Herd immunity** is also viewed as the resistance a population or group (herd) has to the invasion and spread of an infectious disease. Herd immunity relies on the level of resistance a population has to a communicable disease through having a high proportion of the group members unable to get the disease. Immunizations or past experience with a disease reduces the number of susceptibles within a population. Herd immunity is accomplished when the number of susceptibles are reduced to a limited number and the number of protected or nonsusceptible persons dominate the herd (population). Herd immunity provides barriers to direct transmission of infections through the population. The lack of susceptible individuals halts the spread of a disease through a group (see Figures 2.8 and 2.9).

Figure 2.8 graphically shows how a disease can spread through a population when immunity is low and the number of susceptibles is high. Figure 2.9 shows how barriers to the spread of a disease are developed when susceptible levels are low, and how disease

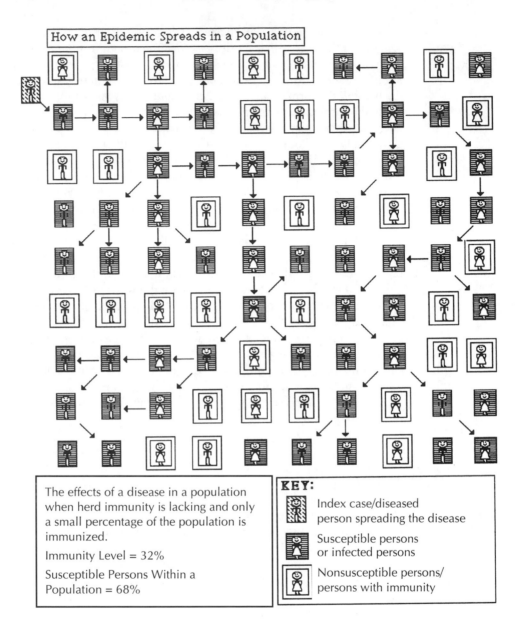

FIGURE 2.8 Diagram of a population, showing a low immunization level which falls short of protecting individuals within the group.

transmission in a population is stopped when an 85% level of immunity exists. With high levels of herd immunity, the ability of a susceptible person to have direct contact with a diseased person is highly limited and the disease transmission is stopped for the most part. Both Figures 2.8 and 2.9 demonstrate the effect that only one diseased person can have on the spread of a disease in a population.

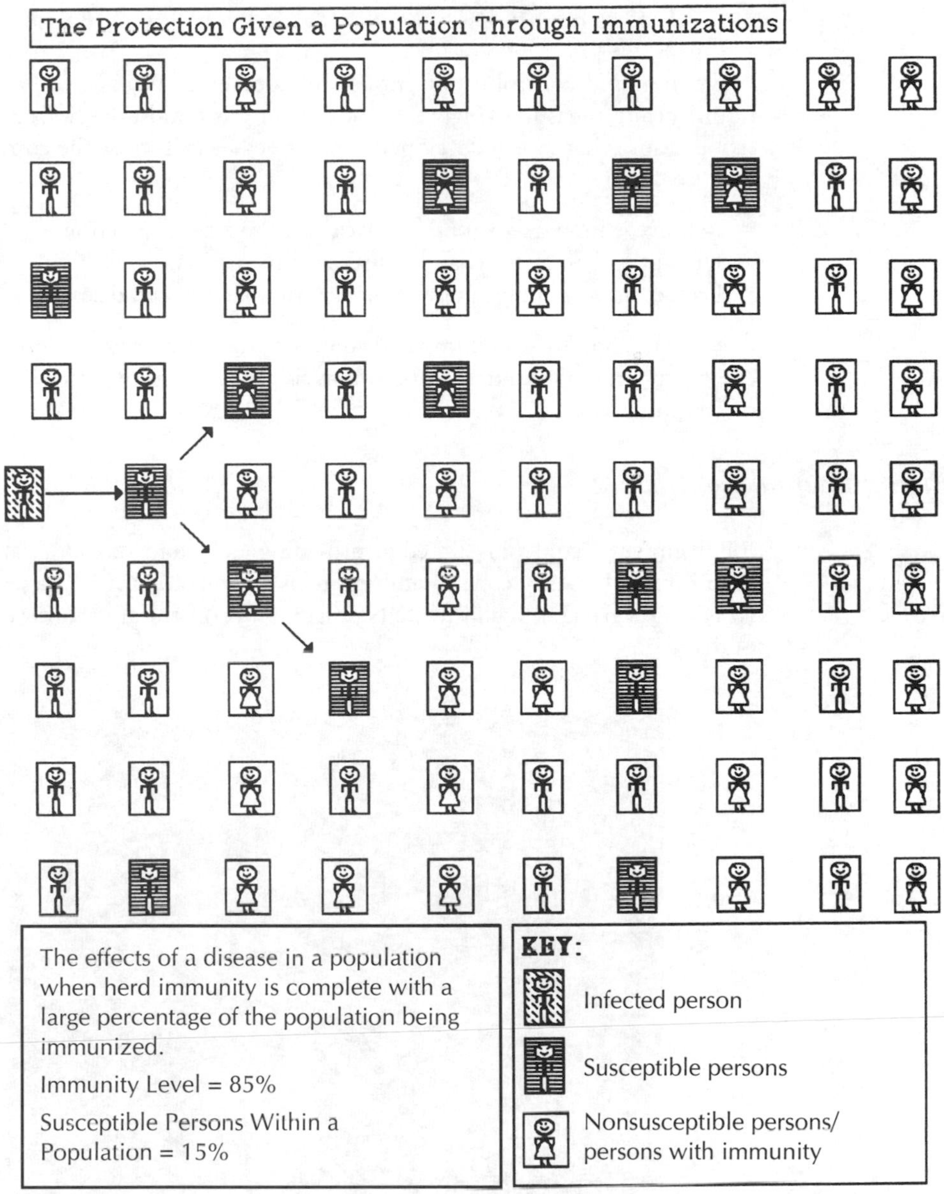

The Protection Given a Population Through Immunizations

The effects of a disease in a population when herd immunity is complete with a large percentage of the population being immunized.

Immunity Level = 85%

Susceptible Persons Within a Population = 15%

KEY:

Infected person

Susceptible persons

Nonsusceptible persons/ persons with immunity

FIGURE 2.9 Diagram of a population showing a high level of immunizations within the group so that it affords a good level of protection to most of the individuals within the group.

One public health immunization goal would be to have close to 100% immunity in a population, so that not even one individual would get the disease. This level of immunity is especially important in life threatening diseases or those diseases which cause extreme disability, such as polio. The goal of any public health immunization program is to reach 100% of the population, even if herd immunity prevents the occurrence of major epidemics.

COMMUNICABLE DISEASE PREVENTION AND CONTROL

Prevention and control of infectious and contagious diseases are the foundation of all public health measures (Figure 2.10). Several prevention methods as well as many control measures have been developed. The three key factors to the control of communicable diseases are

- Remove, eliminate, or contain the cause or source of infection.
- Disrupt and block the chain of disease transmission.
- Protect the susceptible population against infection and disease.[4]

The methods of prevention and control are used on several fronts. The first front is the environment, the second is the person at risk (host), and the third front is the population or community.[4]

Environmental Control

Environmental control is aimed at providing clean and safe air, water, milk, and food. Also involved in the scope of environmental control is the management of solid waste (trash and garbage), liquid waste (sewage), and control of vectors (insects and rodents) of disease.[4]

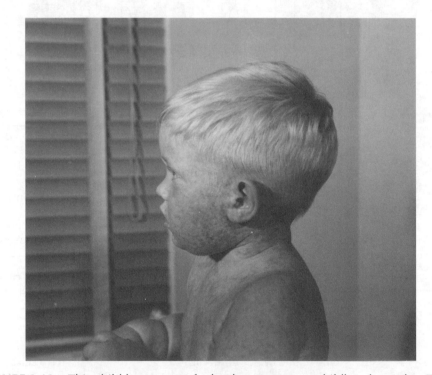

FIGURE 2.10   This child has a case of rubeola, or common childhood measles. This is a preventable disease for which a vaccine [measles/mumps/rubella (MMR)] is widely available. Children should get a vaccination for this disease starting at 12 to 15 months. (Picture courtesy of Centers for Disease Control and Prevention, Atlanta, Georgia)

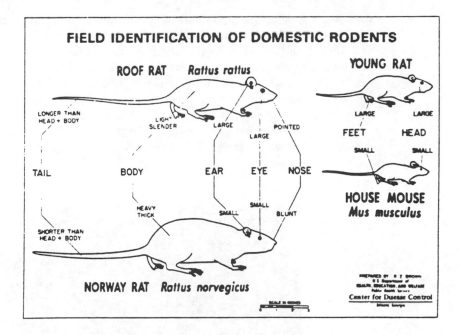

(Source: Centers for Disease Control and Prevention, *Self-Study Course Vector-Borne Disease Control: Control of Commensal Rats and Mice*, U.S. Department of Health and Human Services)

Safe air includes the control of infectious pathogens that are airborne. Toxic fumes, UV light, air pollution, and second-hand smoke are also of concern in air safety control.[4]

Clean and safe water supplies have been key factors in controlling infectious diseases, especially waterborne diseases (enteric or alvine discharge diseases). Maintaining a safe water supply is one of the most basic yet all important public health activities of the modern age.[4]

Liquid waste carries pathogens, fecal material, chemical pollutants, industrial waste, and many other pollutants and waste. Sewage and dirty water run-off must be safely conveyed without exposure to the human population, thus underground sewage systems are of keen importance.[4]

Solid waste management has become one of the greatest public health challenges of modern times. Proper disposal of the massive amounts of garbage and other solid waste such as hazardous and biohazardous materials continues to be a challenge. Control of garbage odors, flies, and insect problems from the garbage can at home to the garbage can sitting at the street curb as well as at the sanitary landfill all help prevent the spread of communicable disease by vectors.[4]

The protection of water, food, and milk are hallmarks of advanced societies. Milk and the cows it comes from must be tested and proved free of infectious diseases. Milk is constantly tested and is treated by heat (pasteurization) to kill pathogens. Proper storage, distribution, transport, and temperature control of milk must be rigorous and continually assured.[4]

Food must be protected from adulteration, contamination, and spoilage.[4] Food must also be properly stored and served. Proper temperatures for refrigeration, cooking, storage, and transport must be maintained without fail. Proper food handling, including hand washing during preparation, is extremely important to infection control. Many bacteria especially staphylococci, salmonella, and shigella can contaminate food and be transmitted to unwary consumers. Foodhandlers must also be checked and screened to protect the general public.[4]

Animals and insects are sources of disease and infection (see Figures 2.11 and 2.12). The control of animals (both domestic and wild) and insects in the community, both rural and urban, are essential to disease control and prevention. Zoonosis was presented earlier in the chapter, as animals are known sources of disease and its transmission. Insects play a passive and active role in the transmission of bacterial and some viral diseases. Proper food storage, refrigeration, water protection, garbage control, and sanitation (including lids on garbage cans as well as screening of windows and doors) all help to control insects and related pathogens.[4]

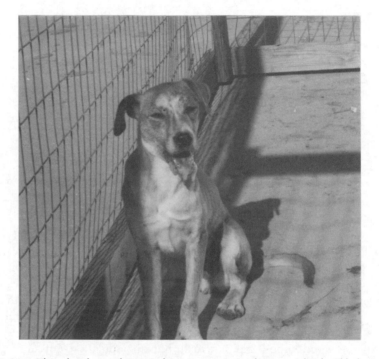

FIGURE 2.11   This dog has rabies. Rabies is a serious disease which, if left untreated in humans, causes a most painful death. Rabies is one of the notifiable diseases and one for which there is a vaccine available. (Picture courtesy of Centers for Disease Control and Prevention, Atlanta, Georgia)

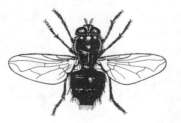

FIGURE 2.12   The common housefly (blue bottle fly) has been shown to be a major source of disease transmission. (Picture courtesy of Centers for Disease Control and Prevention, Atlanta, Georgia)

Host-Related Control and Prevention

The host of a disease can be either human or animal, and both are vulnerable to infectious diseases. (See Chapter 1 for more detail on host concepts.) A goal of public health is to protect the host from contagious diseases and infections by several methods. The protective measures used are quarantine, isolation, sanitation, good hygiene, immunizations, and chemoprophylaxis.

Quarantine has been used throughout history to separate ill people from well people to stop the spread of disease. Quarantine was probably the first public health measure to show a marked level of effectiveness in controlling the spread of disease. In the late 1800s and early 1900s, quarantine activities became an organized effort by government officials and had a major impact on increasing the health status of the community especially in the area of mortality statistics. In modern times quarantine measures are still in use. Currently the World Health Organization evokes quarantine measures on three diseases—cholera, plague, and yellow fever. Some attempts have been made to use quarantine measures against AIDS, but these efforts have been met with much resistance by activist groups.

Isolation is a term that uses quarantine-type activities but is conducted on an inpatient basis in hospitals or nursing homes, as shown in Figure 2.13. Most state laws as well

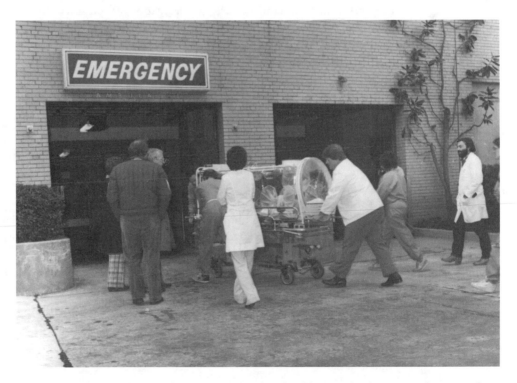

FIGURE 2.13 One form of quarantine used in health care facilities is isolation. When cases of highly contagious diseases enter hospitals, every effort is made to assure that the disease is contained, controlled, and not spread to other patients or to health care workers. Most hospitals have special isolation rooms set up; in serious cases, a Vicker's Isolator unit like this one is required. Vicker's Isolators are also used to transport highly infectious patients. (Picture courtesy of Centers for Disease Control and Prevention, Atlanta, Georgia)

as accrediting organizations require one or two beds to be kept, designated, and equipped in a hospital or nursing home as isolation beds. The isolation beds are used to segregate and isolate any patient with a communicable disease, so that disease will not spread throughout the facility. Isolation is an infection control measure, usually done under the direction and control of the hospital epidemiologist (infection control director) and the infection control committee of a hospital. Six variables or levels of isolation are used in a hospital:

1. One or two private rooms are used as isolation rooms.
2. Separate and infection controlled gowns are used.
3. Staff must wear masks.
4. All staff must be gloved when interacting, treating, or working with or on the patient.
5. Hand washing is required upon entering and leaving the patient's room.
6. All contaminated articles or possibly contaminated articles including linen, dressings, syringes, instruments, etc., must be disposed of properly.

Levels of Quarantine

There are four levels of quarantine used in public health. The four levels of quarantine range from moderate to severe. They are: (1) segregation, (2) personal surveillance, (3) modified quarantine, and (4) complete quarantine. **Segregation** is the control and observation of a group of persons who are separated and have minimum contact with others in order to control and reduce the spread of infection. **Personal surveillance** includes some separation without restricting movement, but patients are under close medical supervision in order to quickly discover any infection or disease. **Modified quarantine** is a partial restriction of movement based on knowledge of susceptibility in the group and an infection affirmed in the host with disease transmission imminent. The most serious level is **complete quarantine** as full limitation of freedom is required in order to protect well individuals. Quarantine takes into consideration incubation periods, communicability of the disease, mode and vehicles of disease transmission, types and levels of contact, and the potential for disease transmission.

Special isolation concerns arise when it comes to dealing with HIV/AIDS patients. The Centers for Disease Control and Prevention issued procedures for the control of infections including AIDS. Universal blood and body-fluid precautions or "universal precautions," are to be applied to all patients from the emergency room, to outpatient clinics, to the dentist office, to the isolation room in the hospital. Barrier techniques are to be implemented which include gloves, masks, gowns, protective eyewear, and hand washing when in contact with all patients. Gloves are to be used when touching blood or body fluids. Proper disposal of all articles that could be contaminated must be done with care. Care to avoid accidental self-punctures with contaminated needles must be taken. High-risk patients for AIDS need to be tested. High-risk hospital and clinic personnel also need to be tested for HIV/AIDS on a regular basis.[4]

Infection Control and Prevention Measures

Personal hygiene is the process of maintaining high standards of personal body maintenance and cleanliness. Cleanliness and health maintenance activities include frequent bathing, regular grooming, teeth cleaning and maintenance, changing clothes frequently, and hand washing. Family beliefs and practices, food preparation and protection, home environment and living spaces all contribute to infection control and prevention and are a benefit to hygienic practices.

Immunizations are for the protection of each person and family from disease and infection. Immunizations are key preventive medicine and public health measures against disease spread in populations or groups.

Chemical and antibiotic prophylaxis have shown great success in treating certain infections since 1945 when penicillin was finally mass produced and made available for wide use in the population. In the 1800s, arsenic, a poisonous chemical, was found somewhat effective in treating syphilis, if used in low doses. Sulfa drugs were also found to be effective against many infectious diseases. Chemical prophylaxis became less of a focus with the

NEWS FILE

Disease Transmission and Universal Precautions

Hand Washing Remains Key to Reducing Disease Transmission

Hand washing has long been recognized as one of the most effective ways to reduce the transmission of disease in laypeople and professionals alike. Many serious and life-threatening diseases are caused by transmission through not washing one's hands, especially disease transmitted through the fecal-oral route. Feces remaining on the hands after toilet use may then enter the body by putting the hands in the mouth or by contaminating food during food preparation. *E. coli 0157-H7*, cholera, typhoid fever, salmonella food poisoning, poliomyelitis, and hepatitis A are but some of the diseases transmitted by the oral-fecal route. Dr. Gail Casell, professor and chair of the Department of Microbiology at the University of Alabama, Birmingham, conducted a national survey, in Chicago, Atlanta, San Francisco, New Orleans, and New York, of 6,333 people, both women and men, directly observed in bathrooms. Although 94 percent of people asked by telephone say that they always wash their hands after going to the bathroom, direct observation found that only 68 percent actually did. Generally, women washed their hands more often than men, with women washing 74 percent of the time and men, only 61 percent of the time (presentation, American Society for Microbiologists, 1996, New Orleans). With the onset of the AIDS/HIV epidemic in the mid 1980s, universal precautions were developed to protect health care professionals, police, and others who come in direct contact with people who could infect them, especially by blood. Universal precautions are aggressive, standardized approaches to infection control, in which all human blood and certain body fluids are treated as if they are known to contain HIV, HBV, or other bloodborne pathogens. In universal precautions, hand washing is not enough protection, so personal protective equipment, such as gloves, masks, eye protection, and special equipment for mouth-to-mouth resuscitation and CPR, might be needed for exposure to blood or body fluids.

development of antibiotic medications. With the development of both specific antibiotics and broad spectrum antibiotics, the treatment of individuals and the practice of medicine has greatly changed. The impact of chemical and antibiotic prophylaxis on the health status in the world has been outstanding. Infants and mothers no longer die due to the childbirth process in the numbers they formerly did. Wounds heal, surgery is completed without the patient dying later from an infection, strep infections are quickly halted and no longer turn into rheumatic fever, and now it has been shown through research that antibiotics administered within 2 hours of surgery can help prevent surgical wound infections. Many lives have been saved and much suffering has been eliminated due to the development and effective use of chemical and antibiotic prophylaxis.[4]

NONCOMMUNICABLE DISEASES AND CHRONIC DISEASE CLASSIFICATION

The first set of diseases that come to mind which are of the noninfectious and noncommunicable type are mental and psychiatric disorders and conditions. Understanding psychiatric disorders and behavioral problems has greatly grown over the last 30 to 40 years. In 1975, a rough draft of the DSM-III was presented at a special session of the annual American Psychiatric Association conference. Several additional drafts and meetings were held over the next five years. Field trials of the suggested new classifications were made. In 1980 a newly developed classification of psychiatric disorders was made available from the American Psychiatric Association, titled, DSM-III, short for Diagnostic and Statistical Manual of Mental Disorders, Third Edition. This revision was a major advancement in the structure and classification of mental conditions. The concept of neurosis was removed from the classification and stress (post-traumatic) related issues were included. In 1987 a revised addition of the book was released titled DSM-IIIR.[17]

Sixteen diagnostic categories for mental conditions and disorders were set forth. A "V" code section for conditions not attributable to a mental disorder but a focus of the treatment process was included, plus a list of additional codes. Tables 2.10 and 2.11 give the classification listings by general category as presented in DSM-IV. For detailed information on any of the conditions or disorders, the DSM-IV manual should be consulted.[17]

TABLE 2.10   Diagnostic categories of mental conditions from DSM-IV

DSM-IV multiaxial system of classification mental disorders:

Axis I   Clinical disorders and other conditions that may be a focus of clinical attention
Axis II   Personality disorders, mental retardation
Axis III   General medical conditions related to psychiatric disorders
Axis IV   Psychosocial and interpersonal environmental problems
Axis V   Global assessment of functioning

Diagnostic categories of mental conditions:

1. Disorders usually first evident in infancy, childhood, or adolescence
2. Delirium, dementia, and amnestic and other cognitive disorders

TABLE 2.10 *(Continued)*

3. Mental disorders due to a general medical condition not elsewhere classified
4. Substance-related disorders
5. Schizophrenia and other psychotic disorders
6. Mood disorders
7. Anxiety disorders
8. Somatoform disorders
9. Factitious disorders
10. Dissociative disorders
11. Sexual and gender identity disorders
12. Eating disorders
13. Sleep disorders
14. Impulse-control disorders not elsewhere classified
15. Adjustment disorders
16. Personality disorders
17. Other conditions that may be a focus of clinical attention
18. Medication-induced movement disorders
19. Relational problems
20. Problems related to abuse and neglect
21. Additional conditions that may be a focus of clinical attention
22. Additional codes for unspecified mental disorders (nonpsychotic)

TABLE 2.11 "V" Codes for behavioral conditions and related disorders

Malingering

Borderline Intellectual Functioning

Adult Antisocial Behavior

Childhood or Adolescent Antisocial Behavior

Academic Problem

Noncompliance with Medical Treatment

Phase of Life Problem or Life Circumstance Problem

Marital Problem

Other Specified Family Circumstance

Other Interpersonal Problem

Additional codes are for unspecified mental disorders (nonpsychotic), and the failure to diagnose a condition by the above classification.[17]

(V codes for conditions not attributable to mental disorders that are a focus of attention or treatment[17])

NUTRITIONAL DEFICIENCY DISEASES AND DISORDERS

Nutritional deficiency diseases and disorders could possibly be classified under chronic diseases and conditions. There is some overlap between the two classifications. However, a separate listing is warranted. Three general use classifications of nutritional disorders are used: malnutrition, undernutrition, and overnutrition. **Malnutrition** literally means bad nutrition; it is faulty nutrition resulting from poor diet, bad assimilation of nutrients, lack of sufficient calories, or undereating or overeating. Malnutrition is generally thought to be poor health caused by the lack of food. **Undernutrition** is having enough food to eat but failing to eat the correct types and amounts of the proper variety of food stuffs, resulting in poor health. **Overnutrition** is the consumption of too much food along with too little activity and exercise, resulting in obesity.

Obesity seems to have many different classifications and approaches to describing it. The most common classifications of obesity are

1. Simple (due to calorie intake exceeding need, or energy expended)
   • alimentary (excessive food intake/low activity)
   • exogenous (excessive food intake/low activity)
2. Endogenous (caused by endocrine and metabolic disorders)

A second approach to obesity classification that is sometimes used is as follows: **Juvenile onset obesity** and **adult onset obesity** are alternative classifications sometimes used.

A third approach to classifying obesity is based on pathogenesis:

• Regulatory (defect in intake control) or reactive, occurs by overeating when reacting to stress.
• Metabolic (physiological defect in using food), also called constitutional obesity.

Other factors listed as contributing to obesity include social, endocrine, psychological, genetic, developmental, activity, and brain damage factors.[8,18]

Primary deficiency diseases can contribute to malnutrition and can result directly from the dietary lack of specific essential nutrients. For example, scurvy results from a dietary

TABLE 2.12   Malnutrition syndromes

Kwashiorkor (protein deficiency)
Marasmus (protein-calorie malnutrition, chronic undernutrition)
Iron-deficiency anemia
Folic acid-deficiency anemia
Vitamin B_{12} deficiency anemia
Xerophthalmia (vitamin A deficiency)
Endemic goiter (iodine deficiency)
Beriberi (thiamin deficiency)
Ariboflavinosis (riboflavin deficiency)
Pellagra (niacin and amino acid tryptophan deficiency)
Scurvy (vitamin C deficiency)
Rickets (vitamin D deficiency)
Tetany (mineral deficiency)
Osteomalacia and osteoporosis (impaired calcium and phosphorus metabolism affecting bone formation)

deficiency of vitamin C. (See Chapter 1 for the historical discovery and the treatment of scurvy.) Secondary deficiency diseases result from inability of the body to use specific-nutrients properly; for example, the food cannot be absorbed into the body while in the alimentary tract or the food stuff cannot be metabolized.

Undereating or being underweight, like obesity, can be caused by either psychological/behavioral problems or some physiological disorder. Anorexia nervosa and bulimia are examples of psychological/behavioral undereating problems. Endocrine problems usually are the source of physiological based underweight problems. Overall, two general categories of nutritional diseases and disorders are used. One is the malnutrition syndromes and the second one is the nutritional deficiency conditions. Listings of both categories together are presented in Table 2.12.

CHRONIC DISEASES AND CONDITIONS

A disease or condition is usually considered chronic if a person indicates the disorder was first noticed more than 3 months before the reference date and if the type of condition usually has a duration of more than 3 months. Any prolonged condition, disorder, or disease that is of a long duration is considered chronic. Generally, infectious or communicable diseases are acute in nature, of short duration, and are usually caused by a pathogen. Chronic diseases are not often caused by a pathogen or infection, but are a result of lifestyle, risk-taking behaviors, occupational exposure, or the aging process. Another way these two classes of diseases are referred to is *infectious disease* and *noninfectious disease*. A noninfectious disease is usually referred to as a chronic disease. However, an infectious disease is considered contagious, as it is easily spread in a population. Some acute conditions that affect one's health status may not be infectious and some chronic diseases can result from infectious diseases.[19]

Another term associated with chronic disease is **impairment**—a chronic or permanent defect, usually static in nature, that results from a disease, condition, injury, or congenital malformation. Impairment is also associated with chronic disease, as it represents a decrease in or loss of ability to perform various functions, particularly those of the musculoskeletal system and the sense organs. Impairments are grouped by type of functional impairment and etiology.[19]

To help clarify the differences between acute and chronic diseases and conditions as well as infectious and noninfectious conditions, Figure 2.14 provides a comparison of the four different states of diseases or conditions.

Prevention and Control of Chronic Diseases

The development of many chronic diseases is preventable and some chronic diseases could also be minimized in their severity by changing behavior and exposure to certain risk factors in life. For example, lung cancer and chronic obstructive pulmonary disease (COPD) could be almost eliminated if no one smoked. Certain liver diseases could be greatly reduced if alcohol consumption were curtailed. Lifestyle, behavior, and unnecessary exposure to risk factors in life continue to contribute to many chronic diseases in our society. Cardiovascular disease and cancer could be reduced if nutritional and dietary factors were altered. These diseases are also affected by smoking and alcohol.

Acute   versus   Chronic

	Acute	Chronic
Infectious	Flu Lyme disease Mumps Measles Cholera	Tuberculosis Polio Leprosy Schistosomiasis Syphilis
Noninfectious	Suicide Homicide Accidents CVA (Stroke) Drug Abuse	Heart Disease Cancer Alcoholism Paralysis/CVA Diabetes

versus

FIGURE 2.14   Samples of acute, chronic, infectious, and noninfectious diseases and conditions compared.

The main lifestyle and behavior changes needed to prevent and control chronic disease include the reduction of and possibly the elimination of the use of tobacco and smoking (which includes the second-hand smoke risks); the use of alcohol, and drug abuse. Additional changes include dietary changes (a reduction of fat in the diet, empty calories, and cholesterol; maintaining proper calcium levels, limiting certain kinds of protein and red meat), increased fitness and exercise, proper weight maintenance, stress reduction, and increased safety measures.

Prevention measures have made great strides in the area of cancer. Efforts to detect breast cancer at early stages are critical in reducing breast cancer associated mortality. Early Detection Programs (EDP) have been found to be most effective as cancer prevention and control measures. Primary care centers have used EDP in order to facilitate cancer screening services. Mammography screening has been done at centers located in shopping centers and mobile mammography vans have also been used.

Table 2.13 presents the results of an Early Detection Program breast cancer screening program in Dade County, Florida in a hispanic population. From the screening of the 9,434 patients, 274 biopsies were performed with 57 of the tests being positive for cancer. Late-stage diagnosis of cancer contributes to the 10–15% lower survival rates among women of low socioeconomic status. Early diagnosis and early treatment are the key hallmarks to prevention and control in cancer.[20]

Disability

One of the unfortunate and devastating aspects of some acute and some chronic diseases is that the end result can be a handicap or disability. Polio can cause a whole range of paralysis from a mild weakness in a leg or arm to complete loss of function of legs and arms, to

TABLE 2.13   Characteristics of 9,434 patients and results from the Early Detection Program for breast cancer among hispanics, Dade County, Florida, 1987–1990

Patient Characteristic	%	Result	%
Race/Ethnicity		**Mammography finding ($n = 11,632$)[†]**	
Hispanic	52.8	Not suspicious for cancer	68.0
Non-Hispanic black	40.8	Additional evaluation	27.7
Non-Hispanic white	6.1	Suspicious for cancer	4.3
Unknown	0.3		
		Biopsy result ($n = 274$)	
Age (yrs)		Negative	79.2
<40	15.2	Positive	20.8
40–49	29.0		
50–69	50.1	**Histologic result ($n = 57$)**	
>70	5.7	In situ	17.5
		Local	36.8
Previous mammogram ($n = 8,397$)*		Regional	35.1
No	74.0	Distant	5.3
Yes	26.0	Unstaged	5.3

*This question was not asked of women during the beginning of the program.

[†]Includes screening, repeat, and follow-up mammograms.

(Source: Centers for Disease Control and Prevention, "Increasing Breast Cancer Screening Among the Medically Underserved—Dade County, Florida, September 1987–March 1991, *Morbidity and Mortality Weekly Report*, Vol. 40, No. 16, April 26, 1991)

loss of ability to breathe. The level of disability can range from a mild weakness to serious paralysis of limbs, yet leaving the person with a degree of function; a most devastating result. Reye's syndrome can leave a person with neurological and muscular deficits and disability. Cerebral Vascular Accidents (stroke; or CVA) can leave a person paralyzed. Diabetes can lead to amputation of parts of fingers, hands, and limbs, again causing a disability. These acute and chronic diseases are but a sample of some of the diseases and conditions leading to disability.

The level of disability in our society is of serious consequence due to the cost of medical care, inability to work, inability to be economically productive, lack of being self-sufficient, lack of mobility, and being a burden on family members. Several measures of disability have been developed and used in public health and social services. **Disability** refers to any long- or short-term reduction of a person's activity as a result of an acute or chronic condition. **Limitation of activity** refers to any long-term reduction in a person's capacity to perform the average kind or amount of activities associated with his or her age group. **Restriction of activity** is any particular kind of behavior usually associated with a reduction in activity due to either long- or short-term conditions. Limitation of activity refers to what a person is generally capable of doing, but restriction of activity ordinarily refers to a relatively short-term reduction in a person's activities below his or her normal capacity. Five of the most common measures of disability are

1. Days of work lost
2. Days of school missed
3. Days of being confined to bed
4. Cut-down days
5. Days of restricted activity

Work-loss, school-loss, and cut-down days refer to the short-term effects of illness or injury. Bed-days are a measure of both long- and short-term disability. A chronically ill bedridden person and a person with a cold could both report having spent more than half-a-day in bed due to illness.

Restricted activity days relies on the number of days of restriction a person experiences and includes at least one of the five types of activity restriction mentioned above. Restricted-activity days may be associated with either persons or conditions. **Person days** are the number of days during which a person restricted his or her activity. **Condition days** are the number of days during which a condition caused a person to restrict his or her activity. A person day of restricted activity can be caused by more than one condition;

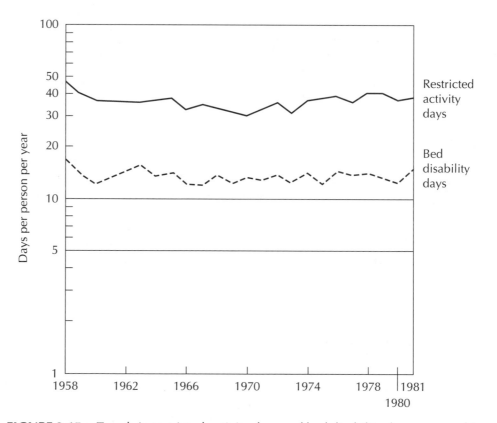

FIGURE 2.15   Trends in restricted activity days and bed disability days among older adults from 1958–1981. (Source: Office of Disease Prevention and Health Promotion, *Prevention 84/85*, Public Health Service, U.S. Department of Health and Human Services, Washington, D.C. 1986)

the number of condition days of restricted activity may exceed the number of person days of restricted activity.[19]

Figure 2.15 illustrates the number of bed disability days and restricted activity days for a 23-year period in the United States.

Activities of Daily Living: A Measure of Chronic Disease and Disability

Another measure of disability is found in the independence one has or lacks as measured by the **Activities of Daily Living** (**ADL**) scale. This index measures the severity of chronic illness and is used to evaluate the effectiveness of treatment programs. The ADL has also been used to provide predictive information on the course of specific illnesses. The ADL index is based on basic psychosocial and biological functioning and reflects the health status and adequacy of organized neurological and locomotor responses.[22] Following is a list of the factors, traits and skills measured by the ADL.[22]

- Bathing
- Toileting
- Continence
- Dressing
- Transfer
- FeedingFeeding

A person who is assessed by the ADL is given a rating by a letter grade that indicates the level of functioning. The letter "A" is for being independent on all six items and is a top grade as found in academic settings. At the other extreme is the letter "G" which indicates a person is dependent in all six functions and needs assistance. The letters between A and G provide a continuum of increasing severity of the disability and loss of ability to perform in six areas. Specific definitions of the six areas have been developed to assist in the assessment.[22]

HEALTH GOALS FOR THE YEAR 2000

The United States has the ability to save many lives lost prematurely and needlessly, to reduce injuries, disabilities, and illnesses. Thus, the development and implementation of goals for the year 2000 for the nation was undertaken. Saving lives was not enough, so *Healthy People 2000: National Health Promotion and Disease Prevention Objectives* was developed and published. The challenge of *Healthy People 2000* is to use scientific knowledge, professional skill, individual commitment, community support, and political will to enable people to achieve their potential to live full and active lives. Means were set forth for preventing premature death, preventing disability, preserving a physical environment that supports human life, cultivating family and community support, enhancing inherent abilities and assuring that all Americans achieve and maintain a maximum level of functioning and overall well-being. Table 2.14 shows the *Healthy People 2000* priority areas. The objectives in each of the priority areas are numerous and the publication itself must be consulted.[23]

TABLE 2.14   *Healthy People 2000*: Priority areas [23]

Health Promotion	Preventive Services
1. Physical Activity and Fitness	14. Maternal and Infant Health
2. Nutrition	15. Heart Disease and Stroke
3. Tobacco	16. Cancer
4. Alcohol and Other Drugs	17. Diabetes and Chronic Disabling Conditions
5. Family Planning	18. HIV Infection
6. Mental Health and Mental Disorders	19. Sexually Transmitted Diseases
7. Violent and Abusive Behavior	20. Immunization and Infectious Disease
8. Educational and Community-Based Programs	21. Clinical Preventive Services
	Surveillance and Data Systems
Health Protection	22. Surveillance and Data Systems
9. Unintentional Injuries	**Age-Related Objectives**
10. Occupational Safety and Health	Children
11. Environmental Health	Adolescents and Young Adults
12. Food and Drug Safety	Adults
13. Oral Health	Older Adults

EXERCISES

Key Terms

Define and explain the following terms.

acquired immunity	etiology	pathogenicity
active immunity	fastigium period	personal surveillance
Activities of Daily Living (ADL)	herd immunity	person days
acute	immunity	prodromal period
adult onset obesity	immunization	quarantine
antibiotics	impairment	restriction of activity
antibodies	infective	segregation
antigen	invasiveness	subacute
antigenicity	isolation	subclinical
chronic	juvenile onset obesity	toxicity
communicability	limitation of activity	toxin
complete quarantine	malnutrition	undernutrition
condition days	modified quarantine	vaccine
convalescence	overnutrition	viability
defection	passive immunity	virulence
defervescence	pathogen	zoonosis
disability	pathogenesis	
disease	pathogenic	

Study Questions

2.1   Using the proposed immunization schedule in Table 2.15, complete the shot record provided in Table 2.16. You may use your own child, a child of a friend or a relative, or yourself to acquire the information. Make a list of recommended immunizations needed in order to have a complete shot history and for the person to be totally immunized.

TABLE 2.15 Recommended ages for administration of currently licensed childhood vaccines—July 1995

Vaccines are listed under routinely recommended ages. Solid bars indicate range of acceptable ages for vaccination. Shaded bars indicate new recommendations or vaccines licensed since publication of the *Recommended Childhood Immunization Schedule* in January 1995.

Hepatitis B vaccine is recommended at 11–12 years of age for children not previously vaccinated. Varicella zoster virus vaccine is recommended at 11–12 years of age for children not previously vaccinated, and who lack a reliable history of chickenpox.

Vaccine	Birth	2 mos	4 mos	6 mos	12[1] mos	15 mos	18 mos	4–6 yrs	11–12 yrs	14–16 yrs
Hepatitis B[2,3]	Hep B-1									
		Hep B-2		Hep B-3					Hep B[3]	
Diphtheria, Tetanus, Pertussis[4]		DTP	DTP	DTP	DTP[1,4] (DTaP at 15+ m)			DTP or DTaP	Td	
H. influenzae type b[5]		Hib	Hib	Hib[5]	Hib[1,5]					
Polio		OPV	OPV	OPV				OPV		
Measles, Mumps, Rubella[6]					MMR[1,6]			MMR [or][6] MMR		
Varicella Zoster[7] Virus Vaccine					VZV[7]				VZV[7]	

[1] Vaccines recommended in the second year of life (12–15 months of age) may be given at either 1 or 2 visits.

[2] **Infants born to HBsAg-negative mothers** should receive 2.5 µg of Merck Sharp & Dohme (MSD) vaccine (Recombivax HB) or 10 µg of SmithKline Beecham (SKB) vaccine (Engerix-B). The 2nd dose should be given between 1 and 4 months of age, if at least one month has elapsed since receipt of the first dose. The 3rd dose is recommended between 6 and 18 months of age.

Infants born to HBsAg-positive mothers should receive immunoprophylaxis for hepatitis B with 0.5 ml Hepatitis B Immune Globulin (HBIG) within 12 hours of birth, and either 5 µg of MSD vaccine (Recombivax HB) or 10 µg of SKB vaccine (Engerix-B) at a separate site. In these infants, the 2nd dose is recommended at 1 month of age and the 3rd dose at 6 months of age. All pregnant women should be screened for HBsAg during an early prenatal visit.

[3] Hepatitis B vaccine is recommended for adolescents who have not previously received 3 doses of vaccine. The 3-dose series should be initiated or completed at the 11–12 year-old visit for persons not previously fully vaccinated. The 2nd dose should be administered at least 1 month after the 1st dose, and the 3rd dose should be administered at least 4 months after the 1st dose.

[4] The 4th dose of DTP may be administered as early as 12 months of age, provided ≥6 months have elapsed since DTP3. Combined DTP-Hib products may be used when these 2 vaccines are to be administered simultaneously. DTaP (diphtheria and tetanus toxoids and acellular pertussis vaccine) is licensed for use for the 4th and/or 5th dose of DTP vaccine in children ≥15 months of age and may be preferred for these doses in children in this age group. Td (tetanus and diphtheria toxoids, adsorbed, for adult use) is recommended at 11–12 years of age if ≥5 years have elapsed since the last dose of DTP, DTP-Hib, or DT.

[5] Three *H. influenzae* type b conjugate vaccines are available for use in infants: HbOC [HibTITER] (Lederle Praxis); PRP-T [ActHIB; OmniHIB] (Pasteur Mérieux, distributed by SmithKline Beecham; Connaught); and PRP-OMP [PedvaxHIB] (Merck Sharp & Dohme). Children who have received PRP-OMP at 2 and 4 months of age do not require a dose at 6 months of age. After the primary infant Hib conjugate vaccine series is completed, any licensed Hib conjugate vaccine may be used as a booster dose at age 12–15 months.

[6] The 2nd dose of MMR vaccine should be administered EITHER at 4–6 years of age OR at 11–12 years of age, consistent with state school immunization requirements.

[7] *Varicella zoster* virus vaccine (VZV) is routinely recommended at 12–18 months of age. Children who have not been vaccinated previously and who lack a reliable history of chickenpox should be vaccinated by 13 years of age. VZV can be administered to susceptible children any time during childhood. Children <13 years of age should receive a single 0.5 mL dose; persons ≥13 years of age should receive two 0.5 mL doses 4–8 weeks apart.

This schedule indicates new recommendations for vaccines licensed since publication of the *Recommended Childhood Immunization Schedule* in January 1995. The Recommended Childhood Immunization Schedule is reviewed and published annually by the Advisory Committee on Immunization Practices, the American Academy of Pediatrics, and the American Academy of Family Physicians. After review and revision, this schedule will be published in the MMWR in January 1996 as the "Recommended Childhood Immunization Schedule, United States—January 1996."

TABLE 2.16 Shot record

	2 months (Date)	4 months (Date)	6 months (Date)	12 months (Date)	15 months (Date)	4–6 yrs (Date)
POLIO						
DTP						
MMR						
HIB meningitis						

Tetanus and diphtheria, adult type are to be given at 14 to 16 years and every 10 years thereafter. If exposed to Hepatitis B, a shot at birth, 2, 6 and possible 15 months.

2.2   Briefly list and explain briefly the different general classifications of diseases.

2.3   Briefly list, explain and provide an example of each of the 5 classifications of the modes of transmission of infectious diseases.

2.4   Briefly list and give examples of the various causes and sources of infectious diseases.

2.5   Briefly list and give examples of the causes and sources of 10 noncommunicable diseases or conditions from inanimate sources.

2.6   Choose 10 infectious diseases, and explain, discuss and give an example of incubation periods in these infectious diseases.

2.7   Draw a graph of the course of the infectious respiratory disease tuberculosis, detail the specific phases and aspects of each stage of the disease, and explain them.

2.8   Explain the concept of notifiable diseases, then select rabies as a specific notifiable disease and explain the reporting system using this disease.

2.9   Explain and discuss herd immunity. Draw a brief graphic presentation of how herd immunity works to protect a population based on Figure 2.9.

2.10 List the different classifications of noncommunicable diseases and chronic diseases presented in the chapter.

2.11 What are the activities of daily living and what role does ADL play in assessing disability?

REFERENCES

1. Sheldon, H. 1984. *Boyd's Introduction to the Study of Disease*. Philadelphia: Lea and Febiger.
2. Crowley, L.V. 1988. *Introduction to Human Disease*, 2nd edition. Boston: Jones and Bartlett Publishing Inc.
3. Timmreck, T.C. 1997. *Health Services Cyclopedic Dictionary*, 3rd edition. Sudbury, MA: Jones and Bartlett Publishing Inc.

4. Evans, A.S. and P.S. Brachman. 1991. *Bacterial Infections of Humans: Epidemiology and Control*, 2nd edition. New York: Plenum Medical Book Company.

5. Bickley, H.C. 1977. *Practical Concepts in Human Disease*, 2nd edition. Baltimore: Williams and Wilkins.

6. Green, L.W. and C.L. Anderson. 1982. *Community Health*, 4th edition. St. Louis: C.V. Mosby.

7. Wigley, R. and J.R. Cook. 1975. *Community Health*. New York: D. Van Nostrand Co.

8. Berkow, R. (Editor). 1982. *The Merck Manual of Diagnosis and Therapy,* 14th edition. Rahway, NJ: Merck and Co.

9. Grant, M. 1987. *Handbook of Community Health*, 4th edition. Philadelphia: Lea and Febiger.

10. Acha, P.N. and B. Szyfres. 1989. *Zoonoses and Communicable Diseases Common to Man and Animals*, 2nd edition. Washington, D.C.: Pan American Health Organization.

11. Olishifski, J.B. and F.E. McElroy. 1975. *Fundamentals of Industrial Hygiene*. Chicago: National Safety Council.

12. Thygerson, A.L. 1986. *Safety*, 2nd edition. Englewood Cliffs, NJ: Prentice Hall.

13. Youmans, G.P., P.Y. Paterson, and H.M. Sommers. *The Biologic and Clinical Basis of Infectious Diseases*. Philadelphia: W.B. Saunders.

14. Summary of Notifiable Diseases in the United States, 1990. *Morbidity and Mortality Weekly Reports*. Centers for Disease Control and Prevention, Vol. 39, No. 53, Oct. 4, 1991.

15. Last, J.M. 1980. *Public Health and Preventive Medicine*. New York: Appleton-Century-Crofts.

16. Vaccinia (Smallpox) Vaccine: Recommendations of the Immunizations Practices Advisory Committee (ACIP), *Morbidity and Mortality Weekly Reports*. Centers for Disease Control and Prevention, Vol. 40, No. RR-14, Dec. 13, 1991.

17. American Psychiatric Association. 1987. *DSM-III: Diagnostic and Statistical Manual of Mental Disorders*, 3rd edition (R). Washington, D.C.: American Psychiatric Association.

18. Williams, S.R. 1989. *Nutrition and Diet Therapy*, 6th edition. St. Louis: Times Mirror/Mosby.

19. National Center for Health Statistics, *Vital Statistics in the United States—1990*. Public Health Service, Washington, D.C.: U.S. Department of Health and Human Services.

20. Increasing Breast Cancer Screening Among the Medically Underserved—Dade County, Florida, September 1987–March 1991, *Morbidity and Mortality Weekly Report*. Centers for Disease Control and Prevention, Vol. 40, No. 16, April 26, 1991.

21. Office of Disease Prevention and Health Promotion. 1986. *Prevention 84/85*, Public Health Service. Washington, D.C.: U.S. Department of Health and Human Services.

22. McDowell, I. and C. Newell. 1987. *Measuring Health: A Guide to Rating Scales and Questionnaires*. New York: Oxford University Press.

23. Public Health Service, U.S. Department of Health and Human Services. 1992. *Healthy People 2000: National Health Promotion and Disease Prevention Objectives*. Boston: Jones and Bartlett Publishing Inc.

3

Selected Historical Developments of Epidemiology

CHAPTER OBJECTIVES

This chapter on historical developments of epidemiology

- presents several key historical events that contributed to the development of the field of epidemiology;
- reviews some introductory concepts and principles of epidemiology;
- presents several scientists who contributed historically to the field of epidemiology;
- reviews several historical epidemiological occurrences that helped establish some of the principles of epidemiological study still in use today;
- reviews several historical disease/epidemic cases and their study that changed the face of medicine and epidemiology;
- presents key terms and study questions for review of chapter concepts.

INTRODUCTION

Men of medicine and epidemiology have studied diseases and how epidemics went through groups of people since the beginning of recorded time. Minor discoveries had to occur in order for major contributions to be made later. Much interconnectedness of events across time happened in order for the causes of diseases to be discovered. These events did not always occur in a neat, chronological order, or in the same country, or even on the same continent. A jigsaw puzzle of discoveries and activities occurred across time and across various countries of the world. The historical developments presented here are not all-inclusive and represent some of the major and a few of the minor events that have influenced the development of epidemiology.

HIPPOCRATES, THE FIRST EPIDEMIOLOGIST

Hippocrates, (460–377 BC) as he saw patients die, must have felt frustrated and discouraged as a physician. If he could only discover the source of the cause of illness and death in his patients. So little was understood and so great was the desire to understand. The Father of Medicine had little knowledge to draw upon in the 5th century BC that would give him the clues needed to search for the true causes of disease. Using his great insights and the knowledge available at the time, Hippocrates compiled and wrote his theory of medicine and treatment of the sick and injured. This misguided theory of medicine was to endure for more than 2,500 years.

Hippocrates' contribution to the field of public health is of importance, as he was the first recorded epidemiologist. Hippocrates' observations about the cause and spread of disease in populations were in many ways more accurate than many of his observations about the medical treatment of illness.[1,2,3,4]

Hippocrates gave advice to persons wishing to pursue the science of medicine, provided insights on the effects of the seasons of the year, and hot and cold winds. The properties of water, he believed, should be examined. He advised one to consider the source of water. Is the water from a marshy, soft-ground source, or is the water from the rocky heights? Is the water brackish and harsh? Hippocrates also made some noteworthy observations on personal behavior of the populace. He believed the effective physician should be observant. The physician should observe if the people are heavy drinkers, inactive, or athletic. Did they eat lunch, eat too much and drink too little, and were individuals industrious?[1,2,3,4]

For traveling physicians, Hippocrates suggested they become familiar with local diseases and with the nature of those prevailing diseases. He believed that as time passed the physician should be able to tell what epidemic diseases might attack and in what season, winter or summer, all of which can be determined by the settings of the stars. He went on to identify those diseases that would be in epidemics due to hot winds and those that would be endemic due to cold winds. Sources of water, how it sets or flows, and smells were always considered in studying disease states.[1,2,3,4]

Hippocrates identified hot and cold diseases, and consequently, hot and cold treatments. Hot diseases were treated with cold treatments and cold diseases required hot treatments. The process of deciding hot and cold diseases is complex. A simple example is diarrhea which is considered a hot disease and is cured with a cold treatment such as eating fruit.[1,2,3,4]

What brought recognition to Hippocrates as the first **epidemiologist** were three books he wrote. The three books were *Epidemic I, Epidemic III*, and *On Airs, Waters and Places*. He recognized that different diseases occurred in different places. He noted that malaria and yellow fever most commonly occurred in swampy areas.

Hippocrates also ascribed to and incorporated into his theory what is now considered the atomic theory, that is, everything is made of tiny particles. He theorized that there were four types of atoms: earth atoms (solid and cold), air atoms (dry), fire atoms (hot), water atoms (wet). Additionally, Hippocrates believed that the body was composed of four humors: phlegm (earth and water atoms), yellow bile (fire and air atoms), blood (fire and water atoms), and black bile (earth and air atoms). Sickness was thought to be caused by an imbalance of humors, while fever was thought to be caused by too much blood. The treatment for fever was to reduce the amount of blood in the body through blood letting or bloodsuckers (leeches). Mucus (phlegm) was considered a cold or wet disease and was treated by applying heat. Imbalances were ascribed to a change in one's "constitution." Climate, moisture, stars, meteorites, winds, vapors, and diet were thought to cause an imbalance and contribute to diseases. Diet was both a cause and cure of disease. Cures to illness or protection from disease came from maintaining a balance and avoiding imbalance in one's "constitution." The essentials of epidemiology noted by Hippocrates included observations on how diseases affected populations and how disease spread. He further addressed issues of diseases in relation to time and seasons, place, environmental conditions, and disease control, especially as it related to water and seasons. The broader contribution to epidemiology made by Hippocrates was that of **epidemiological observation**. His teachings about how to observe any and all contributing or causal factors to a disease are still sound epidemiological concepts.[3,4]

DISEASE OBSERVATIONS OF SYDENHAM

Thomas Sydenham (1624–1689) though a graduate of Oxford medical school, did not at first practice medicine but served in the military and as a college administrator. While at All Souls College where he was a fellow, he became acquainted with Robert Boyle, a colleague who sparked Sydenham's interest in diseases and epidemics. Sydenham went on to get his medical license and spoke out for strong empirical approaches to medicine and close observations of disease. Dr. Sydenham wrote the details of what he observed about diseases without allowing various traditional theories of disease and medical treatment to influence his work and observations. From this close observation process he was able to identify and recognize different diseases. He avoided the Galenic dogma of the time. Sydenham published his observations in a book in 1676 titled *Observationes Medicae*.[4]

One of the major works of Sydenham was the classification of fevers plaguing London in the 1660s and 1670s. Dr. Sydenham came up with three levels or classes of fevers: *continued, intermittent*, and *smallpox*. Some of Sydenham's theories were embraced while others were criticized, mostly because his ideas and observations went against the usual Hippocratic and Galenic approaches. He treated smallpox with bed rest and normal bed covers. The treatment of the time, based on the Hippocratic theory, was to use heat and extensive bed covering. He met with good results but was erroneous in identifying the cause of the disease.[4]

Dr. Sydenham was persecuted by his colleagues, who at one time threatened to take away his medical license for irregular practice as it did not follow the theories of the time. However, Thomas Sydenham gained a good reputation with the public and some young, open-minded physicians agreed with his empirical principles. Sydenham described and distinguished different diseases including some psychological maladies. He also advanced useful treatments and remedies including exercise, fresh air, and a healthy diet, which other physicians also rejected at the time.[4]

THE EPIDEMIOLOGY OF SCURVY IN 1753

In the 1700s it was observed that armies lost more men by disease than by the sword. Like any good epidemiologist, James Lind in his "A Treatise of the Scurvy in Three Parts, Containing an Inquiry into the Nature, Cause and Cure of That Disease, Together with a Critical and Chronological View of What Has Been Published on the Subject," focused on illnesses in populations. He observed the effect of time, place, weather, and diet on the spread of disease.[3,4]

Lind, an observant surgeon, noticed that while on long ocean voyages sailors would become sick from **scurvy**. He saw that scurvy began to rage after a month to six weeks at sea. Dr. Lind noted that even though the water was good and the provisions were not tainted, the sailors still got sick. On one voyage 80 men out of 350 were afflicted with scurvy. Lind pointed out that the months most common to scurvy were April, May, and June. He also observed that cold, rainy, foggy, and thick weather were often present. Being influenced by the Hippocratic theory of medicine, Lind kept looking to the air as the source of disease. For example, he noticed that the atmosphere at sea is more moist than of that on land, hence, a greater disposition to scorbutic diathesis at sea than in dry land air. Dampness of the air, damp living arrangements, and life at sea were the main focus of the observations of Lind as he searched for an explanation of the cause of disease and most of all the cause of scurvy.[5]

Though not completely correct about the weather and climate at sea, Lind, being a good epidemiologist considered all possibilities and made good epidemiological observations. He looked at all sides of the issue at hand and considered what was happening to the sick as compared to what the healthy were experiencing.

When Lind began to look at the diet of the mariners, he began to make his greatest epidemiological inroads. He observed that the sea diet was extremely gross, viscid, and hard on digestion. Being concerned with the extent of sickness in sailors in large numbers, Dr. Lind set up some experiments with mariners. He took 12 ill patients who had all the classical symptoms of scurvy. As he examined the daily diet of the sailors, he found each of the twelve's diet to be the same as the others. Doctor Lind put the sailors into six groups of two and varied the diet of each group, giving some members foods the others did not receive. Two of the mariners were given two oranges and one lemon each day. Both men ate them in greedy fashion, even on an empty stomach. The most sudden and visible good effects were seen in those eating oranges and lemons. In six days the two eating citrus were fit for duty. All the others had putrid gums, spots, lassitude, and weakness of the knees. All of these symptoms disappeared in the two sailors eating citrus and they were asked to nurse the others who were sick. Doctor Lind observed that of the results of all of his experiments the oranges and lemons were the most effective remedies for scurvy at sea.[5]

The epidemiological contributions of Lind were many. He was concerned with the occurrence of disease in large groups of people. Lind not only participated in the identification of the effect of diet on disease, but made clinical observations, used experimental design, asked classical epidemiological questions, observed the population changes and its effect on disease, and considered sources of causation, place, time, and season.

COWPOX AND ITS EPIDEMIOLOGICAL CONNECTION TO SMALLPOX

In England, Benjamin Jesty, a farmer/dairyman in the mid-1700s, noticed his milkmaids never got **smallpox**. However, the milkmaids did develop cowpox from the cows. Jesty believed there was a link to acquiring cowpox and not getting smallpox. In 1774 Jesty exposed his wife and children to cowpox to prevent them from getting smallpox and it worked. The exposed family members developed an immunity to smallpox. Unfortunately, little was publicized about Jesty's experiment and observations.[4]

The experiment of Jesty and similar reported experiences in Turkey, the Orient, America, and Hungary, were known to Doctor Edward Jenner, an English rural physician (1749–1823). He personally observed that dairymen's servants and milkmaids got cowpox and did not get smallpox. Dr. Jenner made a zoonotic and epidemiological connection between cowpox and smallpox and wanted to make common the use of the inoculation process. For many centuries the Chinese had made observations about weaker and stronger strains of smallpox. They learned that it was wise to catch a weaker strain of the disease. If one had a weak strain of the disease one would not get the full disease later on. This was termed "**variolation**."[3,4]

Men and maid servants in the late-1700s were often the ones who were required to milk the cows. One servant was required to tend to the sores on the heels of a horse affected with cowpox. The pus and infectious fluids were referred to as "the grease" of the disease. Being unconcerned about sanitation and cleanliness the disease was passed on to the cows from "the grease" from the servants' hands in the process of milking the cows. The cowpox in turn was transmitted to the dairymaids. Jenner observed that when a person had cowpox, this same person would not get smallpox if exposed to it. Jenner attempted to give a dairymaid, exposed to a mild case of cowpox in her youth, a case of cowpox by cutting her arm and rubbing some of the infectious "grease," into the wound. She had little response to the disease and did not get ill. In other cowpox outbreaks a man got cowpox three different times. A few years later there was an attempt to give this man cowpox by an inoculation, but he was immune. Cowpox was found to shield against smallpox.[3,4] Dr. Jenner invented a vaccination for smallpox from this knowledge. The vaccine was used to protect populations from smallpox.[3,4,7]

Note: On October 26th, 1977, World Health Organization workers tracked down, supposedly the world's last case of smallpox. The patient was 23-year-old Ali Maow Maalin, a hospital cook in Merka, Somalia. Two exceptions occurred which were two cases of smallpox in 1978. Because it was believed that smallpox had been eradicated from the earth, vaccinations have been halted. However, some public health and health care professionals are skeptical and fear that such acts may set the stage for an unexpected future epidemic of smallpox, as the pathogen still exists. Military and government labs retain the smallpox pathogen. As unvaccinated persons proliferate, so does the risk of future smallpox epidemics.

THE EPIDEMIOLOGY OF CHILDBED FEVER IN A LYING-IN HOSPITAL

Historically, epidemiology was centered upon the study of the great epidemics: cholera, **bubonic plague**, smallpox, and **typhus**. As the diseases were identified and differentiated, the focus of epidemiology changed. Such a change in focus came through the work of another physician-epidemiologist, Ignas Semmelweis in the early- to mid-1800s.[9]

In the 1840s one the greatest fears a pregnant mother had was dying of **childbed fever** (**puerperal fever**). Babies were born to the pregnant mother with the usual risks that warranted obstetric assistance and often resulted in an uneventful birth. But upon the birth of the child, the mother would get an infection and die of childbed fever, a streptococcal disease. Many times the child would become infected and die as well. After many years of observing the course of the disease and the symptoms associated with childbed fever, Dr. Semmelweis began a series of investigations reminiscent of classical retrospective epidemiological studies.[9]

The Viennese Maternity Hospital (called a **lying-in hospital**) in which Dr. Semmelweis was clinical director, was divided into two clinics. The difference in mortality between the two clinics was great. Clinic one, consistently had greater numbers of maternal deaths than clinic number two. In 1846 the maternal mortality rate of clinic one was five times greater than in clinic two, and over a 6-year period it was three times as great. Dr. Semmelweis observed that the mothers became ill either immediately during birth or within 24 to 36 hours after delivery. The mothers died quickly of rapidly developing childbed fever. Often the children would soon die as well. This was not the case in clinic number two.

Dr. Semmelweis observed it was not the actual labor that was the problem, but that it started during dilation. The examination of the patients seemed to be connected to the onset of the disease. Through clinical observation, retrospective study, collection and analysis of data on maternal deaths and infant deaths, clinically controlled experimentation, he was able to ascertain that the communication of childbed fever was due to germs being passed from patient to patient by the physician in the process of doing pelvic examinations. Dr. Semmelweis discovered that the medical students would come directly from the death house after working at autopsy of infected and decaying dead bodies and then would conduct pelvic exams on the mothers ready to give birth. Handwashing or any form of **infection control** was not a common practice. Unclean hands with putrefied cadaver material on student doctors' hands were used to conduct the routine daily pelvic exams and the practice was never questioned. There was no reason to be concerned about clean hands, as the theory of medicine that was accepted at the time relied upon spontaneous development for the occurrence of disease and the Hippocratic theory of medicine. Dr. Semmelweis observed that patients became ill sporadically or that whole rows would become ill without a single patient in the row in the ward staying healthy.[9]

Dr. Semmelweis believed that childbed fever was more **endemic** to the hospital and its activities than could be found in the surrounding community. The community identified the disease as an epidemic. Dr. Semmelweis said that the course of the disease of childbed fever did not meet the classic parameters of an epidemic. Most physicians were influenced by the traditional medical theory based on the Hippocratic theory. Dr. Semmelweis pointed out that the traditional beliefs about epidemics was based on the theory that puerperal fever was induced by atmospheric-cosmic-terrestrial influences. Semmelweis disagreed and felt childbed fever was endemic and could be identified as an epidemic in the surrounding community population. Epidemic implies that large populations are affected across a large geographic area. However, because of the numbers of deaths involved in childbed fever at the time, the medical professionals considered the disease to be an epidemic. Dr. Semmelweis was convinced that of the large numbers of deaths most occurred in the hospital and especially in clinic one of his hospital and were endemic, but the cause was unknown.[9]

It was discovered that the cause of the increased mortality rate of the mothers in the first clinic was due to the cadaverous matter adhering to the hands of the physicians who then infected the ward patients who were mothers in the last stages of the birth process. He also discovered that any infected or putrefied tissue, whether from a living patient or a cadaver, could cause disease to spread.[9]

In order to destroy the cadaverous or putrefied matter on the hands, it was necessary that every person, physician, or midwife examining females, wash their hands in chlorinated lime upon entry into the labor ward—clinic one. At first Dr. Semmelweis said it was only necessary to wash upon entry to the labor ward. A cancerous womb was discovered to also cause the spread of the disease. Thus, Dr. Semmelweis required washing with chlorinated lime between each examination. He also discovered that the means of communication was not only person-to-person, but that disease could be transmitted through the air.[9]

Upon requiring strict adherence to hand washing by all medical personnel who examined patients in the maternity hospital, mortality rates fell at unbelievable rates. In 1842 a death rate of 12.11 or 730 out of 6,024 was reduced to 1.28 or 91 out of 7,095 by 1848.[9]

At this time in the history of public health the causes of disease (**pathogens**) were unknown yet suspected. However, it was assured that hand washing with chlorinated lime between each examination would reduce the illness and deaths from childbed fever. Even with the evidence and assurance of the success in reducing mortality of childbed fever in hospitals, Dr. Semmelweis's discovery was discounted by most of his colleagues.[9]

Dr. Semmelweis assessed mortality data, compared treatment and nursing care practices, activities, approaches, and treatment methodologies, made experimental trials, and assessed and compared data and statistics of clinic one with clinic two. As a result of his epidemiological investigations Dr. Semmelweis was able to develop control methods and slowed the death rates from puerperal fever in selected populations.[9]

Note: Today it is known that hand washing is still one of the best sanitation practices for medical and lay people alike. What Ignas Semmelweis discovered is still one of the easiest disease and infection control methods known. Even though AIDS has alerted health care providers to use disposable gloves, hand washing is widely practiced and constantly encouraged in health care facilities and among all health care practitioners in order to control disease and avoid infecting patients.

HISTORICAL EPIDEMIOLOGICAL ASSESSMENT OF CHOLERA IN LONDON

Dr. John Snow (1813–1858) in the 1850s was a respected physician and the anesthesiologist to Queen Victoria of England. He is noted for his medical work with the royal family including the administering of chloroform at the birth of the Queen's children.[6,7,8]

However, John Snow is most famous for his pioneering work in epidemiology. Among epidemiologists Dr. Snow is considered to be one of the most important contributors to the field of epidemiology. Many of the tactics, approaches, concepts, and methodologies used by Dr. Snow in his epidemiological work are still found useful and of value in epidemiological work today.[6,7,8]

Dr. Snow studied **cholera** throughout his medical career. From his studies he established sound and useful epidemiological methodologies. Dr. Snow observed and recorded important factors related to the course of the disease, causation, transmission, and sources of cholera.

In the later part of his career, Dr. Snow conducted two major investigative studies of cholera. As a part of his epidemiology career Snow studied cholera outbreaks in the SoHo District of London in the Broad Street area. Later in his career as an epidemiologist, Dr. Snow studied a cholera **epidemic** in which he compared death rates from cholera with sources of water from two different water companies in London, the Lambeth Water Company and the Southwark and Vauxhall Water Company.[6,7,8]

In the mid 1840s in London in the SoHo and Golden Square districts, on Broad Street, a major outbreak of cholera occurred. Within two hundred and fifty yards of the intersection of Cambridge Street and Broad Street about five hundred fatal attacks of cholera occurred in ten days. Many deaths were averted due to the flight of most of the population. Dr. Snow was able to identify incubation times, length of time from infection until death, modes of transmission of the disease, the importance of the flight of the population from the dangerous areas, and he plotted statistics based on dates and mortality rates. He studied sources of contamination of the water, causation and infection and flow of the water within the underground aquifer by assessing water from wells and pumps. He found that nearly all deaths had taken place within a short distance of the Broad Street pump. Dr. Snow observed that in the SoHo District there were two separate populations of persons not so heavily affected by the cholera epidemic nor were death rates equal to those of the surrounding populations. A brewery with its own wells and a work house also with its own water source were the protected populations. Snow used a spot/dot map to identify all deaths and their locations. He plotted data on the progress of the course of the epidemic, new cases, when the epidemic started, peaked, and subsided. Dr. Snow examined the water, movement of people, sources of exposure, transmission of the disease between and among close and distant people, and possible causation. He knew the importance of working with local officials, political implications that are important in controlling diseases, and getting the support of those in authority in the local community.[6,7,8]

Using scientific methods, Dr. Snow made hypotheses about the disease and its spread, transmission, and control. Toward the end of the epidemic, as a control measure, as protection from any reoccurrence, and as a political statement to the community, Snow removed the handle from the Broad Street pump.[6,7,8]

Dr. Snow had become quite an expert on cholera. In his early days as a practicing physician before the Broad Street outbreak, he recorded detailed scenarios of many, many cases of cholera, many of which he witnessed first-hand. Many of the details he chose to record were epidemiological in substance, i.e., various modes of transmission of cholera, incubation times, cause-effect association, clinical observations and clinical manifestations of the disease, scientific observations on water and the different sources including observations made with a microscope, temperature, climate, diet, what the differences were of those who got the disease and the difference of those who did not get the disease, and immigration and emigration differences.[6,7,8]

A more classical experimental design provided by circumstance, allowed a better scientific approach to the study of cholera for Dr. Snow with the cholera epidemic of 1853. London had been without a cholera outbreak for about five years. During this period the Lambeth Water company moved their intake source of water from the Thames River from opposite Hungerford Market up river above the city to Thames Ditton. By moving the source of supply of water up river to a place in the Thames River above the sewage outlets, Lambeth was able to draw water free from London's sewage, contamination, and pollution.

The Southwark and Vauxhall Water Company did not relocate its source of supply of water. Throughout the South District of the city both water companies had pipes down every street and supplied water down to every street equally. The citizens were free to pick and choose which water company they wanted for their household water. The water customers picked their water company at random. Thus, by mere coincidence, Dr. Snow encountered a populace using water randomly selected throughout the South District. Dr. Snow could not have arranged better sampling techniques than those which had occurred by chance.[6,7,8]

The Registrar General in London published a "Weekly Return of Births and Deaths." On November 26, 1853, the Registrar General observed from a table of mortality that mortality rates were fairly consistent across the districts supplied with the water from the Hungerford market area. The old supply system of Lambeth and the regular supply of the Southwark and Vauxhall Company were separate systems but drew water from the same area in the river. The Registrar General also published a mortality list from cholera. Dr. Snow developed comparison tables on death by source of water by sub-districts. Snow was able to conclude that the water drawn up river solely by Lambeth Water Company caused no deaths. The water drawn downstream, in areas that were below the sewage inlets, mostly by Southwark and Vauxhall Water Company, had very high death rates.[6,7,8]

Gaining cooperation and permission from the Registrar General, Snow was supplied with addresses of persons who died from cholera. He went into the sub-district of Kennington One and Kennington Two and found that 38 out of 44 deaths in this sub-district received their water from Southwark and Vauxhall Company. Each house had randomly selected different water companies and many households did not know from which one they received water. Dr. Snow developed a test using chloride of silver to identify which source each household had by sampling water from within the houses of those he contacted. Dr. Snow got so he could tell the source of water by appearance and smell.[6,7,8]

Vital statistics data, death rates, and location, when compared to water supply sources presented conclusive evidence as to source of contamination. A report to the Parliament showed that in the 30,046 households that were supplied water by the Southwark and Vauxhall Company, 286 persons died of cholera. Of the 26,107 houses supplied by Lambeth, only 14 died of cholera. The death rate was 71 per 10,000 in households supplied with water by Southwark and Vauxhall Company and 5 per 10,000 for Lambeth Company. The mortality at the height of the epidemic in households supplied with water by Southwark and Vauxhall Company was eight to nine times greater than those supplied by Lambeth Company. Dr. Snow was finally able to prove his hypothesis, that is, the circumstance of the cholera-poison passing down the sewers into the river, being drawn from the river and distributed through miles of pipes into peoples' homes produced a specific disease throughout the community. Dr. Snow showed that cholera was a waterborne disease that traveled in both surface and ground water supplies.[6,7,8]

Dr. Snow laid the groundwork for many epidemiological approaches found useful in epidemiology today; i.e., he identified various modes of transmission, incubation times, cause-effect associations, use of comparison groups, clinical observations and clinical manifestations of the disease, scientific observations on water and the different sources for the disease including observations made with a microscope, temperature, climate, diet, the differences between those who get the disease and those who do not, immigration and emigration differences, water as a source of communicating disease by both surface and ground water supplies, sewage (a main contributor to disease), and the importance of the evaluation and assessment of vital statistics in epidemiological work. It was not until Koch's work in 1883 in Egypt when he isolated and cultivated *Vibrio cholerae* that the accuracy and correctness of Snow's work proved and accepted.[3,4,6,7,8]

To control the disease in communities and for all populations, water supplies have to be controlled, cleaned up, protected and kept free of contamination. In 1990 the first outbreak of cholera of major proportions in one hundred years occurred in Lima, Peru. The main cause of the outbreak was uncontrolled dumping of sewage into rivers used as water supplies. Lima grew from 600,000 to 7,000,000 people in just a few years. Building and development failed to keep up with the growth. Shantytowns grew at uncontrolled rates, as did the demand for housing, drainage control, potable water, protected water supplies, sewage systems, and garbage collection and control. The cholera epidemic spread up the coast of South America, Central America and into the Southern coast of the United States and Mexico in 1990 through 1993.[9]

NEWS FILE

Cholera Epidemic

First Cholera Outbreak in 100 Years Hits Peru

In early February of 1991, the first cholera epidemic to hit the world in more than 100 years struck in Lima, Peru. A Valentine's Day flight from South America to Los Angeles with 386 people on board made its last stop in Lima, Peru. Five of those passengers came down with cholera. By the end of February more than 26,000 cases of cholera had been confirmed and 134 people had died. Six months into the outbreak more than 230,000 cases and 2,300 deaths had occurred.

Cholera causes severe diarrhea, dehydration, vomiting, and cramps. This disease has one of the shortest incubation periods of all diseases and can cause death within 48 hours if not treated. The cholera bacterium is highly contagious and is carried in water and food contaminated with human feces. In cholera-stricken areas, one must avoid tap or pump water, ice, and fresh and raw fruits and vegetables.

The Lima epidemic was traced back to streams of raw sewage running through the shantytowns on the outskirts of Lima, especially Acapulco. Garbage was not picked up on a regular basis and the water supply for the shantytown was highly limited. What little potable water was available was hauled in by tank trucks. Cholera bacteria was found in the water systems and in the fish of the coastal cities. Public health measures included restricting imports and travel from Peru, and cleaning up the water supply. Health education efforts were made through radio, television, loudspeakers, newspapers, health workers, government officials, group health talks, and personal contact. Citizens were instructed to boil their drinking water, treat water with chlorine, drink only treated water, wash their produce with treated water, eat cooked food hot, make drinks with treated water, cover stored food, wash and clean utensils in treated water, wash hands after toileting, and wash hands before eating. Cholera moved up the coast of Central America and has been found in several provinces in Central Mexico on its east coast. The local U.S. public health departments along the border of Mexico continue to monitor water and streams in order to prevent the disease from crossing into the United States.

(Source: Quick, R.E., et al., "Using a Knowledge, Attitudes and Practice Survey to Supplement Finding of an Outbreak Investigation: Cholera Prevention Measures During the 1991 Epidemic in Peru," International Journal of Epidemiology, Vol. 25, No. 4, 1996, pp. 872–878, and Barry Lynn, "New Outbreaks of Cholera Reported in Peru," The Sun, Thursday February 20, 28, 1991)

PASTEUR'S AND KOCH'S CONTRIBUTION TO EPIDEMIOLOGY

In the 1870s, if one journeyed into the countryside of Europe it was not uncommon to see dead sheep lying in the fields. Anthrax was a major epidemic that plagued the farmers and destroyed them economically. Being a **zoonotic** disease, anthrax was dreaded because not only sheep were dying from the disease, but humans were also infected. Farmers, not knowing what to do with the dead sheep, would dig large holes in the earth and bury them.[3,4]

By this time, Louis Pasteur, (1822–1895) a French chemist, who was not a physician, had been accepted into France's Academy of Medicine for his work on microbiology. Pasteur had distinguished himself as a scientist and a respected contributor to the field of medicine and public health, (even though not recognized as a separate field at the time). Pasteur had already identified the cause of rabies and many other devastating diseases. Because of his many past successes in microbiology, Pasteur had confidence in his ability to take on the challenge of conquering anthrax.[3,4]

A famous counterpart and Prussian (German) physician competitor in microbial research, Dr. Robert Koch, had previously, in 1876, shown that anthrax was a rod-shaped bacterium and demonstrated the entire life cycle of the bacterium. Both Pasteur and Koch had the goal of linking microbes with disease and bringing recognition to their own countries.[3,4]

Even though the bacteria that causes anthrax had been identified, little was known about how sheep, or man for that matter, contracted the disease. How the tiny bacteria overcame a large animal such as a sheep so quickly was of great interest to the scientists of the time. Though not yet proved, Pasteur was convinced that it was the bacteria identified as anthrax that caused the disease. The anthrax bacteria was always present upon **necropsy** (autopsy) of sheep that died from anthrax. It was unclear why the course of the disease occurred the way it did. The cause-effect association seemed to have some loopholes in it. How did the sheep get anthrax? How were the sheep disposed of? Why did the anthrax occur in some areas and not in others? How was the disease transmitted? How did the disease survive? All were questions that Louis Pasteur sought to answer.

Pasteur observed that the sheep were buried upon dying. The key and insightful discovery was that anthrax spore/bacteria were brought back to the surface by earthworms. Koch had previously shown that the anthrax bacteria existed in silkworms, and that anthrax was an intestinal disease. Pasteur made the earthworm connection.

A mistake led to the development of the very first vaccine from the same bacteria that caused the disease. Some hens were mistakenly vaccinated with old vaccine that had been allowed to sit for a time and inadvertently were immunized against the disease. When injected with the disease, the chickens did not die because of their immunity to the disease.

An anthrax vaccine was discovered in 1881. Pasteur and his assistants had worked on a vaccine for anthrax for months. He had some success in chickens, guinea pigs, and rabbits with a killed vaccine approach and the word of his progress had gotten out into the medical community. After a presentation at the Academy of Science in Paris, Pasteur was challenged to prove that his vaccine was effective. The killed vaccine was somewhat unstable in changes of temperature. Rhou, a physician and assistant created a more stable chemical-based alternative. Pasteur put his career and reputation at stake to prove that his vaccine would work, that disease was caused by microorganisms and that a cause-effect association exists between a particular microbe and a certain disease.

Pasteur agreed to a challenge in a public demonstration to prove his vaccination process could prevent sheep from getting anthrax. He went to a farm in rural France where 60 sheep were provided for the experiment. He was to vaccinate 25 of the sheep with his new vaccine.

After the proper waiting time, Pasteur was then to inoculate 50 of the sheep with a virulent injection of anthrax. Ten sheep were to receive no treatment and were used to compare to the survivors of the experiment (a control group). If the 25 sheep that were not vaccinated died and the 25 that were vaccinated lived Pasteur would have proved that vaccinations work to prevent disease in sheep. Association is that part of epidemiology that scientific experimental design serves as a valuable method in proving effectiveness of preventive medicine measures. Pasteur was successful. The inoculated sheep lived, the unvaccinated sheep died, the control group had no changes. Pasteur was successful in demonstrating that his methodology was sound, that vaccinations were sound approaches in disease control and that bacteria were indeed causes of disease. Both Pasteur and Koch were successful in putting to rest a major misguided notion of medicine at the time; that disease and its causes occurred by "spontaneous generation," that is, organisms would simply appear out of other organisms, a fly would spontaneously appear out of garbage, etc.[8,10]

Historically many scientists have contributed to the methodology used in epidemiology. Robert Koch (1843–1910) lived in Wollstein, a small town near Breslau, in rural Germany (Prussia). Dr. Koch was a private practice physician and district medical officer. Through his compelling desire to study disease experimentally, he set up a laboratory in his home, and purchased equipment, including photography equipment out of his meager earnings. Robert Koch became a key medical research scientist in Germany in the period of the explosion of knowledge in medicine and public health, and used photography to take the first pictures of microbes in order to show the world that microorganisms do in fact exist and that they are what cause diseases.[3,4,15]

Between patients and in the evenings, Koch would investigate diseases, at first anthrax. He discovered the lifecycle of rod-shaped organisms, the anthrax bacilli. Koch showed that anthrax was transmissible and reproducible in experimental animals (mice). He identified the spore stage of the growth cycle of microorganisms. The epidemiological significance was that Koch demonstrated that the anthrax bacillus was the only organism that caused anthrax in a susceptible animal. After several other reports on the etiology of infectious diseases, Koch was appointed to the Imperial Health Department of Prussia. In 1882 Koch discovered the tubercle bacillus by special culturing and staining methods. Koch and his assistant also perfected the concept of steam sterilization. In Egypt and India he and assistants discovered the cholera bacteria and proved that it was transmitted by drinking water, food, and clothing. Incidental to the cholera investigations, Koch also found the microorganisms that cause infectious conjunctivitis. He received the Nobel Prize in 1905 for his work in microbiology. A major contribution to epidemiology by Koch was a paper on **waterborne** epidemics. He showed how they may be largely prevented by proper water filtration.[3,4,15]

Dr. Koch, with beginnings as a country family physician, pioneered the identification of microorganisms and many different bacteria that caused different diseases and pure culturing techniques to grow microorganisms in laboratory conditions. Some of the major public health contributions that Koch made were the identification of the tuberculosis and cholera microorganisms and the importance of water purification in disease prevention.[3,4,14,15]

THE MICROSCOPE AND ITS CONTRIBUTION TO EPIDEMIOLOGY

The important discoveries of Koch, Pasteur, and Snow as well as many others in the sanitation and microbe discovery era would have been difficult without the use of the microscope. Koch's camera would not have been invented if the microscope had not been developed and its lenses adapted to picture taking.

The microscope found first scientific use in the seventeenth century through the work of Cornelius Drebel (1621), the Janssen brothers of the Netherlands (1608), and Antony Van Leuwenhoek (1632–1723). The microscope was used for medical and scientific purposes by Athanasius Kircher of Fulda (1602–1680), and he is thought to be the first to use the microscope for investigating the causes of disease. In 1658 in Rome he wrote his publication *Scrutinium pestis*. He conducted experiments upon the nature of putrification and showed how microscopic living organisms and maggots develop in decaying matter. He also discovered that the blood of plague patients was filled with countless "worms," not visible to the naked eye.

Most of the credit goes to Leuwenhoek for the advancement, development, and perfection of the use of the microscope. He was the first to effectively apply the microscope in the study of disease and medicine, even though he was not a physician. Because of a driving interest in the microscope, Leuwenhoek was able to devote much time to microscopy, owning over 247 microscopes and over 400 lenses (many of which he ground himself). He was the first to describe the structure of the crystalline lens. Some of his contributions to epidemiology include the morphological study of red corpuscles of the blood. He described protozoa and bacteria and made the connection of arterial circulation to venous circulation in the human body through the microscopic study of capillary networks. Chemistry and histology were also developed because of the advent of the microscope, which influenced advances in the study and control of diseases and epidemiology. Leuwenhoek contributed indirectly to epidemiology through microbiology by use of the microscope and the discovery of "animalcules," (microscopic organisms, later called microbes, bacteria, and microorganisms).[4,16]

JOHN GRAUNT AND VITAL STATISTICS DEVELOPMENT

Another major contributor to epidemiology but in a different manner was John Graunt, (1620–1674). In 1603 in London, a systematic recording of deaths was commenced and was called the "Bills of Mortality," summarized in Figure 3.1. This was the first major contribution to record keeping on a population and was the beginning of the vital statistics aspects of epidemiology. Graunt, when he took over the work, systematically recorded, age, sex, who died, of what, and where they died, and when. Graunt also recorded how many persons per year died of what kind of event or disease. (See Figure 3.1)[4,15]

Through the analysis of the Bills of Mortality already developed for London, Graunt summarized **mortality data** and developed a better understanding of diseases as well as sources and causes of death. Using the data and information he collected, Graunt wrote a book: *Natural and Political Observations Made Upon the Bills of Mortality*. From the Bills of Mortality Graunt ascertained important epidemiological information such as: A person was more likely to die when young than old, males died sooner than females, more males are born than females. Graunt was the first to develop and calculate life tables and life expectancy. He divided deaths into two types of causes: (1) acute (struck suddenly, i.e., cholera) and (2) chronic (lasted over a long period of time, i.e., emphysema).[4,15]

When Graunt died, little was done to continue his good work. Two hundred years later, William Farr (1807–1883) was appointed Registrar General in England and built on the ideas of Graunt. The concept of "political arithmetic" was replaced by a new term,

The Diseases And Casualties This Year Being 1632

Abortive and Stillborn	445	Jaundies	43
Afrighted	1	Jawfaln	8
Aged	628	Impostume	74
Ague	43	Kil'd by Several Accident	46
Apoplex, and Meagrom	17	King's Evil	38
Bit with a mad dog	1	Lethargie	2
Bloody flux, Scowring, and Flux	348	Lunatique	5
Brused, Issues, Sores, and Ulcers	28	Made away themselves	15
Burnt and Scalded	5	Measles	80
Burst, and Rupture	9	Murthered	7
Cancer, and Wolf	10	Over-laid/starved at nurse	7
Canker	1	Palsie	25
Childbed	171	Piles	8
Chrisomes, and Infants	2,268	Plague	8
Cold and Cough	55	Planet	13
Colick, Stone, and Strangury	56	Pleurisie, and Spleen	36
Consumption	1,797	Purples, and Spotted Fever	38
Convulsion	241	Quinsie	7
Cut of the Stone	5	Rising of the Lights	98
Dead in the street and starved	6	Sciatica	1
Dropsie and Swelling	267	Scurvey, and Itch	9
Drowned	34	Suddenly	62
Executed and Prest to death	18	Surfet	86
Falling Sickness	7	Swine Pox	6
Fever	1,108	Teeth	470
Fistula	13	Thrush, Sore Mouth	40
Flox and Small Pox	531	Tympany	13
French Pox	12	Tissick	34
Gangrene	5	Vomiting	1
Gowt	4	Worms	27
Grief	11		

Christened
Males 4,994
Females 4,590
In All 9,584

Buried
Males 4,932
Females 4,603
In All 9,535

Increased in the Burials in the 122 Parishes, and at the Pesthouse this year - 993

Decreased of the Plagues in the 122 Parishes, and at the Pesthouses this year - 266

FIGURE 3.1 Selections from *Natural and Political Observations Made Upon the Bills of Mortality* by John Graunt (First Edition 1662). (Source: Johns Hopkins Press: Baltimore, 1937)

"statistics." Farr advanced the use of vital statistics and organized and developed a modern vital statistics system, much of which is still in use today. Edmund Halley (1656–1742) compiled the Breslau Table of Births and Funerals in 1693 in order to estimate mortality rates and was also a major contributor to vital statistics.[3,4,15]

RAMAZZINI AND THE EPIDEMIOLOGY OF OCCUPATIONAL HEALTH AND INDUSTRIAL HYGIENE

Bernardino Ramazzini (1633–1714) was born in Carpi near Modena, Italy. He received his medical training at the University of Parma and postgraduate studies in Rome. Ramazzini eventually returned to the town of Modena where he became a Professor of Medicine at the local University. He was interested in the practical problems of medicine and not in the study of ancient theories of medicine, a fact not well received by his colleagues. Through Ramazzini's continuous curiosity and his unwillingness to confine himself to the study of ancient medical theories, he became recognized for his innovative approaches to medical and public health problems.[3,4,15,16]

In 1692, at the age of 60, Ramazzini was climbing down into 80-foot wells, taking temperature and barometric readings, trying to discover the origin and rapid flow of Modena's spring water. He tried to associate barometric readings with the cause of disease by taking daily readings during a typhus epidemic.[3,4,15,16]

Ramazzini came upon a worker in a cesspool. In his conversation with the worker, Ramazzini was told that if one continued to work in this environment the worker would go blind. Ramazzini examined the worker's eyes after he came out of the cesspit and found them bloodshot and dim. Upon inquiry about other effects of working in cesspools and privies, he was informed that only the eyes were affected.[3,4,15,16]

The event with the cesspool worker turned his mind to a general interest in the relation of work to health. He began work on a book that would become influential in the area of occupational medicine and provided related epidemiological implications. The book titled *The Diseases of Workers* was completed in 1690 but not published until 1703. It was not acceptable to pity the poor or simple laborers in this period of time, which caused Ramazzini to delay the publication, as he thought it would not be accepted.[3,4,15,16]

Ramazzini observed that disease among workers arose from two causes. The first he believed was from the harmful character of the materials that workers handled as the materials often emitted noxious vapors and very fine particles which could be breathed in. The second causes of disease were ascribed to certain violent and irregular motions and unnatural postures imposed upon the body while doing work.[3,4,15,16]

Ramazzini described the dangers of poisoning from lead used by potters in their glaze. He also identified the danger posed by the use of mercury as used by mirror-makers, goldsmiths, and others. He observed that very few of these workers reached old age. If they did not die young, their health was so undermined that they prayed for death. He observed that many had palsy of the neck and hands, loss of teeth, vertigo, asthma, and paralysis. Ramazzini also studied those who used or processed organic materials such as mill workers, bakers, starchmakers, tobacco workers, and those who processed wool, flax, hemp, cotton, and silk—all of whom suffered from inhaling the fine dust particles in the processing of the materials.

Ramazzini further examined the harmful effects of the physical and mechanical aspects of work such as varicose veins from standing at work, sciatica caused by turning the potter's wheel, ophthalmia found in glassworkers and blacksmiths. Kidney damage was seen to be suffered by couriers and those who rode for long periods, and hernia appeared among bearers of heavy loads.[3,4,15,16]

Major epidemiological contributions made by Ramazzini were not only his investigation into and description of work-related maladies, but his great concern for prevention. Ramazzini suggested that the cesspool workers fasten transparent bladders over their eyes to protect them, take long rest periods, or if their eyes were weak, get into a different line of work. In discussing the various trades, he suggested changing posture, exercise, well-ventilated workplaces, and that temperature extremes be avoided in the workplace.

Ramazzini was an observant epidemiologist, and described the outbreak of lathyrism in Modena in 1690. He described the malarial epidemics of the region and the Paduan cattle plague in 1712.[3,4,15,16]

TYPHOID MARY

An Irish cook, Mary Mallon, referred to as Typhoid Mary, was believed to be responsible for 53 cases of typhoid fever in a 15-year period. In the early 1900s, 350,000 cases of typhoid occurred each year in the United States.[14]

George Soper, a sanitary engineer, studying several outbreaks of typhoid fever in New York City in the 1900s, found the food and water supply no longer suspect as the means of transmission of the **typhoid** disease. Soper continued to search for other means of communication of the disease. He began to look to people instead of the **fomites** and the food and water.

He discovered that Mary Mallon had served as a cook in many homes that became typhoid-stricken. The disease always seemed to follow but never preceded her employment. Bacteriological examination of Mary Mallon's feces showed that she was a chronic **carrier** of typhoid. Mary seemed to sense that she was giving people sickness, because when typhoid appeared she would leave with no forwarding address. Mary Mallon illustrated the importance of concern over the chronic typhoid carrier causing and spreading typhoid fever. Like 20% of all typhoid carriers, Mary suffered no illness from the disease. Epidemiological investigations have shown that carriers might be overlooked if epidemiological searches are limited to the water, food, and those with a history of the disease.[14,17]

From 1907 to 1910 Mary was confined by health officials until released through legal action taken by her. The New York Supreme Court upheld the community's right to keep her in custody and isolation. Typhoid Mary was released in 1910 and she disappeared almost immediately. Two years later typhoid fever occurred in a hospital in New Jersey and in a New York Hospital. More than two hundred people were affected. It was discovered that Typhoid Mary had worked at both hospitals as a cook, but under a different name. This incident taught public health officials and epidemiologists that close supervision and keeping track of carriers is essential. It also showed that typhoid carriers should never be allowed to handle food or drink intended for public consumption. In later years Typhoid Mary voluntarily accepted isolation. Should she have wished, Mary could have had her gall bladder removed, which provides a cure in 60% of all typhoid carriers. Typhoid Mary died at age 70.[14,17]

The investigating, tracking, and controlling of certain types of diseases which can affect large populations were epidemiological insights gained from the Typhoid Mary experience. The protection of public food supplies was again reinforced as were investigative aspects of disease control and both were made more justified and important to public health.

THE EPIDEMIOLOGY OF VITAMINS IN CURING NUTRITIONAL DISEASES

In the mid- to late-1800s bacteria were being identified as the major causes of disease. However, the discovery of microorganisms and their connection to disease causation clouded the discovery of the cause of other life-threatening diseases. Beriberi, rickets, and pellagra were still devastating the populations around the world. It was believed in 1870, that up to one-third of the poor children in the inner city areas of major cities in the world suffered from serious rickets. Biochemistry was being advanced with new lines of investigation being opened up. In the 1880s it was observed that when young mice were fed purified diets they died quickly. When fed milk they flourished. A Naval surgeon, T.K. Takaki, in 1887 eradicated beriberi from the Japanese Navy by adding vegetables, meat, and fish to their diet, which was mostly rice. In 1889 at the London Zoo it was demonstrated that rickets in lion cubs could be cured by feeding them crushed bone, milk, and cod-liver oil.[15,18,19]

The first major epidemiological implications discovered in deficiency illnesses came in 1886 when the Dutch commissioned the firm of C.A. Pekelharing and Winkler who sent Dr. Christian Eijkman (1858–1930), an Army Doctor, to the East Indies to investigate the cause of beriberi. Dr. Eijkman observed that chickens fed on polished rice developed symptoms of beriberi and recovered promptly when the food was changed to whole rice, but he mistakenly attributed the cause of the disease to a neurotoxin. Eijkman and G. Grijns (1865–1944), a physiologist, suggested that the beriberi was due to the lack of some essential substance in the outer layer of the rice grain. In 1905, Pekelharing conducted a series of experiments based on Eijkman's observations, was more thorough in his work, and came to the same conclusions.

In 1906 Frederick Gowland Hopkins (1861–1947), a British biochemist, did similar studies with a concern for the pathogenesis of rickets and scurvy. Hopkins suggested that other nutritional factors exist beyond the known ones of protein, carbohydrates, fat, and minerals, and these must be present for good health.

In 1911 Casimir Funk, a Polish chemist, isolated a chemical substance that he believed belonged to a class of chemical compounds called "amines." Funk added the Latin for life, *vita*, and invented the term "vitamine." In 1916, E.V. McCollum showed that two factors were required for the normal growth of rats, a fat-soluble "A" factor found in butter and fats, and a water-soluble "B" factor was found in nonfatty foods like whole grain rice. These discoveries set the stage for labeling **vitamins** by letters of the alphabet. McCollum in the United States and E. Mellanby in Great Britain showed that the "A" factor was effective in curing rickets. It was also demonstrated that the "A" factor contained two separate factors. A heat-stable factor was identified and found to be the one responsible for curing rickets. A heat-labile factor that was capable of healing xerophthalmia (dryness of the conjunctiva leading to a diseased state of the mucous membrane of the eye due to Vitamin A deficiency) was discovered. The heat-stable factor was named Vitamin D and the heat-labile factor was termed Vitamin A.[7,15,18,19]

The discovery of Vitamin D connected observations about rickets and cod-liver oil. Cod-liver oil cured rickets, as it contains Vitamin D. It was observed that children exposed to sunshine were less likely to get rickets. In 1919 Kurt Huldschinsky in Germany, showed that exposing children to artificial sunshine also cured rickets. It was shown that Vitamin D was produced in the body when sunshine acted on its fats. It was later discovered that the anti-beriberi substance, Vitamin B was also effective against pellagra.[15,18,19]

In this era the role of social and economic factors was observed to contribute much to the causation of disease, especially poverty conditions, which clearly contributed to nutritional deficiencies.[15]

THE BEGINNING OF EPIDEMIOLOGY IN THE UNITED STATES (1793–1913)

In 1850 Lemuel Shattuck published the first report on sanitation and public health problems in the Commonwealth of Massachusetts. Shattuck was a teacher, sociologist, statistician, and he served in the state legislature. He was chair of a legislative committee to study sanitation and public health. The report set forth many public health programs and needs for the next century. Of the many needs and programs suggested, several of them were epidemiological in nature. One of the things needed for epidemiology, its investigations, and the all-important control and prevention aspects to work was to have an organized and structured effort. The organized effort has to come through an organization sponsored by a government.

Shattuck's report set forth the importance of establishing state and local boards of health. Secondly, the report recommended that an organized effort to collect and analyze vital statistics be established. He also recommended the exchange of health information, sanitary inspections, research on tuberculosis, and the teaching of sanitation and prevention in medical schools. The health of school children was also of major concern. As a result of the report, boards of health were established, with state departments of health and local public health departments soon to follow, through which epidemiological activities took place.[21,22]

Quarantine conventions were held in the 1850s. The first in the United States was in Philadelphia in 1857. The prevention of typhus, cholera, and yellow fever were discussed. Port quarantine and the hygiene of immigrants were also of concern. Public health educational activities began at this time. In 1879 the first major book on public health, which included epidemiological topics, was published by A.H. Buck. The book was titled *Hygiene and Public Health*.[21,22]

The infectious nature of yellow fever was established in 1901 (see Figure 3.2). In 1902 the U.S. Public Health Service was founded and in 1906 the Pure Food and Drug Act was passed. Standard methods of water analysis were also adopted in 1906. The pasteurization of milk was shown to be effective in controlling the spread of disease in 1913, and in this same year the first school of public health, the Harvard School of Public Health, was established.[21,22]

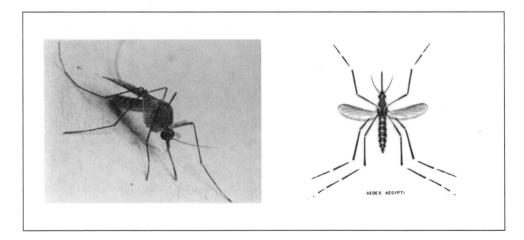

FIGURE 3.2   It has been said "that of all the people who ever died, half of them died from the bite of the mosquito." For thousands of years it was not known that the mosquito was responsible for diseases such as yellow fever and malaria. These two diseases are still not fully contained in many parts of the world. In 1900, Walter Reed, M.D., a U.S. Army physician working in the tropics, made the epidemiological connection between the mosquito (*Aedes aegypti* species) and yellow fever. (Pictures courtesy of Centers for Disease Control and Prevention, Atlanta, Georgia)

HISTORICAL DEVELOPMENTS OF MORBIDITY IN EPIDEMIOLOGY

One epidemiology professional of the early 1900s who helped advance the study of disease statistics or morbidity was Edgar Sydenstricker. The development of a morbidity statistics system in the United States was quite slow. One problem was that the assessment and analysis of morbidity statistics cannot be done in the same manner that death (mortality statistics) are done. Sydenstricker struggled with the mere definition of sickness and recognized that to all persons, disease is an undeniable and frequent experience. Birth and death comes to a person but once while illness comes often, especially in this era when sanitation, public health, microbiology, and disease control and prevention measures were still being developed.[23]

In the early 1900s morbidity statistics of any given kind were not regularly collected on a large scale. Interest in disease statistics came only when the demand for them arose from special populations and the importance that different uses of the statistics would play socially and economically. Additionally Sydenstricker noted that the differences in data collection, definitions, cases of illness, the existence of peculiar factors that affect the accuracy of records, and time elements all were barriers to collecting homogeneous morbidity data in large amounts.[23]

Sydenstricker suggested that morbidity statistics be classified into five general groups in order to be of value. The five groups were

1. **Reports of communicable disease**—Notification of those diseases for which reasonably effective methods of administrative controls have been devised.

2. **Hospital and clinical records**—These records were viewed as being of little value in identifying incidence or prevalence of illness in populations. (At this time most people were treated at home unless they were poor and in need of assistance.) Such records are only of value for clinical studies.

3. **Insurance and industrial establishment and school illness records**—The absence of records of illnesses in workers in large industries in the United States were of concern for defining and explaining work-related illness. Criteria for determining disability from illness or injury at work and when sick benefits should be allowed were not well-developed. Malingering was also considered and how it would affect the workers' illness rates. It was suggested that if illness records showing absence from school were kept with a degree of specificity they could be of value to the understanding of the effect of disease on these populations.

4. **Illness surveys**—Illness surveys have been used by major insurance companies to determine the prevalence of illness in a specific population. House-to-house canvass approaches have been used. Incidence of diseases within a given period are not revealed by such methods, whereas chronic type diseases are found to be of higher incidence (which should be expected and predicted).

5. **Records of the incidence of illness in a population continuously or frequently observed**—To benefit epidemiological studies two study methods were employed (1) to determine the annual illness rate in a representative population, and (2) to develop an epidemiological method whereby human populations could be observed in order to determine the existence of an incidence of various diseases as they were manifested under normal conditions within the community.[23]

A morbidity study by Sydenstricker and his colleagues under the direction of the U.S. Public Health Service in Hagerstown, Maryland in 1921–24 was conducted. The study involved 16,517 person-years of observation or an equivalent population of 1,079 individuals who were observed for 28 months beginning in 1921. Illnesses discovered in field investigations from family members being sick or observing a sick person were recorded from each family visit. A fairly accurate record of actual illness was obtained by a community interview method. Some findings included were that only 5% of illnesses were of short duration of one day or less; 40% were not only disabling but caused bed confinement as well. An accurate data-gathering process was developed from the experience.[23]

In the study 17,847 cases of illnesses were recorded in a 28-month period. An annual rate of 1,081 per 1,000 years of life were observed; about one illness per person year. The illness rate was 100 times the annual death rate in the same population.[23]

The most interesting results of this first morbidity study were the variations of incidence of illness according to age. The proportion of frequent attacks of illness, four or more a year was highest (45%) in year 2–9-year-olds, lowest in 20–24-year-olds (11%) and rising to 21% by age 35. When severity of illness was looked at, it was found that the greatest resistance to disease was in childhood; 5–14 years. The lowest resistance to disease was in early childhood; 0–4 years and toward the end of life.[23,24]

THE TUSKEGEE SYPHILIS STUDY

Many epidemiology professionals find the Tuskegee Syphilis Experiment interesting to discuss. However, this unfortunate and prejudicial set of occurrences was not an epidemiological study and lacked the credibility of a respectable public health research study or of biomedical research. Instead the events of the Tuskegee Study have become an embarrassment to the field of public health and a medical ethics concern.[25]

In the early 1900s the poverty-stricken blacks in the Southern United States were referred to as a "syphilis-soaked race." Macon County was one of the worst. This eastern Alabama county was economically depressed, even though the rich soil made it one of the best agricultural areas in the south, with cotton as its most common crop. In this rural setting much of the agriculture activity was tied to poor black sharecroppers. In 1930 Macon County's population was just over 27,000 and 82% were black. The demographics remained mostly the same into the 1970s. Food was scarce and malnutrition was common. The most primitive living conditions were commonplace and extremely poor sanitation conditions existed including unprotected water wells. Illiteracy was widespread among adults and children, educational endeavors were meager, which went hand in hand with the dire poverty. The big issue of concern was a high incidence rate of syphilis among black males and because it was so common it was referred to among the black community as "bad blood."[25]

Some official reports claimed that the blacks were told that they had syphilis. Most personal interviews with physicians and subjects showed a different story. Various physicians involved with the study said that the black subjects were not told what was being done, and some thought they were being treated for rheumatism or bad stomachs. One subject said that when he went to the public health clinic he was only told that he had "bad blood."[25]

Medical facilities were meager and access to physicians and medical care was almost nonexistent except for the public health venereal disease (VD) clinics. The physicians expected full payment in cash. Blacks only used physicians in extreme emergencies, while conditions like syphilis were simply endured.[25]

The Tuskegee study had nothing to do with medical experiments and no treatment was offered for syphilis. No new drugs were tested, nor were there efforts made to establish the efficacy of older chemical treatments, such as Salvarsan (an arsenic derivative) used to treat syphilis for years. The three stages of syphilis were clearly understood as were the incubation periods of each. The mode of transmission of the syphilis spirochete pathogen was also well-understood. Still, the Public Health Service never established a formal protocol for this study and withheld treatment. The Wassermann test for syphilis was developed in 1907. Salvarsan was available and moderately successful in treating syphilis. Penicillin was made readily available in 1945, yet no treatment with this antibiotic was attempted, Figure 3.3.[25]

One report states that the Tuskegee study involved 399 black men who had syphilis and 201 who were free of the disease and were used as controls. A variety of tests and medical exams were given to these black males, yet they were never allowed treatment in order that the full course of the disease could run without interference. The men were denied enlistment in the military and arrangements were made to exclude them from being drafted into the military in World War II in order to assure that they would not receive treatment, which they would most assuredly get in military service.[25]

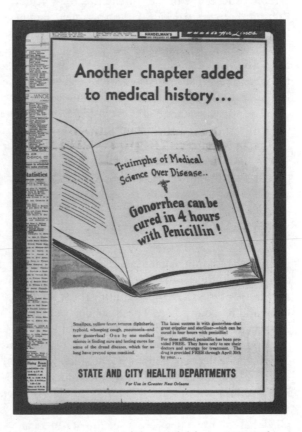

FIGURE 3.3 Penicillin was made widely available in 1945. This antibiotic became known as the "miracle drug," with promises of rapid cures of many infectious diseases, including gonorrhea. (Picture courtesy of Centers for Disease Control and Prevention, Atlanta, Georgia)

The tracking, examining, and withholding of treatment and autopsy of the syphilis-infested males continued by the government doctors until the early 1970s. News reporters in the early 1970s began to investigate this study and wondered why the black men went along with the study. The subjects received free exams, free rides to the clinics, hot meals on the exam days, and a burial stipend paid to their survivors. It was disclosed that the venereal disease branch of the Centers for Disease Control and Prevention was in charge of the Tuskegee study. Local health departments were also involved with the study.

The Alabama State Board of Health began its campaign against venereal disease in 1918. Since the venereal disease control task was more difficult than expected, federal support was welcomed. By 1930 about 175 clinics had agreed to accept some of the black syphilis subjects. Health officials, due to their stereotyping and bias were misled, even in their clinical judgment about how diseases afflicted black people. Physicians at the time believed that syphilis in blacks was different from the disease in whites. It was hoped the study would show the differences.[25]

In the late 1960s, meetings and a blue-ribbon panel were convened to discuss the Tuskegee Syphilis Study. The racial composition of the study and the fact that "Negroes" had long been used in medical experiments and as teaching subjects added concern to the greater issue. Some of the conferences were held at the Centers for Disease Control and Prevention to try to decide if the experiment should continue. In 1969 it was disclosed that the Tuskegee Study started in 1932 and had 412 black men with syphilis and 204 controls and that 373 men in both groups had died, 36 controls and 56 syphilitic subjects remained alive. The ages of the survivors ranged from 59 to 85. Moral and ethical issues about treatment were raised and discussed. Some still wanted the study to continue, others thought it was unethical to not treat the syphilis-infested subjects.[25]

The story broke in the press in 1972. A year later a class-action law suit was filed in the United States District Court for the Middle District of Alabama. The case never came to trial. In December of 1974, the United States government agreed to pay approximately $10 million in out-of-court settlements to the untreated survivors and heirs of the deceased syphilitics.[25]

THE FRAMINGHAM HEART STUDY

In 1948 the Framingham, Massachusetts cardiovascular disease study was launched. The aim of the study was to determine which of the many risk factors contribute most to cardiovascular disease. At the beginning the study it involved 6,000 persons between the ages of 30 and 62 years of age. These persons were recruited to participate in the study over a 20-year period. Eventually the study spanned 30 years, with 5,100 residents completing the study. In each of the 30 years, medical exams and other related testing activities were conducted with the participants. The study was initially sponsored by the National Health Institute of the U.S. Public Health Services and the Massachusetts Department of Public Health, along with the local Framingham Health Department.[26,27,28]

The site for the Framingham Heart Study was determined by several factors which implied that this town was a cross-section of Americana and was a typical small American city. Framingham had a fairly stable population, one major hospital used by most all in the community, an annual updated city population list was kept and a broad range of occupations, jobs, and industries were represented. The study approach used in the Framingham Study was a prospective cohort study, also called a longitudinal study. (See Chapter 8 for explanation of prospective cohort and longitudinal studies.)[26,27,28]

The diseases of most concern in the study included, coronary heart disease, rheumatic heart disease, congestive heart failure, *angina pectoris*, stroke, gout, gallbladder disease, and eye conditions. Several clinical categories of heart disease were distinguished in this study which included: myocardial infarction, *angina pectoris*, coronary insufficiency, and death due to coronary heart disease as shown by a specific clinical diagnosis.[25,26,27]

Many prospective and longitudinal study methods and approaches were advanced in the study such as cohort tracking, population selection, sampling, issues related to age of the population, mustering population support, community organization, a specific chronic disease focus, and analysis of the study findings.[26,27,28]

THE EPIDEMIOLOGY OF CIGARETTE SMOKING AND CANCER

Epidemiology progress was slow from the late 1800s to the mid-1900s. As World War II ended, more and more lung cancer cases were being diagnosed. Physicians were taking notice and were curious as to the reason why. In the early 1950s a number of studies on the cause of the increase in lung cancer rates were begun, with cigarette smoking being a prime suspect.[29,30]

Several types of studies were developed, setting the stage for future epidemiological investigations, such as the case-control study and the cohort study. In the case control study, factors associated with one or more diseases developing were looked at, therefore persons with lung cancer and persons without lung cancer were questioned about past habits including smoking. In the cohort study, diseases associated with one or more causative factors were assessed, and smokers and nonsmokers were followed over a period of time. Disease rates including lung cancer were developed and measured.

One classic case-control study was conducted by Doll and Hill in 1947. The research study was planned to determine whether patients with lung cancer differed from others without the disease with respect to their smoking habits. Subjects of the study were patients admitted to a hospital in London with cancer of the lung, stomach, colon, or rectum, as well as persons with no cancer. The findings showed that cigarette smokers had more lung cancer than nonsmokers.[29,30]

In this study, Doll and Hill asked solid and basic epidemiological questions.

- Were the subjects of the study the same for both groups?
- Do those persons with the disease and those without the disease differ in any way other than by the disease state and their smoking behavior?
- Was the data collected in a standard manner for subjects and the control group?
- Is the difference between diseased and nondiseased persons great enough to be meaningful?

Doll and Hill, in 1951, sent a questionnaire to all British physicians to determine their smoking habits. A cohort study was used. (A cohort is a group of persons who were born in a certain time period and are identified by birth years.) A **cohort study** follows the cohort group over time. Over a 25-year period, death certificates were collected on this same group of physicians. Diseases recorded on the death certificates were studied and associated with the physician's smoking habits. A cause-effect relationship was found between the cigarette smoking physician and having lung cancer. The death rate for lung cancer in smokers was found to be ten times the rate of nonsmokers. Doll and Hill provided epidemiological insights and typical questions that are useful in epidemiology studies even today.[29,30]

EXERCISES

Key Terms

Define and explain the following terms.

bubonic plague	mortality data
carrier	necropsy
childbed fever	pathogens
cholera	puerperal fever
cohort	scurvy
cohort study	smallpox
endemic	transmission of disease
epidemic	typhoid
epidemiological observation	typhus
epidemiologist	variolation
fomites	vitamin
infection control	waterborne
lying-in hospital	zoonotic

Study Questions

3.1   What contributions did Leuwenhoek make to epidemiology?

3.2   a.   On what disease did Dr. Semmelweis do his epidemiological investigations? Give the common name and the medical term.
        b.   What were the causes of the disease?
        c.   What control approaches did he find effective?

3.3   a.   For what zoonotic disease did Louis Pasteur develop a vaccine?
        b.   Explain the investigative approaches used to prove that the vaccines worked.

3.4   What were several contributions made by Hippocrates to the field of epidemiology?

3.5   What were three major contributions made by Koch to epidemiology?

3.6   Explain briefly two major classical epidemiological investigations made by Dr. John Snow.

3.7   Explain the contributions made to epidemiology by John Graunt.

3.8   What were the epidemiological methods used by James Lind?

3.9 **a.** What were the major deficiency diseases that were causing a great deal of disease in the 1800s?

b. Explain briefly the epidemiological methods used in identifying nutritional deficiency diseases.

3.10 Explain how the work of Doll and Hill on cigarette smoking contributed to epidemiology. Give specific examples.

3.11 Explain the contributions of Lemuel Shattuck to the advancements of epidemiology in the United States.

REFERENCES

1. Hippocrates. 1988. "Airs, Waters, Places," in *The Challenge of Epidemiology: Issues and Selected Readings* by Buck, C., Llopis, A., Najera, E., and Terris, M. Washington, D.C.: Pan American Health Organization, Pan American Sanitary Bureau, pp. 18–19.
2. *Dorland's Illustrated Medical Dictionary*, 25th edition. 1974. Philadelphia: Saunders.
3. Cumston, C.G. 1926. *An Introduction to the History of Medicine*. New York: Alfred A. Knopf.
4. Garrison, F.H. 1926. *History of Medicine*. Philadelphia: Saunders.
5. Lind, J. 1988. "An Inquiry into the Nature, Causes and Cure of the Scurvy," in *The Challenge of Epidemiology: Issues and Selected Readings* by Buck, C., Llopis, A., Najera, E., and Terris, M. Washington, D.C.: Pan American Health Organization, Pan American Sanitary Bureau, pp. 20–23.
6. Jenner, E. 1988. "An Inquiry into the Causes and Effects of the Variolae Vaccine," in *The Challenge of Epidemiology: Issues and Selected Readings* by Buck, C., Llopis, A., Najera, E., and Terris, M. Washington, D.C.: Pan American Health Organization, Pan American Sanitary Bureau, pp. 31–32.
7. Clayton, T. (Editor). 1981. *Taber's Medical Dictionary*, 14th edition. Philadelphia: Davis, p. 762.
8. Benenson, A.S. (Editor). 1990. *Control of Communicable Diseases in Man*, 15th edition. Washington, D.C.: American Public Health Association, pp. 367–373.
9. Semmelweis, Ignas. 1988. "The Etiology, Concept, and Prophylaxis of Childbed Fever," in *The Challenge of Epidemiology: Issues and Selected Readings* by Buck, C., Llopis, A., Najera, E., and Terris, M. Washington, D.C.: Pan American Health Organization, Pan American Sanitary Bureau, pp. 46–59.
10. Snow, J. 1936. *On the Mode of Communication of Cholera* (2nd edition, 1855), reprinted by Commonwealth Fund, New York.
11. Snow, J. 1988. "On the Mode of Communication of Cholera," in *The Challenge of Epidemiology: Issues and Selected Readings* by Buck, C., Llopis, A., Najera, E., and Terris, M. Washington, D.C.: Pan American Health Organization, Pan American Sanitary Bureau, pp. 42–45.
12. Shindell, S., Salloway, J.C., and Oberembt, C.M. 1976. *A Coursebook in Health Care Delivery*. New York: Appleton-Century-Crofts.
13. Nash, N. "Cholera Epidemic Strains Peru's Limited Medical, Financial Resources," *New York Times*, reprinted in *The Sun*: San Bernardino, CA, Feb. 17th, 1991.
14. Nester, E.W., McCarthy, B.J., Roberts, C.E., and Pearsall, N.N. 1973. *Microbiology: Molecules, Microbes and Man*. New York: Holt, Rinehart and Winston.
15. Rosen, G. 1958. *A History of Public Health*. New York: MD Publications.
16. Seelig, M.G. 1925. *Medicine: An Historical Outline*. Baltimore: Williams and Wilkins.
17. Medical Milestone: Mary Mallon, "Typhoid Mary," *Health News*. New York Department of Health, November, 1968.
18. Krause, M.V. and Hunscher, M.A. 1972. *Food, Nutrition and Diet Therapy*, 5th edition. Philadelphia: Saunders.

19. Guthrie, H.A. 1975. *Introductory Nutrition.* St. Louis: Mosby.
20. Doll, R., and Hill, A.B. 1950. "Smoking and Carcinoma of the Lung" *British Medical Journal,* 2, p. 739.
21. Green, L., and Anderson, C. 1986. *Community Health,* 5th edition. St. Louis: Times Mirror/ Mosby.
22. Picket, G., and Hanlon, J. 1990. *Public Health: Administration and Practice,* 9th edition. St. Louis: Times Mirror/Mosby.
23. Sydenstricker, E. 1926. "A Study of Illness in a General Population," *Public Health Reports,* Vol. 61, No. 39, p. 12.
24. Sydenstricker, E. 1928. "Sex Difference in the Incidence of Certain Diseases at Different Ages," *Public Health Reports,* Vol. 63, No. 21, pp. 1269–1270.
25. Jones, J.H. 1993. *Bad Blood: The Tuskegee Syphilis Experiment.* New York: The Free Press.
26. Miller, D.F. 1992. *Dimensions of Community Health,* 3rd edition. Dubuque, IA: William C. Brown.
27. Hennekens, Ch. H., and Buring, J.E. 1987. *Epidemiology in Medicine.* Boston: Little, Brown and Company.
28. Dawber, T.R., Kannel, W.B., and Lyell, L.P. 1963. "An Approach to Longitudinal Studies in a Community: The Framingham Study," *Annals New York Academy of Sciences,* 107, pp. 539–556.
29. Monson, R.R. 1990. *Occupational Epidemiology,* 2nd edition. Boca Raton, FL: CRC Press.
30. Doll, R., and Hill, A.B. 1976. "Mortality in Relation to Smoking: Twenty Years' Observations on Male British Doctors, *British Medical Journal,* Vol. 2, p. 1525.

4

Epidemiological Measures of Health Status: Mortality— Rates and Ratios

CHAPTER OBJECTIVES

This chapter on epidemiological mortality

- reviews mortality statistics as used in epidemiology;
- presents the basic and general concepts of rates and ratios and the specific mortality rates and ratios;
- defines terminology related to rates, ratios, mortality, and epidemiology;
- presents the formulas of mortality vital statistics and epidemiology;
- reviews basic vital statistics and concepts that relate to death in populations;
- presents and reviews the different mortality statistics that affect the health status of populations;
- provides exercises that help review rates and ratios, and mortality concepts of the chapter.

INTRODUCTION

It is estimated from the current rate of births as compared to deaths, that every five days over one million people are added to the world's population, with between 75 and 80 million people added each year. At the current pace of increase, in about 41 years the entire population of the world will double. Population growth in underdeveloped countries, at their current pace of increase, will double in only 20 to 25 years.[1] On the other hand, if the spread of AIDS continues, these figures may be altered significantly. The South African government is concerned about the spread of AIDS in the Zulu tribe. One hospital in Pietermaritzburg, South Africa that tests Black patients for AIDS, reported that in 1989, 1 in 3,000 tested HIV positive and in 1990, 1 in 500 tested HIV positive. By 1991, 1 in 186 were testing HIV positive, and by January of 1992, 1 in 4 had tested HIV positive. It was concluded that at this rate of increase by the year 2007 the 7 million strong Zulu nation would be almost extinct. It is also predicted that by the year 2012, AIDS could reduce the South African population to 3 million blacks and one million whites. The country of Malawi, in Africa, has 32% of its 8.5 million infected with AIDS, and the statistics for Botswana, Tanzania, Zambia, and Zimbabwe are almost as serious. In the United States the cost to treat all AIDS patients was set at 5.8 billion. Since 1981, 145,000 people in the United States have died of AIDS.[2]

A worldwide concern exists about public health measures, including the use of epidemiology in tracking diseases and assessing data about populations. Vital statistics, as well as disease, disability, injury, and other related population issues need to be understood and investigated. Tracking the various factors affecting the health status of populations is done best using standardized measures and statistics, with results presented in a standardized manner. This chapter presents the standardized epidemiological approaches to the tracking and analysis of public health as well as population data and vital statistics.

MORTALITY STATISTICS

Mortality is a term which means "death," or describes death and related issues. Statistics on death are one part of and basic to vital statistics, epidemiology, and demographic data. Mortality statistics are reported from information contained in death certificates filed in death registration areas. A death registration area is a geographic area, a city, county, or state for which mortality data are published.

Public health agencies and the National Center for Health Statistics produce tables of mortality, which are published on a regular basis. Published tables of mortality provide actual numbers of deaths and death rates by age, sex, and cause of death. Special death tables present these variables as well as other vital statistics descriptors such as race, religion, occupation, education, etc., related to death rates (see Table 4.1 and Table 4.2).

TABLE 4.1   Mortality table for the United States–1990

Age	Total Deaths	Rate per 100,000 Population		
		Both Sexes	Male	Female
All ages	2,175,000	867.7	922.0	816.1
Under 1 year	38,200	944.0	1,042.9	839.7
1–4 years	6,859	45.7	50.7	40.4
5–14 years	8,600	24.1	28.8	19.2
15–24 years	37,280	103.7	154.3	51.7
25–34 years	60,910	139.2	204.4	73.9
35–44 years	83,790	221.9	307.2	138.5
45–54 years	118,550	465.4	603.6	334.4
55–64 years	253,280	1,181.7	1,516.7	880.8
65–74 years	483,490	2,624.8	3,384.1	2,013.4
75–84 years	611,220	6,137.4	7,992.3	4,999.8
85 and older	471,090	14,974.3	17,743.4	13,897.8
Not stated	1,440	—	—	—

(Source: National Center for Health Statistics, Monthly Vital Statistics Report, U.S. Department of Health and Human Services, April 8th, 1991)
Note: For the 12 months ending November 1990, data are provisional, estimated from a 10% sample of deaths.

TABLE 4.2   Table of selected mortality rates for the United States

Selected Mortality Statistics	1980	1986	1988
Deaths (in thousands)	1,990	2,105	2,168
Death rate, crude (per 100,000)	878.3	873.2	882.0
Death rate, adjusted (per 100,000)	585.8	541.7	535.5
Infant mortality (per 1,000 live births)	12.6	10.4	10.0
Fetal death rate (per 1,000 live births)	9.1	7.7	7.5
Life Expectancy at birth (in years)	73.7	74.8	74.9

(Source: National Center for Health Statistics, *Health—United States, 1990*, Public Health Service, U.S. Department of Health and Human Services, Vol. 40, No. SS–2, July 1991)

RATES

Basic to epidemiology is the need to assess the amount of growth, disease, disability, injury, and death in populations. Equally important is the need to study and analyze any or all factors affecting these measures of health status. However, basic to understanding the data and statistics is the understanding of how much disease, injury, illness, disability, or death is regularly occurring in the population.

It is also important to present the data and statistics in a manner that makes sense and is comparable from one population group to another. It is common to see in newspapers or magazines stories reporting disease outbreaks or other health problems. It is not unusual in newspaper stories to see statements like, "58 students were reported to be sick with the measles," or "70% of poverty level children interviewed have dental caries." These statements provide no comparison and offer little meaning as much information is lacking.

The problem with such statements is the reader is left not knowing what the numbers are being compared to: "58 out of how many students?" or "70% of how many children?" The problem is trying to get a true picture of the illness or injury, because a total population is not presented for comparison. If the statistic on measles was given as 58 out of 100 it has a different meaning than 58 out of 280,000. The same goes for percentages. If figures were 70% of 10 children interviewed, that would mean a narrow sampling of children, which may not represent all poverty level children, and that few children were actually at risk. If the study was 70% of 1,000 poverty level children selected at random from welfare recipient rolls, the meaning of the findings changes greatly and many people are at risk. If a date or time were included with the data, then even more significance would come to the meaning of the statistics. The shorter the time period the greater the concern and higher the risk. If a standard time period such as *1 year* is used, then comparisons with other statistics or populations using the same standardized measures are possible.

If an epidemiologist wishes to compare one town, county, or state, one to another, then percentages are not enough. Thus, a rate is needed so that one population can be compared accurately and correctly to another. Defined in a generic manner, **rate** is the amount or number of one thing measured in units of another; the amount or degree of a thing in relation to units of something else. Rate is the measure of an event, condition, injury, disability, or death with a unit of a population, and within a time period.[3,4,5]

A rate, as used in epidemiology, is the number of or frequency of a disease per unit size of population of group. The unit size is presented as 100, 1,000, 10,000, or 100,000. For example, the homicide rate for 1993 the United States is 8.7 per 100,000 population. In charts and graphs on vital statistics and epidemiological data distributed by government agencies and other organizations producing vital statistics reports, the hundreds approach is used. Usually it is stated on the margin, side, top, or bottom, of the chart, "per 100,000 population" (see Tables 4.1 and 4.2 and Figure 4.1). A time period is also included as part of the rate. Time periods are clearly stated in the charts and data by the epidemiologist.[3,4,5]

A rate measures the amount of disease, injury, or death in a population, group, community, or geographical area by relating cases of the disease to the population base. A basic formula for a rate includes a *numerator* (the number of *cases* with the disease), a *denominator* (the *population* of the area) and a time period. The rate formula is presented as a fraction.

There are three basic factors needed to develop rates. First, the numerator of the rate formula (which includes the number of individuals affected, ill, exposed, etc.). Second, the denominator of the formula (the total population of the study, the total number in the group

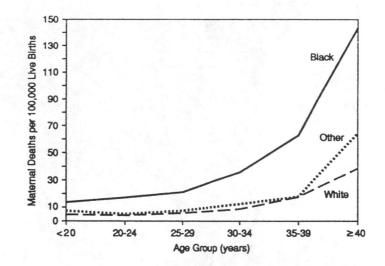

FIGURE 4.1   Maternal mortality by age group and race in the United States for 1979–1986. (Source: Centers for Disease Control and Prevention, "Special Focus on Reproductive Health Surveillance—Maternal Mortality Surveillance, United States, 1979–1986," *Morbidity and Mortality Weekly Report*, Public Health Service, U.S. Department of Health and Human Services, Vol. 40, No. SS-2, July 1991)

among whom the affected persons are derived), and third, a specific time period (usually year). The results are usually multiplied by 100 or 1,000 to complete the rate. The numerator is confined to a specific set of characteristics such as age, sex, race, occupation, religion, etc. The denominator is limited to the population of the study group or the total population; i.e., the city, school, state, county, age group, total population of a nation, etc.

If the numerator is limited to males, then the denominator is limited to males, if the numerator is used to study a condition of pregnant women, the denominator is restricted to all pregnant women in the population, etc. Equal and balanced comparisons must be made in the rate formula. The denominator can set limitations to the formula such as determining the population at risk—those capable of being exposed to the disease. The numerator includes those affected by an exposure to the risk.

From a mathematical perspective, a rate is considered a type of a ratio. The traits of rate are that time is one element and there is a distinct relationship between the denominator and numerator. Time is an element of the denominator.[4,5,6]

Stated in a different way, a rate is a numerical statement, using a formula to determine the frequency of an event derived by dividing the number of cases (the numerator) by the total number capable of experiencing the event (the denominator, or population at risk) and multiplying the results by 100, 1,000 or 10,000 (a constant) in order to arrive at how many cases occurred for that unit of population.[4,5,6]

$$\text{Rate} = \frac{\text{Number of cases}}{\substack{\text{Population of the area} \\ \text{in a specific time period}}} \times 1000$$

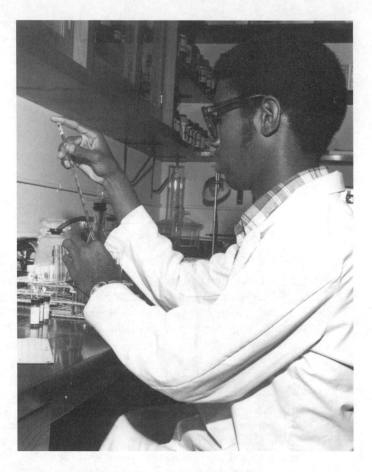

FIGURE 4.2   One of the goals of the Centers for Disease Control and Prevention (CDC) is to reduce mortality rates. A CDC scientist works toward this goal. (Picture courtesy of Centers for Disease Control and Prevention, Atlanta, Georgia)

High rates as well as low rates provide useful information and insights into cause, spread, transmission, and overall effect of a disease on a population (see Figure 4.2). Well groups can be compared to sick groups living in the same area that otherwise should be affected equally with a disease but are not. From this, the epidemiologist gains much insight into the transmission of the disease as well as how to develop control measures for it. The high rate of AIDS found in homosexuals and a low rate of AIDS found in monogamous people all living in the same community helped in the past to point to the cause and transmission of the disease. The transmission of AIDS is related more to sexual behavior, mixing of bodily fluids, especially blood and not the characteristics of the population, and is but one example of how rates are developed and used.[3,4,5]

Rates are expressed in terms of the total population. Rates are also expressed for subgroups of a population. There are three types of rates: crude rates, adjusted rates, and specific rates. Specific rates are for subsets or subgroups of a total population. (These three rates

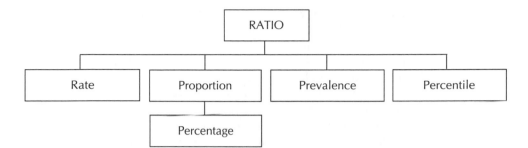

FIGURE 4.3 Diagram of the relationship of ratio to rate, proportion, prevalence, and percentile.

are addressed later in this chapter.)[4,5,6] Figure 4.3 is a graphical representation of the relationship of various epidemiological measures to the *ratio*.

The difference between a proportion and a percentage is that a percentage is a result of multiplying by 100, which moves the decimal point 2 places to the right. The proportion is when the decimal remains and is not moved.

Key to Using Rates

The key to using rates, making new rate formulas, and applying rates to new and different settings or situations is qualifying what you are doing or what you have done. When using a rate that varies from standard usage, be sure to provide a definition or explanation of the numerator and denominator, as well as an explanation of the use and application of the rate. Be sure any new application reflects its being a rate and not a proportion by making sure the number of cases in the numerator is a subset of the population number in the denominator.

RATIOS

As presented in Figure 4.3, the term *rate* is loosely used in epidemiology. Many measures referred to as rates are actually ratios. The generic definition of **ratio** is the relation in number, degree, or quantity, existing between two things; a fixed relationship in number or degree between two similar things, such as 25 males to 30 females. In a mathematical sense, a ratio is the result of one quantity divided by another of the same kind and expressed as a fraction. Ratios are less useful than rates in descriptive statistics and of even less value in inferential statistics (see Chapter 7). A ratio is also a general measure of which a rate, proportion, or percentage are subsets (see Figure 4.3).

In a ratio, the numerator is not included in the population defined by the denominator. No restrictions exist on the ranges or dimensionalities of ratios. There are limitations on rates, percentages, prevalence, proportions, etc. Unlike a percentage, ratios can exceed 100%. Ratios have been expressed as percentages in epidemiology, making for some confusion. Measured and counted values may be included in the denominator and numerator.

Being a more general term, ratio is a relative number that expresses the magnitude of one occurrence in relation to another. All rates can be viewed as ratios, but ratios are not necessarily rates. Ratios are less useful than rates in epidemiology as the time element is missing, making the results a more generalized finding.

Another term and measure used in epidemiology is **rate ratio**, which is a modification of the rate and is the ratio of two rates. (See *ratio, rate,* and odds ratio.) For a better understanding, an example is in order. Rate ratio is not a general ratio but one that has a specific use. It is a ratio of the rate of an "at risk population," to the rate in the "not-at-risk" population, or a group of unimmunized children in a school compared to children who already had measles or immunizations within a specific time period.[4,5,6]

A less rigid view of rate is also used in epidemiology. "True," rates are presented above. Birth rates and death rates are true rates. However, an attack rate is not a true rate. (See *attack rate.*) Neonatal mortality rates, perinatal mortality rates, or any other mortality rates that represent only a part of mortality are not true rates. Any factor that changes or dwindles as time passes cannot be a true rate. Infant mortality, is not a true rate but a proportion. (See *proportion.*) Additionally, cumulative incident rates and prevalence rates are not true rates.[4,5,6]

A **true rate** exists only if the numerator is included as part of the denominator and if the denominator represents the entire population of concern or the entire population at risk. Rates can be expressed as a total group or population or as a subgroup, which are expressed as specific rates, i.e., crude rates, specific rates, and adjusted rates.[4] Rates related to a total population are expressed as crude rates or adjusted rates. Crude, specific, and adjusted rates are presented in detail below.

The terms **odds ratio** (or *risk ratio* or *risk odds ratio*) are terms that are used more in assessing morbidity than mortality and are mentioned only briefly here. (See Chapter 5 and 8 for more on odds ratio, relative risk.) In mortality statistics odds ratio could be the ratio of the odds of death occurring if exposed to a life threatening agent against the odds of no death if not exposed.

Formula for Ratio

Since a ratio is a fixed relation between two similar items or things, a ratio is obtained by dividing one quantity by another. The quotient of one quantity divided by another of the same kind and is usually expressed as a fraction; 5 cases of measles compared to 30 children without measles then becomes:

$$5 \text{ to } 30 \text{ ratio} \quad \text{or} \quad \frac{5}{30}$$

PROPORTIONS

A **proportion** is a form of percentage, with percentages being a special type of proportion. A percentage is a certain part of or a number in each hundred; any part or proportion of a whole. A proportion is the relation between the amount, number, size, or degree of one thing and the amount, number, size, or degree of another. Mathematically, a proportion is a statement of equality between two ratios.

In epidemiology, if the numbers of those people currently with a disease or condition are expressed relative to the total number of all who have had the disease or condition, this is a proportion. If expressed in relation to the total population, it is a rate. In epidemiology one ratio that is used is fetal death ratio, which is usually expressed as the number of fetal deaths relative to the number of live births. The total number of deaths due to a particular cause may be expressed as a proportion of all deaths but not to all births.

In epidemiology, a proportion is a ratio in which the numerator is included as part of the denominator. In the strict definition, a proportion must fall within the range of 0.0 to 1.0. The important difference between a ratio and a proportion is that the numerator of a proportion is included in the population defined by the denominator.

Formula for Proportions (Percentages)

Remember, in proportions one has to compare like populations or like illnesses within populations. To change a fraction into a percentage the numerator is divided by the denominator which produces a decimal × 100; changing the decimal to a percentage. Left as a decimal, this is a proportion. The following example shows how to calculate a proportion and Figure 4.4 is graphic presentation of the use of proportions/percentages.

Example: 40 children are currently ill with the measles, 80 children all together have had the measles.

$$\frac{40 \text{ currently ill}}{80 \text{ total cases of measles}} = 40 \text{ divided by } 80$$

$$= .50 \times 100$$

$$= 50\% \text{ are ill.}$$

(.50 is the proportion. 50% is the percentage)

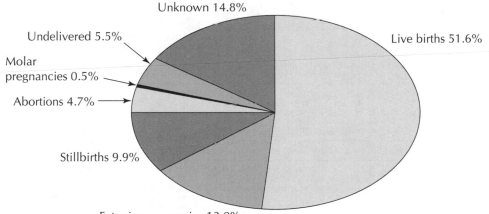

FIGURE 4.4 Maternal deaths by outcome of pregnancy in the United States for 1979–1986. (Source: Centers for Disease Control and Prevention, "Special Focus on Reproductive Health Surveillance—Maternal Mortality Surveillance, United States, 1979–1986," *Morbidity and Mortality Weekly Report*, Public Health Service, U.S. Department of Health and Human Services, Vol. 40, No. SS-2, July 1991)

The Vital Statistics Registration System in the United States

Responsible Person or Agency	Birth Certificate	Death Certificate	Fetal Death Report (Stillbirth)
Hospital authority	1. Completes entire certificate in consultation with parent(s). 2. Files certificate with local office or State office per State law.	When death occurs in hospital, may initiate preparation of certificate: Completes information on name, date, and place of death; obtains certification of cause of death from physician; and gives certificate to funeral director. NOTE: If the attending physician is unavailable to certify to the cause of death, some States allow a hospital physician to certify to only the fact and time of death. With legal pronouncement of the death and permission of the attending physician, the body can then be released to the funeral director. The attending physician still must complete the cause-of-death section prior to final disposition of the body.	1. Completes entire report in consultation with parent(s). 2. Obtains cause of fetal death and other medical and health information from physician. 3. Obtains authorization for final disposition of fetus. 4. Files report with local office or State office per State law.
Funeral director		1. Obtains personal facts about decedent and completes certificate. 2. Obtains certification of cause of death from attending physician or medical examiner or coroner. 3. Obtains authorization for final disposition per State law. 4. Files certificate with local office or State office per State law.	If fetus is to be buried, the funeral director is responsible for obtaining authorization for final disposition. NOTE: In some States the funeral director, or person acting as such, is responsible for all duties shown above under hospital authority.
Physician or other professional attendant	For inhospital birth, verifies accuracy of medical information and signs certificate. For out-of-hospital birth, duties are same as those for hospital authority, shown above.	Completes certification of cause of death and signs certificate.	Provides cause of fetal death and other medical and health information.
Local office* (may be local registrar or city or county health department)	1. Verifies completeness and accuracy of certificate and queries incomplete or inconsistent certificates. 2. If authorized by State law, makes copy or index for local use. 3. Sends certificates to State registrar.	1. Verifies completeness and accuracy of certificate and queries incomplete or inconsistent certificates. 2. If authorized by State law, makes copy or index for local use. 3. If authorized by State law, issues authorization for final disposition on receipt of completed certificate. 4. Sends certificates to State registrar.	If State law requires routing of fetal death reports through local office, the local office performs the same functions as shown for the death certificate.
City and county health departments use data derived from these records in allocating medical and nursing services, following up on infectious diseases, planning programs, measuring effectiveness of services, and conducting research studies.			
State registrar, office of vital statistics	1. Queries incomplete or inconsistent information. 2. Maintains files for permanent reference and is the source of certified copies. 3. Develops vital statistics for use in planning, evaluating, and administering State and local health activities and for research studies. 4. Compiles health-related statistics for State and civil divisions of State for use of the health department and other agencies and groups interested in the fields of medical science, public health, demography, and social welfare. 5. Sends data derived from records or copies of records to the National Center for Health Statistics.		
Public Health Service, National Center for Health Statistics	1. Prepares and publishes national statistics of births, deaths, and fetal deaths; constructs the official U.S. life tables and related actuarial tables. 2. Conducts health and social-research studies based on vital records and on sampling surveys linked to records. 3. Conducts research and methodological studies in vital statistics methods, including the technical, administrative, and legal aspects of vital records registration and administration. 4. Maintains a continuing technical assistance program to improve the quality and usefulness of vital statistics.		

* Some States do not have local vital registration offices. In these States, the certificates or reports are transmitted directly to the State office of vital statistics.

FIGURE 4.5 Vital statistics registration system in the United States. (Source: Medical Examiners' and Coroners' Handbook on Death Registration and Fetal Death Reporting, National Center for Health Statistics, Public Health Service, U.S. Department of Health and Human Services, Oct. 1987)

MORTALITY

In the late 1600s Graunt developed a system of tracking and understanding the cause of death that was called the Bills of Mortality. William Farr (1807–1883), was appointed Registrar General in England and built on the ideas of Graunt. Farr's registration system for vital statistics laid the foundation for data collection and for the use of vital statistics in epidemiology. The foundation of the work of both Graunt and Farr were death related statistics. (See Chapter 3.)

Mortality is the epidemiological and vital statistics term for death. In our society there are generally three things that cause death: (1) degeneration of vital organs and related conditions; (2) disease states; and (3) as results of society or the environment (homicide, accidents, disasters, etc.).[8]

In most industrialized and advanced nations, laws require the registration of vital events: births, marriages, divorces, and deaths. Legally, death is the most protected of all vital events and mortality is the foundation of all vital statistics. All deaths have to be certified by a physician or a coroner. If any foul play is involved in a death, an autopsy is required in most states and the results of the autopsy are recorded. Autopsy findings serve as objective data as certification of the cause of death and are the most accurate. Some diagnoses by physicians as to cause of death are not always completely correct, due to the difficulty of making an accurate cause of death diagnosis without an autopsy. The physician signing the death certificate may not be the attending physician, thus may not have complete information on cause of death and may record only what he or she knows about the death. All deaths are recorded and reported to local health departments and to the state office of vital statistics. Reports of vital event statistics including deaths are reported to the National Center for Health Statistics.[4,5,6,8] (See Figure 4.5.)

The registration of births, fetal deaths, deaths, and other vital events in the United States is a state and local function. The laws of each state provide for a continuous, permanent, and compulsory vital registration system. Each system depends on the conscientious efforts of physicians, hospital personnel, funeral directors, coroners, and medical examiners in preparing or certifying information needed to complete the original death records (see Figure 4.5). The role of the medical examiner and coroner are presented in Chapter 6.

Causes of Death

The National Center for Health Statistics developed and recommends the use of a Standard Certificate of Death in the United States. Each state is expected to include on the death certificate the minimum information set forth on the U.S. Standard Certificate of Death. Some states include additional information deemed important. Death statistics are of great importance to epidemiological activities, thus the information from death certificates is extremely useful. Death certificates provide not only information on the total numbers of deaths, but also provide demographic information and other important facts about each person who dies, such as date of birth (for cohort studies) and death (for accurate age), stated age, place of death, place of residence, occupation, sex, cause of death, marital status. Other information may include, type of injury, and place and time of injury, etc. See the sample certificate of death for the State of California (Figure 4.6). A separate certificate for fetal deaths is used (Figure 4.7).

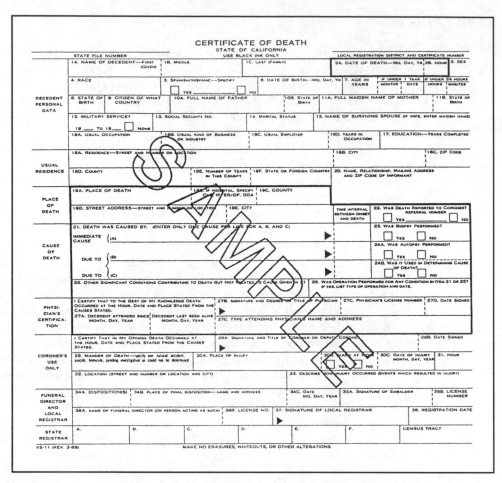

FIGURE 4.6   Example of a standard certificate of death for the state of California. (Revision 3-1989)

Cause of Death on Death Certificates

How the cause of death is presented on the death certificate is of much importance. "Causes of Death and Underlying Causes of Death," are set forth by ICD-9-CM (International Classification of Diseases—9th Edition—Clinical Modification)[9] and are used on the death certificate. The causes of death as entered on the death certificate are all diseases, injuries, and morbid conditions that resulted in or contributed to the death. Also circumstances of any accident or violent act which produced death are recorded.

In 1999 in the United States, causes of death on the death certificate are to be classified using ICD-10-CM codes.

Underlying Cause of Death

Found on the death certificate is a space for the "underlying cause of death." This is stated on a death certificate directly after the main cause of death. The underlying cause is any

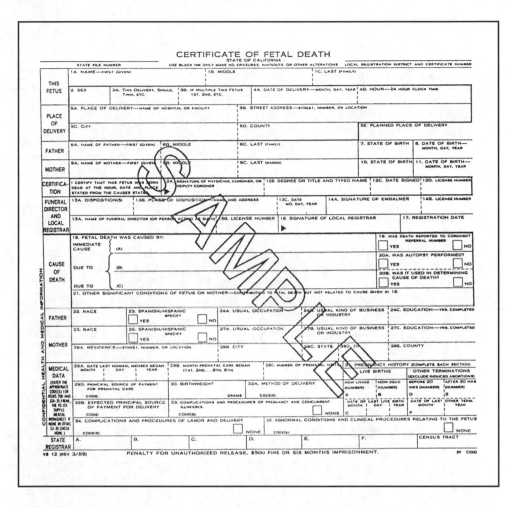

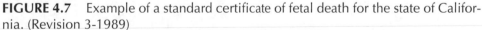

FIGURE 4.7 Example of a standard certificate of fetal death for the state of California. (Revision 3-1989)

disease or injury which initiated the set of events leading to the death. Any violent act or accident that produced the death would be stated on this section of the death certificate.

Death Certificate Data

Data from death certificates and the formal death reporting system provide a database for studying a variety of epidemiological issues and events. The main cause of death is entered first on a death certificate. Two additional or contributing causes can also be listed (see Figure 4.6). Diagnosis of death listings are done according to ICD-9-CM (International Classification of Diseases—9th Edition—Clinical Modification).[9] The existing diseases and conditions at the time of death may hold as much epidemiological value as the listed cause of death.

Top Causes of Death Worldwide

Heart Disease Is Top Killer Across the World

For much of the recent history of the world, the main cause of death in developing nations has been infectious diseases. Chronic and lifestyle diseases were common to advanced nations. Now ischemic heart disease kills 6.2 million people worldwide in both developing and advanced nations. In addition, many chronic diseases are shown to have infections in their origins. A study finished in 1990, reported in the April 28, 1997 issue of *Lancet*, reported the top 30 killers to be

1. Ischemic heart disease, 6.2 million
2. Stroke, 4.3 million
3. Respiratory infections, 4.3 million
4. Diarrheal diseases, 2.9 million
5. Perinatal disorders, 2.4 million
6. Lung disease, 2.2 million
7. Tuberculosis, 1.9 million
8. Measles, 1.1 million
9. Traffic accidents, 999,000
10. Respiratory cancer, 945,000
11. Malaria, 856,000
12. Suicides, 786,000
13. Cirrhosis, 779,000
14. Stomach cancer, 752,000
15. Congenital abnormalities, 589,000
16. Diabetes, 571,000
17. Violence, 563,000
18. Tetanus, 542,000
19. Kidney disease, 536,000
20. Drowning, 504,000
21. War injuries, 502,000
22. Liver Cancer, 501,000
23. Inflammatory heart disease, 495,000
24. Colon and rectal cancer, 472,000
25. Malnutrition, 372,000
26. Esophageal cancer, 358,000
27. Whooping cough, 347,000
28. Rheumatic heart disease, 340,000
29. Breast cancer, 322,000
30. HIV/AIDS, 312,00

THREE LEVELS OF RATES (GENERAL USE)

Rates used to present data or information for a total population or group, are *crude rates*. A mathematical adjustment or transformation of crude rates is an *adjusted rate*. Any rate that expresses information or data on a population subgroup is a *specific rate*.

Crude Rates

Crude rates are based on the number of experiences or events that happen in a total population in a certain period of time. Two crude rates are fundamental to epidemiological methods: (1) crude death rates (presented later in this chapter) and (2) crude birth rates (presented in Chapter 6). The crude birth rate formula is basically the same as the crude death rate except total births are used in the denominator. Overall general statistical and vital event information is derived from crude rates, using the average population as the denominator for each factor of population statistics. The unique differences, characteristics, behaviors, risks, occurrences, experiences, or cultural implications of subgroups or sections of a population are not reflected in crude death rates.

Crude rates are not presented as percentages but as a rate per hundreds of a population. The population size or group size used for comparison usually determines which number is selected for comparison and should closely reflect the size of that population. If it is a small population, the rate for comparison would be per 100. A larger group would be per 1,000 or 10,000. If it was a very large population, 100,000 and in some cases 500,000 or 1,000,000 would be used.

Crude rates are summary rates and are developed from only minimal data and limited information and are good for comparison of one country to another. Crude rates have limitations as they ignore information derived from subgroups and special circumstances, and they fail to show the differences found in or between subgroups.[3,4,7]

Adjusted Rates

When assessing crude rates, it is important to evaluate specific rates and age distributions in order to ascertain if an adjustment is needed. **Adjusted rates** use mathematical calculations and transformations to allow comparisons among and between populations having characteristics or traits that may differ or which may affect risk of injury, disease, disability, or death.[3,4,7] (See adjusted death rates and age adjusted rates on page 120.)

Specific Rates

Specific rates provide detailed information presented as rates for a specific age, religion, race, gender, etc. The denominator of a specific rate uses a specific population or subgroup for a certain geographical area and certain period.[3,4,7]

TYPES OF MORTALITY RATES/RATIOS

Many different death rates are used in epidemiology. The mortality rates/ratios are

- annual death rate
- crude death rates
- infant mortality rates (ratio)
- neonatal mortality rates
- postneonatal mortality rates
- perinatal mortality rates
- fetal death ratios
- fetal death rates
- abortion rates
- maternal mortality rates
- adjusted mortality rates
- standardized mortality ratio

- specific death rates (age)
- proportionate mortality rate—case fatality rate
- mortality crossover—mortality time trends

Annual Death Rate

The first and most basic measure of death is the general mortality rate (death rate). The general death rate has three aspects:

1. a population group exposed to the risk of death
2. a time period
3. the number of deaths occurring in that population group during that period of time.

In the **annual death rate** the numerator contains the number of deaths that occurred in the population and the denominator contains the number of persons in the total population. The denominator is obtained from known sources such as the census or calculated estimates of the population. Some epidemiologists consider this a crude death rate.[10]

$$\text{Annual death rate from all causes} = \frac{\text{Total numbers of death during a specific 12-month time period}}{\text{Number of persons in the total population at middle of the time period}} \times 1,000$$

Crude Death Rate (CDR)

Another basic mortality rate is the **crude death rate**. The term *crude* is used because it does not account for the difference of age, sex, or other variables in any aspects of death. The crude death rate is a summary rate based on the actual number of deaths in a total population over a given time period (see Table 4.3). The crude death rate is used as it only requires three basic pieces of information: (1) total deaths, (2) total population, and (3) a given time period.[4,8,10,11]

The crude death rate is the total number of deaths in a year divided by the average total population times a set part of the population such as 100, 1,000, 10,000, or 100,000. To create a rate it has to be multiplied by 1,000 or one of the other multiples of a population. The time element is determined by the epidemiologist.

$$\text{CDR} = \frac{\text{Total deaths per year}}{\text{Average total population of that year}} \times 100,000$$

$$\frac{2,134,000}{248,709,873} \times 100,000 = 858.0$$

TABLE 4.3 Crude death rates for all causes in the United States for selected years (number of deaths per 10,000 population)

Years	1965	1970	1975	1980	1985	1991
Crude Rate	94.46	84.53	88.85	87.80	87.00	85.80

INFANT MORTALITY

Infant mortality is a major health status indicator of populations and a key measure of health status of a community or population. **Infant mortality rate** (which is not a true rate but a ratio) is a measure of the numbers of deaths in a one-year period.

Infant mortality is significant as a health status indicator, as it reflects the health status of the mother and the child throughout the pregnancy and birth process. There is nothing more fragile than a newborn child who is completely dependent upon an adult for surviving, thriving, and growing to a healthy child. Nothing is more helpless than a child in the mother's uterus depending on her to eat well, be physically fit, and to avoid drugs, alcohol, and tobacco so that the infant may emerge from the womb healthy and normal.

Reflected in infant mortality is prenatal and postnatal nutritional care, or the lack of it. If women have an intake of sufficient calories and nutrients including appropriate weight gain upon becoming pregnant, this will improve infant birthweight and reduce infant mortality and morbidity. Seeking immediate medical care upon becoming pregnant as well as total abstinence from any drugs, chemical, alcohol, and smoking can reduce infant mortality. Proper immunization of newborns at the appropriate time will also reduce infant mortality.[11] Some underdeveloped countries in Africa have more than 150 infants die for every 1,000 births each year and some advanced, industrialized, and homogeneous populated nations have less than 8 infant deaths in 1,000 each year. Prenatal care is often lacking in most underdeveloped countries, as are the basic public health measures of immunizations, sanitation, and infection control, which also contribute to high infant mortality rates. Infants born to Mexican-American parents are more than twice as likely to be born outside of a hospital than any other racial group. It is also reported that statistics for Hispanic populations are not accurate due to some returning to their birthplace to have their babies, or failure to report a birth or death related to birth due to mistrust of United States authorities. It is suggested that the Hispanic population in the United States is quite heterogenic and that infant mortality prevention can be tailored to specific ethnic risk factors and outcomes within this population and thus should easily be reduced.[13]

The United States infant mortality rate for 1990 was 9.2 deaths per 1,000 live births. In 1989 the infant mortality rate was 9.8 per 1,000 live births for all races. For blacks, the rate was 18.6 and for whites it was 8.1 per 1,000. The infant mortality rate in the U.S. has dropped considerably over the years and continues to drop. For every 1,000 live births in 1990 among blacks, 18 died before age one. For whites the infant mortality rate was 7.9 (see Figure 4.8).

The Infant Mortality Rate

A specific definition of infant mortality is necessary in order to correctly calculate infant mortality rates and must be adhered to. Infant mortality includes all deaths of children from the moment of birth up to and including the 365th day of life. Infant mortality is the rate of deaths in newborn children less than one year old. Included in the denominator is the number of live births for the same time period: one year. The goal of the infant mortality rate is to include in the numerator only those deaths occurring in the denominator population. It is assumed that the number of infant deaths takes place within the same time period and within the same population as the numbers of live births. Death rates under one year are based on the total population (denominator) and differ from infant mortality rates which

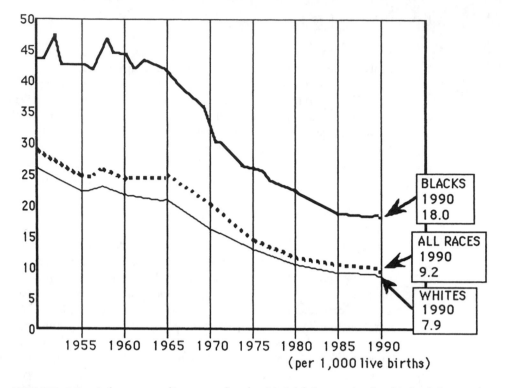

FIGURE 4.8   Infant mortality rates for the United States. In the United States the infant mortality rate for 1990 was 7.9 per 1,000 live births. (Source: Centers for Disease Control and Prevention)

are based on live births (denominator). The numerator includes the number of deaths of children under one year of age. Infant mortality rate lacks meeting the true definition of a rate and is actually a ratio. Nonetheless, the infant mortality rate is presented as follows:

$$\text{Infant mortality rate} = \frac{\text{Number of child deaths less than 1 year old in one year}}{\text{Number of live births in the same year}} \times 1,000$$

$$\text{Infant death rates under one year} = \frac{\text{Number of child deaths less than 1 year old in one year}}{\text{Total population}} \times 100,000$$

San Bernardino County, California, the largest geographical county in the United States, had the following infant mortality rate as shown through the use of the formula.

$$\text{San Bernardino County (1988)} = \frac{291}{28,013} \times 1,000$$

$$= 10.4$$

Neonatal Mortality Rate

The most dangerous time for infants is just prior to and just after birth. Neonatal rates reflect poor prenatal care, low birth weights, infections, lack of proper medical care, injuries, prematurity, and congenital defects. A special concern lies in the proper reporting of neonatal deaths. Some very low birthweight (under 2,500 grams) infant deaths may go unreported, and this may be even more so for very low birthweights: under 1,000 grams.[14]

Neonatal mortality rate is defined as the number of deaths of infants under 28 days of age (the numerator) in a given period of time, usually one year. The denominator includes the total number of live births for the same period. Rates are usually presented as deaths per 1,000 (or 10,000 or 100,000, as specified).

$$\text{Neonatal mortality rate} = \frac{\text{Number of infant deaths under 28 days old}}{\text{Number of live births in the same year}} \times 1,000$$

Postneonatal Mortality Rate

Postneonatal mortality rates are important to track in underdeveloped countries, especially in areas where infants die somewhat later than in their first year of life due to malnutrition, nutrition deficiencies, and infectious diseases. Figure 4.9 is an example of the use of the trend of neonatal and postneonatal rates for the 24-year period of 1960–1984. Neonatal mortality rate is the deaths occurring among infants from 0 to 28 days of age per 1,000

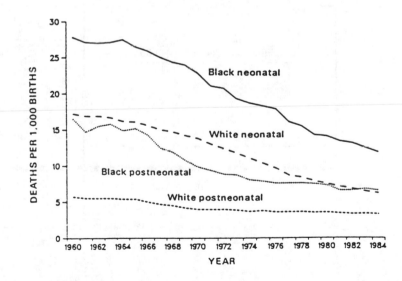

FIGURE 4.9 Neonatal and postneonatal mortality rates among single delivery infants by race and year for the United States, 1960–1984. (Source: *Chronic Disease and Health Promotion Reprints from the MMWR, 1985–1989*, Vol. 4, Center for Chronic Disease Prevention and Health Promotion, Centers for Disease Control and Prevention, U.S. Department of Health and Human Services)

births in a calendar year. Postneonatal mortality rate is the deaths occurring among infants from 28 days to 1 year of age per 1,000 live births in a calendar year. The number of deaths between 28 days and one year of age is the numerator and is for a given period of time, usually one year. The denominator includes the total number of live births for the same period. Rates are usually presented as deaths per 1,000 (or 10,000 or 100,000, as specified).

$$\text{Postneonatal mortality rate} = \frac{\text{Number of infant deaths between 28 days of age and 1 year of age}}{\text{Number of live births in the same year}} \times 1,000$$

Perinatal Mortality Rates

The greatest period of risk of death to all populations is the perinatal period and the period after 60 years. It is of value to clinical medicine to evaluate the loss of a child within a few days and then within a few hours or minutes before and after birth in order to prevent unnecessary deaths and illness at this time. **Perinatal mortality rates** link deaths of late fetal life, birth, and early infancy and are defined by the number of fetal deaths of 20 or more weeks gestation plus all neonatal deaths for a specific period of time. A second way they are determined is by all fetal deaths (28 weeks of gestation) plus postnatal deaths (first week) (numerator). The denominator includes all fetal deaths (28 weeks of gestation) plus live births. Some sources suggest using the two perinatal death periods. Perinatal mortality period I is 28 weeks of gestation up to 7 days post-delivery. Perinatal mortality Period II is 20 weeks of gestation up to 28 days post-delivery (see Figure 4.10).

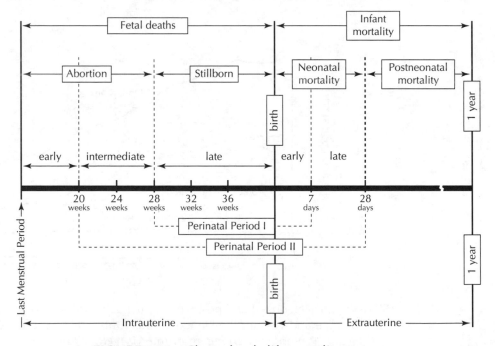

FIGURE 4.10   Chart of early life mortality measures.

(As used in advanced/industrialized nations)

$$\text{Perinatal mortality rate} \text{ (Period I)} = \frac{\text{Number of fetal deaths of 28 or more weeks gestation + postnatal deaths (7 days)}}{\text{Total fetal deaths + live births in the same period}} \times 1,000$$

$$\text{Perinatal mortality rate} \text{ (Period II)} = \frac{\text{Number of fetal deaths of 20 or more weeks gestation + neonatal deaths}}{\text{Total number of births (stillborn and live births) in the same period}} \times 1,000$$

(World Health Organization use for countries with inconsistent or less formalized vital statistics collection and record system)

$$\text{Perinatal mortality rate} \text{ (W.H.O.)} = \frac{\text{Number of fetal deaths of 28 or more weeks gestation + postnatal deaths (7 days)}}{\text{Total live births in the year}} \times 1,000$$

Fetal Death Rate and Fetal Death Ratio

The term fetal death is used synonymously with *stillborn*. Fetal deaths are those deaths that are due to the expulsion or extraction of the fetus from the womb irrespective of the duration of pregnancy. When the fetus does not breathe or shows no signs of life upon leaving the mother's womb it is dead. Signs of life are usually determined by breathing, a beating heart, pulsating umbilical cord, or voluntary muscle movement. The fetal death rate was developed as a measure of risk of the stages of gestation. The fetal death rate is usually defined by death after the 20th week or in some cases after the 28th week of gestation. Different countries and agencies use different lengths of gestation to measure the fetal death rate, making if difficult to compare data.[3,4,14,15]

Fetal Death Rate

The **fetal death rate** is a proportion of the number of fetal deaths in relationship to the number of births for a certain period of time, usually one year. The numerator has the actual deaths reported and the denominator has the number of fetal deaths plus live births for a certain period usually one year.[3,4,14,15]

$$\text{Fetal death rate} = \frac{\text{Number of fetal deaths in a time period (1 year)}}{\text{Total number of fetal deaths + live births in the same period}} \times 1,000$$

Fetal Death Ratio (FDR)

To assist in study and to clarify issues in statistics surrounding the deaths of the unborn fetus, the fetal death ratio is also used. The **fetal death ratio** (FDR) is used as a measure of risk in the last stages of gestation. This ratio measures the fetal loss in relationship to and in comparison with the number of live births. The numerator has the actual numbers of fetal deaths in a certain time period (1 year). The denominator includes the numbers of live births in the same time period (1 year) and is often expressed per 1,000 population, (actually this is not a true a rate as it includes a time element and uses per 1,000 population to express the results). Two approaches/formulas are reported in use.[3,4,14,15]

$$\text{Fetal Death Ratio (1)} = \frac{\text{Number of fetal deaths after 28 weeks or more gestation}}{\text{Total number of live births in the same period (1 year)}}$$

$$\text{Fetal Death Ratio (2)} = \frac{\text{Number of fetal deaths in a certain period (1 year)}}{\text{Total number of live births in the same period (1 year)}}$$

ABORTION

The deliberate termination of a pregnancy before the fetus is capable of living outside the womb is an abortion. Abortion has been legal (with restrictions and limitations in various places and states) in the United States for the most part, since the Supreme Court decision of *Roe v. Wade* in 1973. The Alan Gutmacher Institute and the Centers for Disease Control and Prevention maintain statistics on abortion. According to the Centers for Disease Control and Prevention, the typical woman seeking an abortion is white, unmarried, had no live-born children, and is 24 years of age or younger. The rate of abortion among women in the United States is greater than other industrialized countries. About half of the abortions in 1990 were performed during the first 8 weeks of gestation; with 88% performed in the first 12 weeks. 97% of all abortions were performed with curettage. From 1972 to 1988, between 3.9 to 8.2 percent of abortions were done between 16 and 20 weeks of gestation and between 0.9 to 1.3 percent had abortions past 21 weeks of gestation. A total of 1,371,285 abortions were performed in 1988 or 352 per 1,000 live births, compared to 1,297,606 in 1980 and 359 per 1,000 live births.

Abortion Rate

The **abortion rate** for 1985 was 28 per 1,000 women aged 15–44. Among those who have had a first abortion it is estimated that 76 out of 100 with previous abortions will have another.

$$\text{Abortion rate} = \frac{\text{Number of abortions done per year}}{\text{Total number of women age 15–44 per same year}} \times 1,000$$

MATERNAL MORTALITY RATES

Maternal mortality is one of the major health status indicators of a population. It is common to compare the health status of the United States with other countries using maternal mortality and infant mortality. (See Table 4.4 comparing the United States to other countries on maternal mortality.)

Maternal mortality has been lowest for highly homogeneous, industrialized, and advanced countries. Underdeveloped countries have higher rates where poverty is high and public health measures are lacking. In the United States, maternal mortality is higher for blacks and Hispanics than whites and Asians. Age also has an effect on maternal mortality. Teen mothers and older mothers have higher maternal death rates than mothers in the prime childbearing years of 20 to 35 years. Hospitals and physicians separate the types of maternal deaths into two groups: (1) *direct* obstetric caused deaths, which are related to obstetric and health care provider causes, and (2) *indirect*, which is related to preexisting conditions and deaths are not due to the acts of health care providers.

Maternal mortality is associated with complications of pregnancy and the birth process. Maternal deaths reflect how well medical management of the birth process is handled. It also reflects hemorrhage, toxemia, and infection. Sanitation and public health measures as well as advanced medical treatments, obstetrical care and procedures have helped to reduce maternal mortality rates. Prenatal care, continuity in pregnancy care, as well as laboratory analysis of blood types, medical examinations to eliminate disease, nutrition counseling, smoking and drug and alcohol abuse prevention all contribute to reducing maternal deaths. Education level, poverty level, and socio-economic status are also factors that contribute to maternal mortality. Maternal mortality is viewed as a tremendous loss to society as it disrupts the lives of family members, destroys the structure of young families, cuts short the mother's life at an early age, and leaves young children without a mother. **Maternal mortality rates** are based on the risk of death in mothers as associated with the childbirth process, labor and delivery, obstetric care, pregnancy complications, and puerperium.

TABLE 4.4 Maternal mortality rates of the United States compared to selected other countries (per 100,000, 1982)

Country	*Rate*
Canada	1.9
Israel	3.1
Hong Kong	3.5
Sweden	4.3
Finland	4.5
Ireland	5.6
Netherlands	6.4
England and Wales	6.7
Kuwait	7.4
Belgium	7.5
United States	7.9

(Source: *Demographic Year Book,* Demographic Office of UNICEF, United Nations, 1985)

The World Health Organization defines maternal mortality as the death of a woman who is pregnant or dies within 42 days of ending her pregnancy, with no regard to length of pregnancy or site of the pregnancy. Death of a mother from any cause related to pregnancy and or its management constitutes maternal death. Accidental deaths or any incidents not related to pregnancy, childbirth, or puerperal causes are not included in maternal mortality cases.[3,4,14,15]

The numerator includes those deaths surrounding pregnancy or due to pregnancy or any death from puerperal causes. The number of women who are pregnant establishes the population at risk of dying from puerperal causes. The population group or geographical area such as a city, county, state, or country should be identified and the numbers used in both numerator and denominator should present the same geographical area or population group. Since live births are regularly registered in a standard form, they are easier to track than fetal deaths. As the total number of pregnant women is unknown, maternal mortality rate formulas use live births.

$$\text{Maternal mortality rate} = \frac{\text{Number of deaths from puerperal causes in a given year and population}}{\text{Total number of live births in the same period (1 year) and population}} \times 100,000$$

ADJUSTED DEATH RATES

A basic epidemiological concept is adjustment of rates, a statistical manipulation which is a summarizing process for rates. Many times, when rates are presented, the effects of differences in composition of variables between or among a group or population need to be controlled by a mathematical procedure, thus are in need of adjustment. Adjustment most often is applied to rates or measures of association. If two or more groups need to be compared, and if the groups differ in risk, or a third variable is present that confuses the presentation of the numbers, an adjustment of the data is needed. Adjustment of rates allows comparisons by controlling for differences in select variables. Adjustments most common are age, age-direct, and age-indirect.

Age Adjusted Death Rates or Standardized Mortality Ratio (SMR)

Age adjusted death rates provide a summary approach to the presentation of death data that eliminates some of the limitations of crude death rates. Of all the epidemiological or demographic data that can show differences in subelements or in subgroups of a population, age will show more differences as a means for comparison. An adjusted rate shows a single summary figure for a total group or population. Mathematical adjustments are completed in order to remove differences or the effect of the differences in the variables making up a population. Age is the most common of the variables to be adjusted, because age differences cause the most effect on death and morbidity rates. Adjustments are made for other variables as appropriate: race, religion, sex, marital status, etc.

Direct method   The first method to remove differences of the effect is the *direct method*. A total population or a subgroup of a population is used. Rates observed for subjects in a specific age category are used. Choices of categories and population groups are fairly arbitrarily selected. Age-specific rates of two or more groups are applied to a group with a known age arrangement, which is referred to as a **standard population**.

Once a standard population is determined, then age-specific death rates are used with the two groups and are then compared to the numbers in the same age groups of the selected standard population. This approach provides the numbers of deaths expected in a standard population if the age-specific rates had prevailed. This is basically a projection of what is expected in the population. Rates of certain traits or characteristics of two or more groups are averaged, based on the distribution of a standard population. Once completed, average rates can be compared.[3,4,7,11]

Indirect Method   Indirect adjustment is preferred to direct adjustment if there are small numbers in specific age groups. Sampling problems can occur with small groups. When indirect adjustment is used, the rates are more stable as they are based on a large standard population. Instead of applying the subgroup's age-specific rates to a standard population, age-specific rates of a standard population are used but in portions equal to that of the study group. From this process the number of cases expected in the subgroup are produced, but only if the age specific rates of the standard population are useful in the subgroup. Two populations are compared if in one group the age specific rates are not known or are variable due to small numbers. Large population rates are applied to the smaller population study group, extrapolating a more stable rate from the standard population to the study group.[3,4,7,11]

Standardized Mortality Ratio (SMR)

Another more common approach to age adjustment is the **standardized mortality ratio (SMR)**. The notion of standardization is based on the weighted averaging of characteristics of specific rates according to a standard distribution of age, race, religion, or other categories. A standardized rate is equal to what the crude rate would produce if the group for which the rate is adjusted had common traits and variables for which the adjustment is made. The number of expected deaths in a smaller study group is compared with the number actually observed. The number of deaths occurring in a given group are shown as a percentage of the number of deaths that were expected to occur in the same group if it had experienced that same risk or exposure within each age group having the same rate as that of a standard population. Stated another way, it is the ratio of numbers of deaths in a selected group compared to the number of expected deaths in the same group, if the group had the same rate structure as that of the standard population. This is a ratio of the numbers of deaths compared to the numbers expected if the specific rates in the standard population are applied to the group being studied.

$$\text{Standard mortality ratio} = \frac{\text{Observed deaths}}{\text{Expected deaths}} \times 100$$

Proportionate Mortality Ratio (PMR)

Some cohort study records are not complete and fall short in assisting the determination of years at risk and work history for cohort occupation epidemiology studies. In some cases only death certificates are available. Under such circumstances SMRs are reliable and **proportionate mortality ratios (PMRs)** are used. In occupational health studies PMR is used based on deaths from a specific cause in a cohort group. Expected deaths are also considered. The formula for PMR is presented below. The numerator is the same as the SMR. Expected deaths are included in PMR and calculated by using the proportion of total deaths due to a specific cause compared to total deaths of the study population. PMR is the numbers of deaths from a specific cause in a given period per 100 or 1,000 deaths that occur in the same time period. PMR must use the study (cohort) population not the general population and should not be compared to deaths from different distributions. (See cohort studies and cohort occupational studies in Chapter 11.)

$$PMR = \frac{\text{Observed deaths from a specific cause}}{\text{Expected deaths from the same cause}} \times 100$$

Specific Mortality Rates

One of the most common specific mortality rates is **age specific mortality rate.** When age across the life span is plotted and a line graph is used, based on death rates, it produces a J-shaped curve which is referred to as Gompertz's Law. (See Figure 4.11.) Demographic components such as age, sex, race, religion, occupation, etc., are used in specific death rates. Death rates are also used for select or specific groups or subgroups of the population. Specific death rates provide a broader view of a group or subgroup and give more meaningful data and information than a crude death rate. The most common specific death rates are age, race, and sex. Specific death rates are defined in the same manner as crude death rates, with some minor changes and with a specific focus. The numerator and denominator are limited to a specific group, such as an age group. For example, the formula for the death rate of youth under age 14 is presented below, showing the differences in the numerator and the denominator of a specific mortality rate. A second example of an age specific mortality rate formula for persons age 55+ is also presented. Using the formula examples below as models, the epidemiologist can easily determine and plug in the correct population for the numerator or the denominator. The epidemiologist must feel free to correctly identify the appropriate subgroup and plug into the formula the information needed to assess the death rates of a specific subgroup, whether it be for gender, race, religion, heart disease deaths, cancer deaths, etc.[4,7,10,14]

$$\text{Age specific mortality rate} = \frac{\text{Number of deaths of persons age 1–14 in a given year}}{\text{Total persons aged 1–14 in the same period (1 year)}} \times 100,000$$

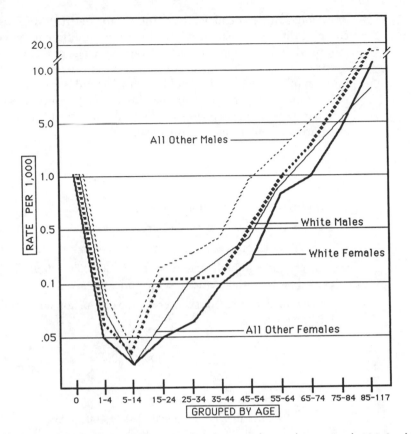

FIGURE 4.11 Specific mortality rates by age, gender and race, in the United States. Presented in semilogarithmic scale. (Source: Adapted from data from *Vital Statistics of the United States*, The National Center for Health Statistics, 1980)

$$\text{Age specific mortality rate} = \frac{\substack{\text{Number of deaths of} \\ \text{rural elderly age 55+ in a given year}}}{\substack{\text{Average population of rural} \\ \text{elderly in the same period}}} \times 100,000$$

Figure 4.11 is an example of Gompertz's law. Deaths are higher in the first year of life and drop off to the lowest level in the first years of childhood and gradually climb in the later decades of life. After about age 40 the death rate increases in a logarithmic fashion for the remainder of life. Benjamin Gompertz developed survival curves for populations in English villages in the mid-1800s.

Proportionate Mortality Rate (Ratio) (PMR)

The **proportionate mortality rate (PMR)** is stated as the number of deaths from a specific disease or cause in a certain time period per 100 or 1,000 or 10,000 deaths in the same year or period. Some epidemiologists caution as to how the PMR is used. If the PMR is used to compare differences between different groups or different time periods it has some limitations. If different populations have varying causes of disease which lead to death and if mortality rates are compared using PMR it can provide distorted findings. Being a proportion, to make it a rate it is multiplied by 100 and is presented as a percentage. The PMR is not a measure of risk or of probability of dying from a specific cause within a group. Comparing percentages is always risky, and is true for PMR. Rates instead of proportions are more accurate means of comparison.[4,7,10,14]

Example of PMR

- Two cities had a population of 1,000,000.
- Death rates from all causes in Metro City was 400 or 40 per 100,000.
- Death rates from all causes in Suburban City was 900 or 90 per 100,000.
- Cancer deaths in both cities were 4 per 100,000 or 40 deaths per city. Risk of a cancer caused death for both cities was the same.
- Percent of all deaths from cancer are the proportionate mortality rates (ratio). For each city the PMR was

$$\text{Metro City} \;=\; 40 \text{ over } 400 \times 100 \;=\; 10\% \qquad \frac{40}{400} \times 100 = 10\%$$

$$\text{Suburban City} \;=\; 40 \text{ over } 900 \times 100 \;=\; 8\% \qquad \frac{40}{900} \times 100 = 4\%$$

The difference due to percentages of the PMR fails to reflect the risk of a cancer death in these two cities, even though the actual numbers are the same. Deaths from all causes are different. PMR can be useful in determining within a given subgroup or a population the extent to which a specific cause of death contributes to the overall mortality. This proportion can assist health planners or epidemiologists to ascertain which causes of death and related diseases lead to death and which are in need of further investigation.

The numerator of PMR includes death for a certain disease or for a specific cause of death. The denominator includes death from all causes multiplied by 1,000, 10,000 or 100,000.[4,7,10,14]

$$\text{Proportional mortality rate} \;=\; \frac{\begin{array}{c}\text{Number of deaths}\\ \text{from a specific cause/disease}\end{array}}{\text{Total deaths in the same population}} \times 1,000$$

Cause Specific Mortality Rate

Cause specific mortality rate is a death rate that targets death by specific cause or source. Mortality rates for any specific disease such as heart disease, can be presented for a specific cause of death, any subgroup, or for any age, race, gender, religion, or for an entire

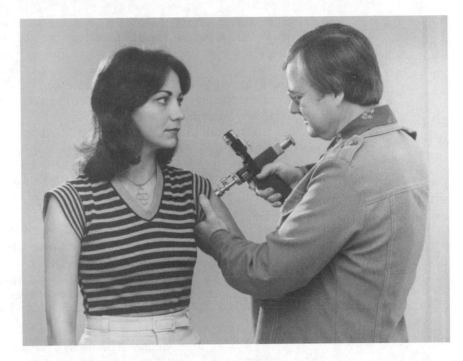

FIGURE 4.12 Mortality rates have been greatly reduced by mass immunizations against life-threatening diseases, all made available through the cooperative efforts of biomedical research, medicine, public health, and epidemiology. (Picture courtesy of Centers for Disease Control and Prevention, Atlanta, Georgia)

population. The numerator of the cause specific death rate includes deaths for a certain disease for the subgroup for a certain time period (see Figure 4.12). The denominator is for the total subgroup population for the same time period and is usually expressed in hundreds, such as 100, 1,000, 10,000, or 100,000. Age adjusted rates are also used in cause specific mortality rates. Age patterns of deaths for a disease such as cancer show distinct changes from one age group to the next.

$$\text{Cause specific mortality rate} = \frac{\substack{\text{Number of deaths by a certain} \\ \text{disease for a select subgroup in a given year}}}{\substack{\text{Total mortality cause population (or sub-} \\ \text{group) in the same period (1 year)} \\ \text{(population at risk)}}} \times 100{,}000$$

Case Fatality Rate (Ratio)

Case fatality rate is used to link mortality to morbidity. In the modern era of environmental and occupationally caused diseases, this ratio may have wider application than for infectious diseases. Chemicals, injury, or disasters can cause acute deaths and need to be measured.

Case fatality rate is the rate or the proportion of persons dying from a certain disease or occurrence within the same time period. The time period may be related to an epidemic or a geographical outbreak or could cover extended periods of time with an endemic disease or occurrence. One function of the case fatality rate is to measure various aspects or properties of a disease such as its pathogenicity, severity, or virulence.

In the past the case fatality rate was used more for acute infectious diseases. However, it can also be used in poisoning or chemical exposures or other short-term, non-disease caused deaths. Case fatality rate has had limited use in chronic diseases as time of onset may be hard to determine and date of diagnosis to death are longer in duration. The number of deaths that occur in a current time period may have little relationship to the number of new cases that occur. Prevention and control measures may already be in place for new cases, but long-term and past exposed cases may still die. Whenever using the case fatality rate, it is good to make a statement regarding the time element. If case fatality rate is used for chemical or hazardous waste, or occupational health exposure, the time dimension has some limitations and may vary. Occupational or chemical exposures may have some acute deaths while also having many chronic disease occurrences causing death years later. In case fatality rates, the numerator includes the total number of deaths by a specific disease within a set time period. The denominator includes the total number of cases that occurred in the same time period.[4,6,7,10,14,16]

$$\text{Case fatality rate (1)} = \frac{\text{Number of deaths by a certain disease in a given time period}}{\text{Number of diagnosed cases in the same period}} \times 100$$

$$\text{Case fatality rate (2)} = \frac{\text{Number of deaths by a certain disease or cause in a specified time period}}{\text{Number of cases which occurred in the same period}} \times 100$$

MORTALITY CROSSOVER

Mortality crossover is based on the concept that life expectancy for certain races may change as age progresses. Certain races may change from having higher death rates at an early age to lower death rates later in life or vice versa. It is thought by some that blacks do not live as long as whites. Such ideas imply a mortality disadvantage for blacks.

It is falsely assumed that disadvantages in youth carry over in the later years of life while compounding the problems. Life expectancy for black males is 69 years and for white males is 72 years. However, when approaching 75 years of age, blacks "cross over" moving from death rates that are higher than whites to death rates that are lower than whites. At age 75 blacks have a longer life expectancy than whites. Mortality crossover is not a phenomenon of bad data but a fact observed in many populations. One observation seeming to hold true, at least to an extent, is the fact that the longer one lives the longer they can hope to live, at least up to a point.[8]

MORTALITY TIME TRENDS

As time passes the trends of some diseases change. This is most prominently seen in chronic diseases, such as cancer and heart disease. Why and to what extent changes occur is sometimes difficult to determine. Diagnostic improvement, changes in public health and sanitation knowledge, behavioral patterns, cultural changes, medical care knowledge and technique, and advances in technology all contribute to the changes in mortality trends over time, or **mortality time trends**. Another concern is that mortality trends can be affected by a decrease or increase in another disease or another population. The decrease in lung cancer in males has been off-set by the increase of lung cancer in females.

YEARS OF POTENTIAL LIFE LOST (YPLL)

Years of potential life lost (YPLL) is a concept of public health related to the value of human life and the economic implications of the loss of individuals in a society. The improvements in death rates can cause an increase in an available work force which in turn benefits society by increased productivity. A count of the number of deaths occurring early in life show that such occurrences remove more years of life one could possibly live than does a death occurring later in life. A 20-year-old who dies in an automobile accident due to drinking and driving, could theoretically have lived to average life expectancy of 72 years of age, thus 52 years of productive life are lost. This life that was lost is a waste to society as it could have been prevented. When 2,000 deaths like this result, 104,000 potential years of life are lost. Some sources calculate years of potential life lost based on the retirement age of 65, as this concept can have a strictly economic point of view. However, the social and humane aspects need to be considered, thus the example uses average life expectancy rather than age of retirement. Questions such as "What is life worth?" are often raised. The loss to society in the cost of training, manpower, and tax dollars not paid are often considered. Prevention and the decrease of the loss of unnecessary death is a major concern of public health. The value of human life is an underlying goal of public health, as are economic factors, as both issues have long-reaching societal implications.[17]

Rate for Years of Potential Life Lost (YPLL)

The YPLL rate represents years of potential life lost per 1,000 population for the healthy productive work years of life, usually below the age of retirement, with age 65 often used. As retirement age is pushed to 70 in many industries, this age may be used as the end year. The average life expectancy also has been used for YPLL rates, depending on the issue being addressed. The YPLL rate is used to compare premature deaths in different populations. YPLL for an individual is found by subtracting the age at death from an end point such as age 65. Exclude all persons over age 65 from consideration and sum all YPLLs.

$$\text{YPLL rate} = \frac{\text{Years of potential life lost}}{\text{Population under age 65}} \times 1,000$$

A concept related to years of potential life lost is that of Quality-Adjusted Life Years (QALY), which is a measure of well-being that measures mental, physical, and social functioning. By multiplying the measure of well-being by the number years of life remaining at each age interval, an estimate of the years of healthy life for a population can be determined. The calculation of years of healthy life uses life tables and the average number of years of life remaining at the beginning of each age interval. Also needed are age specific estimates of the well-being of a population, compared to the population of the life table. See Chapter 12 for additional information on Quality-Adjusted Life Years.[18]

EXERCISES

Key Terms

Define and explain the following terms.

abortion rate	neonatal mortality rate
adjusted rate	odds ratio
age specific mortality rate	perinatal mortality rate
annual death rate	postneonatal mortality rate
case fatality rate (ratio)	proportion
cause specific mortality rate	proportionate mortality rate (PMR)
crude death rate	proportionate mortality ratio (PMR)
fetal death rate (FDR)	rate
fetal death ratio	rate ratio
infant mortality	ratio
infant mortality rate	specific rate (age)
maternal mortality rate	standardized mortality ratio (SMR)
mortality	standard population
mortality crossover	true rate
mortality time trends	years of potential life lost (YPLL)

Study Questions

4.1   **Crude Death Rate.** In 1990 Idaho had a crude death rate of 13.7 per 1,000 and Alaska had a crude death rate of 21.9 per 1,000. Idaho had a total population of 1,006,749. Alaska had 550,043.

In the United States, the crude death rate is 8 per 1,000 and in Malaysia the crude death rate is 5 per 1,000.

Crude birth rate for Malaysia = 25 per 1,000.
Crude birth rate for the U.S. = 12 per 1,000.
Life expectancy for Malaysia = 70 years.
Life expectancy for the U.S. = 76 years

a.   Can the difference in crude death rates of Idaho as compared to Alaska be explained by the fact that Alaska has a larger land mass? Why? Because Idaho has a larger population? Why?

b. Can a lower crude death rate in Malaysia (as compared with the U.S.) be explained by the fact that the U.S. has a larger population and Malaysia has a smaller population? What factors could explain differences in life expectancy? Birth rate differences?

4.2   Table 4.5 gives the mortality statistics for a fictitious county in a rural state for the period of July 1st to June 30th (1 year).

   After reviewing the health status indicators and mortality data, calculate the following mortality rates.

1. Crude death rate.
2. Maternal mortality rate.
3. Infant mortality rate.
4. Neonatal mortality rate.
5. Perinatal mortality rate.
6. Age specific mortality rate for persons age 55 years or older.
7. Cause-specific mortality rates for those who died from heart disease.
8. Cause-specific mortality rates for those who died from stroke.

4.3   Two cities had a population of 3,000,000.

   Death rates from all causes in Metro City was 500 or 50 per 100,000.

   Death rates from all causes in Suburban City was 800 or 80 per 100,000.

   Cancer deaths in both cities were 4 per 100,000 or 40 deaths per city. Risk of cancer caused death for both cities were the same.

   Calculate the proportionate cancer mortality rates for each city.

TABLE 4.5   Mortality statistics, July 1–June 30

Total one-year population	160,000
Population of 55 years of age and older	44,000
Number of live births	3,300
Number of fetal deaths	66
Number of maternal deaths	5
Total deaths	1,444
Number of infant deaths	88
Number of deaths under 28 days old	4
Number of deaths between 20 weeks gestation to 28 days old	8
Number of deaths of persons 55 and older	848
Number one cause of death in the county is heart disease—deaths from heart disease	133
Number two cause of death in the county was from cancer—deaths from cancer	66
Number three cause of death in the county was from cerebral vascular accident (stroke)	56
Number four cause of death in the county was accidents.	45
Number of deaths from cancer age 55 years and older	44
Number of persons diagnosed with heart disease	5,600
Number of deaths from other causes	504
Number of persons diagnosed with high blood pressure, artheriosclerosis, and artherosclerosis (precursors for a stroke)	1,200

4.4   Using the Standard Death Certificate fill it in with the following information: Mr. Captain J. C. Hook, was born on October, 31st 1790, in Seaside City, Ocean County, Never-Never Land, to Mr. and Mrs. Pegleg Hook. His mother, Lisa, died in childbirth. His first name was John. Captain Hook listed his official occupation as earning his living as a ship's captain. He died in Seaside City, in Ocean View Regional Medical Center and the cause of death was stated as multiple puncture wounds due to crocodile bites, but the autopsy report listed the actual cause of death as drowning. A distinguishing clinical identifying mark on Mr. Hook was that his left hand was amputated just above the wrist. John Hook had only completed 3rd grade and spent 46 years of his life in Never-Never Land and was captain of a ship for 25 years. Mr. Hook was never married, but had one survivor, a 22-year-old daughter, named Ruby, who lives in Havana, Cuba. The attending physician's name was Sharp E. Blade, D.O. The coroner who did the autopsy was Dr. Cutt M. Upp. Captain Hook served in Her Majesty's Navy from 1808 to 1812. The funeral director who signed the death certificate was Barry M. Deep. He was buried on Friday, Dec. 13th, 1836, 5 days after his death. Witnesses stated that the crocodile attack occurred at noon during lunch, in a rowboat near the ship.

4.5   List and explain the 7 different steps required to file a death certificate with the Vital Statistics Registration System in the United States.

4.6   Infant mortality and maternal mortality are two of the most commonly used health status indicators. What is the significance of infant mortality to public health and epidemiology? What is the significance of maternal mortality to public health and epidemiology?

4.7   Compare and contrast the differences between neonatal, postneonatal, and perinatal mortality and how they are determined and used as rates.

REFERENCES

1. Hartley, S.F. 1982. *Comparing Populations*. Belmont, CA: Wadsworth.
2. *The McAlvany Intelligence Advisor*, Phoenix, AZ, Jan. 1992, p. 12.
3. McMahon, B. 1970. *Epidemiology: Principles and Methods*. Boston: Little, Brown and Company.
4. Mausner, J., and Bahn, A. 1983. *Epidemiology, An Introductory Text*, 2nd edition. Philadelphia: Saunders.
5. Slome, C., Brogan, D., Eyres, S., and Lednar, W. 1982. *Basic Epidemiological Methods and Biostatistics: A Workbook*. Monterey, CA: Wadsworth.
6. Rothman, K.J. 1986. *Modern Epidemiology*. Boston: Little, Brown and Company.
7. Friedman, G.D. 1981. *Primer of Epidemiology*. New York: McGraw-Hill.
8. Weeks, J.R. 1981. *Population*, 2nd edition. Belmont, CA: Wadsworth.
9. *International Classification of Diseases, 9th edition, Clinical Modification* (ICD-9-CM, 2nd edition), U.S. Department of Health and Human Services, U.S. Public Health Service, Health Care Financing Administration: Washington, D.C. 1980.
10. Lilienfeld, A.M. and Lilienfeld, D.E. 1980. *Foundations of Epidemiology*. New York: Oxford University Press.
11. Hartley, S.F. 1982. *Community Populations*. Belmont, CA: Wadsworth.
12. Surgeon General's Report. 1988. *Nutrition and Health*. U.S. Department of Health and Human Services, Public Health Service.

13. Becerra, J.E., Hogue, C.J.R., Atrash, H.K., and Perez, N. 1991. "Infant Mortality Among Hispanics: A Portrait of Heterogeneity," *Journal of The American Medical Association*, Jan. 9, Vol. 265, No. 2, pp. 217–221.

14. Fox, J.P., Hall, C.E., and Elveback, L.R. 1970. *Epidemiology: Man and Disease*. New York: Macmillan.

15. Green, L., and Anderson, C.L. 1986. *Community Health*, 5th edition. St. Louis: Times Mirror/Mosby.

16. Selvin, S. 1991. *Statistical Analysis of Epidemiologic Data*. New York: Oxford University Press.

17. Pickett, G., and Hanlon, J.J. 1990. *Public Health: Administration and Practice*. St. Louis: Times Mirror/Mosby.

18. Public Health Services. 1990. *Healthy People 2000: National Health Promotion and Disease Prevention Objectives*. U.S. Department of Health and Human Services, Washington, D.C. Boston: Jones and Bartlett Publishing Inc.

5

Epidemiological Measures of Health Status: Morbidity— Rates and Ratios

CHAPTER OBJECTIVES

This chapter on morbidity rates and ratios

- presents the rates and ratios used in incidence, prevalence, and related morbidity concepts;
- defines terminology related to morbidity;
- presents incidence, incidence rates and formulas, and related information;
- presents prevalence, prevalence rates and formulas, and related information;
- reviews sources of morbidity information and data;
- presents exercises and questions that assist in the review of chapter concepts and material.

INTRODUCTION

Any disturbance in the function or structure of one's body is considered a disease. Disease, illness, injury, disorders, and sickness are all categorized under the single term *morbidity*. **Morbidity** is the extent of illness, injury, or disability in a defined population. Morbidity is also any deviation from a state of health and well-being, or the presence of a morbid condition. Morbidity is usually expressed in general or specific rates of incidence of prevalence. Morbidity also refers to sickness rates; the number of ill persons compared to a certain population, which is often a well or at-risk group.[1,2]

Mortality and mortality rates as presented in Chapter 4 are used as health status indicators. Sickness or morbidity rates are also used as health status indicators.

In 1959, the World Health Organization set forth three measures of morbidity in a report of the Expert Committee on Health Statistics. The first measure was numbers of persons who were ill, the second was the period or spells of illness experienced, and the third was the duration (time = hours, days, weeks, months) of the illness. In epidemiology the main measures of morbidity are incidence and prevalence rates and the various submeasures of each. Each occurrence of disease, condition, disorder, or illness can be measured by incidence and prevalence rates.

INCIDENCE AND INCIDENCE RATES

Three key morbidity rates are used in epidemiology: (1) incidence, (2) prevalence, and (3) attack rates. Subcategories or specific rates which help with clarity or provide further information about the three key rates are used to describe certain or specific outbreak situations. Incidence is used as a measure of the rate at which new cases of disease, disorders, or injury occur in a population. The term *incidence* is sometimes used interchangeably with **incidence rates.**[2,3]

When it comes to understanding the basics of epidemiology methods, the student must learn to study closely each word and phrase of the definitions of all of the terms and rates. Each word of a definition in epidemiology is important. Each key word in a definition provides a clue as to what to look for and how to use a rate formula. The definition of *incidence* is a prime example. **Incidence** is the number of *new cases* of a disease which came into existence within a *certain period of time* per *specified unit of population*. Stated differently, it is the number of *new* cases of a disease occurring in a *specific population* in a *specified time period*.

In the actual application of incidence rates to outbreaks, it may be somewhat challenging to determine incidence, as the time of onset of an outbreak may be unclear. Time of diagnosis, date of reporting, time of appearance of symptoms, visit to physician, appearance at the emergency room or other time element factors that identify the beginning of an outbreak may have to be used. Incidence is not the onset of the outbreak but the frequency of new cases or events in the time period and in a specific population. On occasion, an individual may be the victim of more than one disease or occurrence within the same time period. Thus, more than one type of incidence rate can be used with the same set of data and each rate presents a different picture of the data.[3,4,5]

$$\text{Incidence rate} = \frac{\text{Number of new cases of a disease within a population in a given time period}}{\text{Number of persons exposed to risk of developing the disease in the same time period}} \times 1{,}000$$

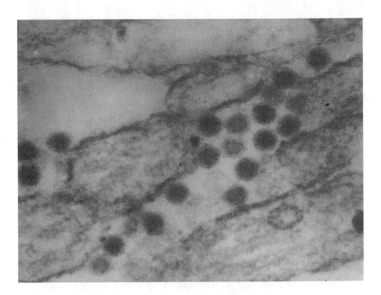

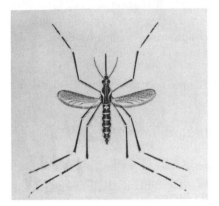

FIGURE 5.1   The top picture shows the virus that causes St. Louis encephalitis. The bottom picture is of the *Aedes* mosquito, which is the reservoir and vector responsible for the transmission of this disease. (Pictures courtesy of Centers for Disease Control and Prevention, Atlanta, Georgia)

Incidence Rates Denominator/Numerator Issues

The denominator as used in incidence rates, should accurately set forth the numbers at risk or under study in the group or population. As time passes the numbers of persons at risk in a population change. Some people come into risk at the end of a period established as the study period, while other people are removed from risk shortly after the defined period starts. To accommodate a transient population problem in larger community populations, the epidemiologist picks the population numbers/cases at a midpoint in the time period to represent the average population at risk. For example, if the incidence study was a one-year study based on the regular calendar year, the population at risk would be determined as it existed on July 1st.[3,4,5,6,7]

Since incidence rate is used to study the new cases of a disease, only those individuals at risk of developing the disease, in other words the *population at risk*, should be included in the denominator. The denominator should exclude individuals with the disease, those who have already had the disease (if they are no longer susceptible), or those not susceptible due to immunizations. However, in larger populations it is best not to try to correct the data in the denominator by excluding those not at risk. When census data are used for the denominator, the diseased cases data should not be removed. For example, if measles cases are being calculated using the census data of a county for the denominator, the cases of those who have had measles are not removed.[3,4,5,6,7]

Numerator in Incidence

The role of the numerator in incidence is to provide specific information about the occurrences of a disease. If the number of cases or persons can vary, the numerator should clearly reflect the differences. The time period length used to calculate incidence should be of enough length to assure stability of the numerator. The numerator is the number of new cases or incidences starting within a time period. In smaller populations, groups such as public schools, industrial plants, universities, and hospitals, the numerator of the incidence rate should be the exact number of new cases or instances of illness commencing or persons falling ill within a time period for a specific group, while the denominator of incidence rates should include only those who are disease free at the beginning of the time period.[3,4,5,6,7]

Person-Time Denominators/Person-Years

In prospective studies, those investigations that track cases forward in time, **person-years** are used in denominators in the calculation of incidence rates. (Prospective studies are presented in Chapter 8.) Person-years are used when many factors come together such as age, sex, race, in varying time periods and when time variation is caused by individuals entering and leaving studies at different times and at different ages, all making the calculation very difficult. In person-years, personal traits and time are used as denominator information in short-term incidence rates. The sum of each unit of time in the study that the individuals of the study group were exposed to are used. Only the total period of time or cumulative years that the person was active in the study are used in the denominator. If a person was in the study for 4 years he contributed 4 person-years. Person-years make it possible to show in one number the period of time that is useful for calculation when a number of persons are exposed to the same risk at various time periods. When sample size is large, risk is low and the time period is long, person-years work best. One problem is that the exposure to risk is unclear when time under study is not constant and activities vary for individuals over the time period. Another problem is that as time passes, age increases, providing a major potential for the data to change. For example: toward the end of a longitudinal person-years study, as the subject ages, the probability of an increase in pathology also increases.

For the person-time to be of use and for it to have validity, three conditions must exist. First the probability of disease or risk must be constant in the entire study period. Second, it is assumed that those who drop out will have the same level of pathology as those who remain and complete the study. Lastly, for some subjects, the pathological condition may be so severe and advance so rapidly, that select persons are observed for less than the full time period. Full numerical count is used in the numerator but less than a full measure of time has to be used in the denominator and can distort the findings.[3,4,5,6]

The following list presents a compiled comparison of rates and proportions and time related differences, summarizing morbidity incidence related issues.[3,4,5,6,7]

When comparing disease rates and proportions, it is essential to distinguish between actual differences and what appears to be the basis of differences or apparent differences. When assessing differences the following guidelines are suggested:

Differences in Disease Rates and Proportions That Occur in Study Groups or Exposed Populations. What are the

1. differences in classification of the diseases, conditions, disorders, disabilities or deaths between the study groups?
2. differences in levels of the diseases, conditions, disorders, disabilities or deaths between the study groups, which result from varying levels of exposure across the population?
3. differences in distributions of age in or between study groups?
4. differences in the quality of the measures used in the denominator between the study groups? (Denominator issues and differences)
5. differences in diagnosis between study groups that are used in the numerator? (Numerator issues and differences)

Time Related Differences. What are the

1. differences in the classification of diseases, conditions, disorders, disabilities or deaths over time?
2. differences in the levels of diseases, conditions, disorders, disabilities or deaths over time, that result from varying levels of exposure across the population?
3. differences in distributions of age over time or in different time periods?
4. differences in the quality of the measures used in the denominator over time? (Denominator issues and differences)
5. differences in the quality of diagnoses or the influence of diagnosis trends over time that are used in the numerator? (Numerator issues and differences)

APPROACHES TO INCIDENCE RATES

Incidence rates may be used for short-term, communicable acute diseases (such as cholera or measles) or may be used to measure chronic or long-term conditions (such as cancer or diabetes mellitus). Two approaches to incidence rates are used. **Cumulative incidence rate** is one approach in which the number of persons at risk is used as the denominator. The cumulative incidence rate is useful in longitudinal studies. Rates may change over time and the longer the time period used, the more likely it is that one could mistakenly average different rates. Secular variations in the rates become hard to see or are not clear and the longer the time period, the less clear the changes or differences become. The relationship of incidence to time is not always linear as rates may increase over time and as the cohort gets older things change. Thus, the cumulative incidence is used to study a group of persons followed over the same time period.

The other approach is the **force of morbidity**. In force of morbidity, the population and time element are used in the denominator, whereas the numerator includes the number of new cases of the disease or disorder. This is the number of new cases of a disease which occurs per unit of population and at a point in unit time. It is used to predict the risk that a well person has of getting ill over a certain period of time. Force of morbidity is also referred to as *incidence density*. (See also rate-ratio.) A per-person incidence rate is also occasionally used. **Per-person incidence** rate is expressed in terms of an individual person at risk rather than in terms of a unit of population at risk, such as per 1,000 population, making the measure a proportion.[4,5,6.7]

When dealing with chronic diseases, and if an incidence rate is calculated for one year, the number of previous cases may exceed the number of persons at risk, thus the annual incidence rate is different than the prevalence rate, which is usually lower.[4,5,6]

SOME FUNDAMENTAL CONCEPTS OF INCIDENCE

To determine the incidence of an outbreak, a population or group must be studied prospectively (backward in time) in order to ascertain the extent and the rate at which new cases of a disease occur. The process of new cases occurring as followed over time should produce an epidemic curve (see Figure 5.9 and Figures I.2 and I.3 in Case Study I). Basic to incidence, when an outbreak is suspected, is to confirm a diagnosis of the disease or establish the source of the occurrence of the event if it is non-pathogen in origin. Additionally, sufficient information based on solid biomedical sciences, must be available from which to evaluate the health status of the persons within the at-risk population group. From this information, the epidemiologist should be able to classify the individuals as either infected (diseased) or not infected (not diseased). Information may come from self report, physician, health maintenance organizations, clinic or hospital medical records. Clinical examinations or clinical screenings may be needed to further ascertain or verify the outbreak. When gathering data about an outbreak on more than one population, the information must be comparable between the different populations; the same amounts and types of data must be used in comparing groups or populations. Inconsistent or unverifiable data may have to be disregarded or thrown out.

Another term occasionally seen in the epidemiology literature is *incidence study*, which is similar to a cohort study and is presented under that topic heading elsewhere (see cohort study).[3,4,5,6,7]

"Time" in Incidence

Incidence meets the formal definition of a rate and is expressed as a change per unit of time. Time or date of onset or discovery of an outbreak is essential in the study of and determination of incidence. The first step is to determine a diagnosis or its equivalent; however, without a time of onset, incidence is difficult to determine. Time of onset of some acute diseases, heart attacks or other acute occurrences can be set down to the hour. Other diseases or occurrences may be much more difficult to set an exact time of onset, for example, in the chronic disease emphysema. In circumstances in which time of onset is difficult to determine, the most objective, clear, and earliest verifiable event that can be determined must be used as the time of onset. In many diseases, acute or chronic, the first date of a diagnosis may be the time of onset to be used. In diseases that have a silent development such as cancer or stroke, the earliest verifiable event, diagnosis of cancer or the cerebrovascular accident event in stroke will be the time of onset used in studying and determining incidence of stroke. In slow or silent developing diseases or disorders, such as psychiatric disorders, the time of onset may have to be defined by the epidemiologist. The setting forth in definition form, parameters such as a definition of time of onset by the epidemiologist, standardizes and clarifies issues in a specific study that might cause questions later on. For example, in substance abuse such as cocaine abuse, the occurrence of using would be the date of onset.

In summary the incidence rate is an accurate estimate of the risk or probability of getting a disease within a certain time period and the denominator is to include only the "at risk" population. A population must be followed for a period of time in order to determine the ongoing level of disease within the population, and the rate of appearances of new cases in order to be able to make statements about the probability of risk to the members of the population.[3,4,5,6,7]

Time Periods in Incidence

Incidence rates must include a time period and have specific limitations in the time elements. The time element must have a beginning date and end date, for example, one year. Any length of time can be used for the time period in calculating incidence but should be of enough length to assure stability of the numerator. When faced with the chore of calculating incidence for diseases having low frequency of occurrence, cases may have to be accumulated over a long period of time. The denominator should be drawn from a standardized or commonly used time period.

When the time period of the disease under study spans an epidemic of very short duration, it is called an *attack rate*. Attack rates are used in analyzing epidemics in which smaller select populations are exposed to some disease or injury-causing event, such as food poisoning, chemical exposures or environmentally related occurrences. (See Incidence and Attack Rates in this chapter.)

Some Principles of Incidence Rate Use

- An incidence rate can be used to estimate the probability of, or risk of developing a disease during a specific time period.
- As the incidence rate goes up the risk possibility or the probability of getting the disease goes up.
- Time—If the incidence rate is consistently higher during a specified time of year (such as in winter), the risk of developing that disease goes up at that time; example: influenza is highest in the winter.

CASE FILE

Rubella (Incidence of Disease)

Rubella among the Amish

From January 1 through April 19, 1991 (time period), at least nine outbreaks of Rubella, involving more than 400 cases (number of new cases), were reported in Amish communities (given population), in the United States in New York, Pennsylvania, Tennessee, and Ohio. In general, the cases occurred among unvaccinated children and young adults. Because interstate and intrastate travel to other Amish communities is common among the Amish population, state and local health departments and clinicians were alerted to the risk of local outbreaks among the Amish. Many Rubella infections cause only mild illness; therefore, outbreaks may remain unreported, unless active surveillance for cases is conducted. Vaccination coverage among the Amish is low, yet some health departments report that with vigorous effort, many Amish will accept vaccination.

(Source: Adapted from Morbidity and Mortality Weekly Report, *Centers for Disease Control and Prevention, April 26, 1991, p. 264)*

- Place—If the incidence rate is consistently higher among people who live in a certain place, the risk goes up for developing that disease if one lives in the area; example: valley fever (coccidioidomycosis) is contracted while living in the deserts of the Southwest.
- Person—If incidence rates are consistently higher among individuals with a specific lifestyle factor the risk goes up among that group; example: lung cancer increases among cigarette smokers.
- Higher incidence implies many new cases, thus risk increases.
- When incidence of disease is known to be high, the existence of or potential for an epidemic becomes known and predictable.

Incidence is a bit like a motion picture of the development of a disease in a population. It provides a picture of the measure of the movement of disease through a population; the rate at which people without a disease develop the disease during a specific period of time. In comparison, prevalence is more of a snapshot of the level of disease in a population at a given point in time.

RISK IN MORBIDITY

Risk is the probability that a disease, injury, condition, death, or related occurrence which may have an unfavorable outcome and that will affect health status of a population in a negative fashion will happen.

Population at Risk

The population at risk, is the population group used in the denominator and must be limited to those individuals capable of being exposed to or contracting a disease, condition, injury, disability, or having died. The first concern of the epidemiologist is the population at risk. Determining this population can be quite straightforward. However, simple complexities of the population group should not be overlooked nor any aspect viewed lightly as all facets related to disease occurrence may be of importance to the outbreak investigation.

One problem in determining the population at risk is that the population within the study is often calculated with a yearly time frame. Yet people get disease prior to the time period, infected within the time frame but not diagnosed, and people migrate. Persons who move in or out and spend only part of the year in the population study group throw the figures off. One solution to this problem is to estimate the population at midyear or at a midpoint in the study time period.[3,7]

The epidemiologist has to account for all differences in the characteristics of the study groups. The biases found in sampling and selection of individuals exposed to suspected causes and the various ways of measuring different levels of exposure and risk also need to be accounted for.[3]

Risk Ratio

A major risk concern is that of risk ratio. **Risk ratio** is the ratio of two separate risks. Risk ratio is also referred to as the *cumulative incidence ratio* and is closely associated to rate ratio. Risk ratio is founded on a comparison of probabilities of developing a disease. Risk ratio is useful when the time period of a disease has a set or established duration.[6] For example, cholera, with an established incubation period has an established duration. In diseases with long or variable incubation periods, risk ratio would require long periods of observation. Over short time periods the risk ratio or the ratio of the proportion of each group will be close to 2.0, but as the time period lengthens, all group members will be exposed. Rate ratio may remain constant at 2.0 over the longer observation period but the risk ratio would approach 1.0 as individual risks increase.[6]

$$\text{Risk ratio} = \frac{\text{Probability of a disease exposure}}{\text{Probability of a disease with no exposure}}$$

or

$$\frac{\text{Risk for group of primary study interest}}{\text{Risk for comparison group}}$$

RELATIVE RISK

Epidemiology is interested in the association between the characteristics of group or populations and certain diseases. Relative risk is the traditional measure used to study associations between group characteristics and diseases. **Relative risk** is the ratio of the rate of incidence of the disease among those exposed to a disease as compared to the rate of those not exposed to the disease. The ratio of the probability of getting a disease or a death occurring among those exposed to a disease compared to the risk of those unexposed to the disease is what relative risk deals with. Odds ratio and forces of morbidity and cumulative incidence ratio are terms that seem to be interchanged with relative risk, however, relative risk has a specific formula. The cumulative incidence ratio is the cumulative incidence rate of those exposed to a disease compared to the unexposed cumulative incidence rate.[3,4,5]

In relative risk two assumptions are used. *Assumption 1*: The frequency of the disease or occurrence in a population must be small. *Assumption 2*: The cases of the disease or occurrence should be representative of the cases in the population and study controls are representative of noncases. The formula of relative risk is presented below.[3,4,5,14]

$$\text{Relative risk} = \frac{\text{Incidence rate of disease of exposed within a group}}{\text{Incidence rate of disease of nonexposed within a group}}$$

Relative risk has been used in more complex arrangements as well, such as multiple categories. Epidemiological findings are strengthened if the association between exposure to a disease and certain other characteristics are based on a gradient relationship. Relative risks are computed for each exposure to, or dose of, the risk factor. Data are entered into a table so subjects of the study and controls of the study can be easily compared. Various levels of exposure or dose of risk are presented and then the relative risk for each is calculated.

Relative risk is a measure of association. A 2×2 four-celled grid can be most useful in determining relative risk. The grid allows for analysis of the diseased group and the non-diseased group, and either can be used as a comparison group for the other. (See pages 141 and 161–162.)

Relative risk can be confusing but need not be. Relative risk is used simply to determine chance. It answers the questions, What is the chance that a part of a group of exposed people will or will not get a disease? What is the chance that a part of a group of people will get sick if they are not exposed to a pathogen or some other source of disease? Relative risk is the risk for those *with* the risk factor relative to (ratio to) those *without* the risk factor; it compares the ratios for the two risks. Relative risk uses retrospective information to project future risk. Cases must represent and include the risk in all cases within the outbreaks or study, and controls represent all noncases. The epidemiologist compares existing cases with noncases.

Relative risk, stated in the form of a ratio, is also referred to as risk ratio because it is the ratio of the risk of getting ill if you do not have the disease. Relative risk is used to determine the ratio of the chance of getting ill for those of a group at risk but not yet exposed to the agent (pathogen), compared to those who were exposed. Relative risk is the ratio of incidence of disease in the exposed group divided by the incidence of disease in the non-exposed group, and is found by dividing the incidence of one group (those exposed) by the incidence in the other group (those not exposed).

The ratio of risk is based on a ratio of 1.0. A risk ratio of 1.0 or greater indicates that the risk is increased for those people not exposed. The nonexposed group is the comparison group and is used in the numerator of the formula. Conversely, a risk ratio of less than 1.0 indicates a decreased risk for those people not exposed. The group of people at risk is used in the denominator of the formula.

Relative risk compares two groups or populations and can be applied to a variety of epidemiological situations. Males can be compared to females in a group that is at risk of getting a disease. It can be used to compare exposed people to those not exposed or to compare those infected to those not infected from the same group, such as comparing males to females when investigating smoking as a cause of lung cancer. For example, in a foodborne outbreak at a church picnic, of those persons attending the picnic, who is at risk of getting sick? Who ate the tainted potato salad and got ill, as compared with those who did not eat the potato salad and got ill? Who did not get ill even though they ate the suspected food?

Case Example   A fictional case example using relative risk may help in understanding how to determine the ratio of risk. *Escherichia coli 0157: H7* has been classified as a new emerging infection. This serotype of *E. coli* is different from previously identified *E. coli* strains and propagates slowly, which makes it difficult to detect. Outbreaks of this infection have caused death in a few cases and serious illness in vast numbers of cases exposed to it, especially children. *E. coli* outbreaks have been identified in the western United States, tied to a single fast-food restaurant chain, especially in Washington State, Las Vegas, and California.[15]

A Little League baseball organization decided to have a season-end barbecue. The hamburger was furnished by a local private butcher shop. While butchering a steer, one of the butchers accidentally nicked the large intestine, and some of the animal's feces got into the parts ground into hamburger.

It was a nice day, a family affair, with a large turnout of 275 persons—172 males and 103 females—attending the barbecue. There were 55 people who were part of the Little League who did not attend the barbecue. The total number of children and family members affiliated with the Little League was 330 people.

At the barbecue, two separate grills were used to cook the hamburgers. Two of the fathers volunteered to do the cooking. One father, I. R. Macho, heard many children complaining about being hungry, so he wanted to get their burgers to them as fast as he could. Mr. Macho liked his meat rare, so he seared the extra-thick hamburger patties on one side, flipped them over, and seared them on the other, heating up the meat quite well but not really cooking them all the way through. He failed to make the center of the hamburger reach the required 155°F—proven to be the safe cooking temperature. The second father, R. M. Cooke, liked his hamburgers well done, but not burned. He held them to the grill with the spatula each time, squeezing out the juice and helping the meat cook more. He checked each patty, to ensure that he was cooking the burgers well done, by opening each one with the corner of the spatula to see that each patty was not pink in the middle. Late the next day, on Sunday, several different children from several different families ended up at the emergency room of the local hospital, all with similar symptoms of fever, pain, malaise, stomach ache, and bloody diarrhea. After seven children, all with the same symptoms, were presented at the emergency room, the local public health department and communicable disease epidemiologist were notified.

Several physicians also called the department of public health to report serious diarrhea cases, all of which had bloody stools with the diarrhea. Laboratory results of samples collected from the cases showed that the pathogen was *Escherichia coli 0157: H7*.

In the epidemiological investigation, it was found that, of those who were sick, 46 boys, 22 men, 14 girls, and 16 women got their hamburger patties from I. R. Macho, whereas 6 boys, 4 men, 4 girls, and 2 women got their patties from R. M. Cooke. It was discovered that 123 people in all got their hamburger patties from Mr. Cooke and 152, from Mr. Macho. Relative risk was to be determined by the epidemiologist for the risk of eating hamburgers cooked by Mr. Macho as compared to those cooked by Mr. Cooke. In order to determine relative risk, the matrix in Figure 5.2 was developed by the epidemiologist.

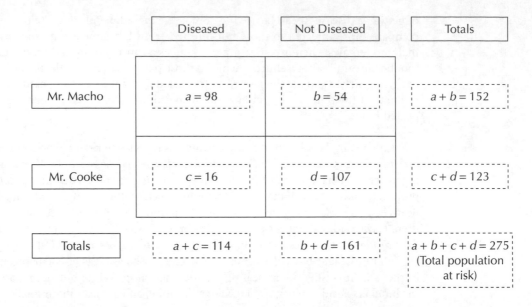

FIGURE 5.2   Number of cases of *E. coli 0157: H7* at Little League barbecue outbreak.

To calculate the risk ratio of the *E. coli 0157: H7* outbreak and cases of illness resulting from the cooking of Mr. Macho or Mr. Cooke, you calculate the risk of getting ill for those who ate Mr. Macho's cooking versus risk for those who ate burgers cooked by Mr. Cooke.

$$\text{Risk of illness from Mr. Macho} = \frac{a}{a+b} = \frac{98}{152} = .645 \times 100 \text{ or } 64.5\%$$

(64.5% risk of getting ill by eating Mr. Macho's cooking)

$$\text{Risk of illness from Mr. Cooke} = \frac{c}{c+d} = \frac{16}{123} = .130 \times 100 \text{ or } 13.0\%$$

(13.0% risk of getting ill by eating Mr. Cooke's cooking)

A comparison group must always be used. For example, the nondiseased group can become the comparison group and be compared to the diseased group. In this case, Mr. Macho's exposure group is compared to Mr. Cooke's exposure group. From this analysis, one can see that the risk of illness from eating Mr. Macho's cooking is 0.645, or 64.5%, and the risk of illness among those eating Mr. Cooke's cooking is 0.130, or 13.0%. To calculate the ratio of risk (risk ratio) for Mr. Macho (0.645) versus Mr. Cooke (0.130), the following steps are taken. First, to assess the ratio of risk, the highest number in the ratio formula is placed in the numerator, and the lesser number is used in the denominator. Thus, the formula is

$$\text{Relative risk} = \text{Risk ratio} = \frac{.645}{.130} = 4.96$$

The risk of getting *E. coli 0157: H7* at the Little League barbecue by eating Mr. Macho's cooking is 4.96—very high compared to that for Mr. Cooke's cooking. Recall that a ratio over 1.0 indicates increased risk. For every 1 person who gets sick from eating Mr. Cooke's cooking, 5 will get sick from eating Mr. Macho's cooking.

Attributable Risk

Attributable risk is the rate of disease in exposed persons that can be directly attributed to the exposure of the disease. Attributable risk is determined by subtracting the incidence rate (or mortality rate) of the disease of the nonexposed individuals from the exposed persons. It is assumed that the cause of the disease had an equal chance of causing the disease outbreak or illnesses in both the exposed and nonexposed individuals. Attributable risk is an individually based risk or risk difference.

If risk factors in a population are modified so as to benefit the population, the risk factor is measured by the *population attributable risk proportion* (also called *population attributable risk fraction*, if not multiplied by 100). Population attributable risk proportion is the proportion of the disease rate in the whole study group or a total population. This is calculated by taking the total population rate minus the rate in the nonexposed group to get the total exposed persons. The result is the proportion of the total rate that represents the population attributable risk proportion ($\times$ 100).[7]

p = proportion of total population with characteristics of the disease
r = relative risk

$$\text{Attributable risk} = \frac{p(r-1)}{p(r-1)+1} \times 100$$

Using the letter symbols found in the 2 $\times$ 2, 4-celled epidemiology grid on page 161, attributable risk is determined using the following method.

Since:

$$r = \frac{ad}{bc}$$

$$d = (1-b)$$

$$c = (1-a)$$

Then:

$$\frac{ad}{bc} = \frac{a(1-b)}{b(1-a)} = \frac{(a-ab)}{(b-ab)}$$

and

$$AR = \frac{b(r-1)}{b(r-1)+1} = \frac{a-b}{1-b}$$

From the above formula the proportion of disease attributable to the behavior among those with the disease characteristics is identified and the proportion of disease in the population that is attributable to the behavior that contributes to the risk is determined.[3,4]

Relative Risk and Attack Rates

Relative risk is a true ratio and is presented as a ratio. If relative risk is calculated using attack rates, the result is a ratio of the attack rates. The best approach is to use the ratio of the "exposed and ill," divided by the "not-exposed and ill."

Relative risk can be used in attack rates for risk of exposure to food poisoning or exposure to chemical or industrial risk. The formula for a food poisoning outbreak and the relative risk is presented below. At a church picnic, 48 people ate the food and got sick and 15 persons did not eat the food and got sick. The relative risk would be calculated using the formula:

$$\text{Relative risk} = \frac{\text{Eating and sick}}{\text{Not eating and sick}} = \frac{48}{15} = 3.2$$

A factor related to relative risk is that of **gradient of risk (infection)**. If an exposure or dose-response related relationship or other cause-effect relationship exists, such as smoking leading to lung cancer, gradient of risk should be considered. Scientifically it is observed that a threshold phenomena response exists in the body when exposed to diseases or chemicals. At first no response is observed until the exposure or dose reaches a certain level, when a reaction is finally seen. Under some circumstance, a gradient of response might not be seen if the dose is small or the threshold is low. Two related but different factors or behaviors, can result in correlation and cause-effect responses. For example, in a smoking caused disease, the role of alcohol as it correlates with cigarette use might show an apparent dose related response.[6,16]

An individual can have a whole range of responses to a disease or an exposure. Some persons with a strong immune system, high nutritional status, low stress, and a high level of well being may have only a short spell of illness when exposed to a cold virus. Another person within the same family might have high stress, be in a run down physiological state, and have a spell of illness for 3 weeks with the same cold infection. If this same person has allergies affecting the upper respiratory tract as does the cold, a correlation between symptoms and two different contributing factors can be seen, showing an apparent dose related response.[6,16]

Occasionally in epidemiology studies-of-risk, risk difference is considered. **Risk difference** is the measure of difference between two risks. In *association*, risk difference is obtained by subtracting the risk of a disease or exposure in an unexposed population from a similar or same risk for the exposed population. Risk difference as a measure is found useful in that it permits a direct calculation of the numbers of excess exposures or cases of a disease associated with the same exposure.

Risk Factors in Health Promotion

One area of risk that has drawn much attention in modern time is that of risk factors in the cause of disease, disability, injury, conditions, disorders, and death. The focus on risk factors is important, as it points the way to intervention, health education, health promotion, prevention, and health protection.

In epidemiology, risk factor has been considered on several different fronts including being used interchangeably with causative agents. The term is used more recently in chronic disease or lifestyle and behaviorally caused maladies. **Risk factors** are those behaviors or exposures associated with increased risk of a disease, injury, condition, or disability which can develop later on in life. If a certain risk is associated with an elevated frequency of occurrence of a disease, disorder, injury, disability, or early death, and the association can be explained on the basis of a cause-effect relationship, it would be considered a risk factor. Not only are risk factors important to identify, but are in need of measurement of health status. Frequently, magnitude, level of exposure to a population, and prevention activities all rely on research data that demonstrate the effect of the risk factor on a group or population. Thus, any factors associated with disease, disability, injury or death by virtue of an elevated relative risk, are risk factors.

If an exposure to a disease or occurrence will cause an increased probability of getting the disease, this could be a risk factor. If any activity, behavior or exposure is experienced which will increase the chance of a negative impact on health status, these are possible risk factors. If a risk related activity or behavior can be prevented or an intervention made, the risk might be reduced and any detriment to health status might be avoided, all being the aim of epidemiology.[3,4,6,11]

Findings about relative risk will show that a benefit might be experienced if a person with the risk stops the behavior or stops participating in the risk. Since risk factors are associated with chronic disease or disorders or diseases caused by a risk-taking lifestyle, intervention and prevention through behavior change is highly probable, such as smoking cessation, not drinking alcohol, using shoulder/seat belts, reducing cholesterol, etc.[3,4,6,11]

Associated with a risk factor is a risk marker. A **risk marker** is a key, obvious or well proven behavior, activity or attribute that has been associated with an increased chance of acquiring a disease. A risk marker is a risk factor which can be used as an indicator of an increased risk and which should be observed and modified in susceptibles, or in an entire population group. A risk factor is similar to a health status indicator, but is more specific to one disease or condition and can be changed or reduced. Some risk factors that have become risk markers which have an impact on overall health status include[3,4,6,11]

smoking	drinking alcohol
high-speed driving (especially teens)	drinking and driving
lack of exercise	not using seat belts
overweight	high blood pressure
elevated cholesterol/high fat diet	living alone
low levels of education	high levels of stress
lack of adequate nutrition	lack of proper rest

A population at risk can fall within both prevalence and incidence considerations. However, populations at risk are mostly calculated within incidence rates. When considering incidence, the **population at risk**, should be included in the denominator. The denominator should include those with the disease, those who have had the disease (if they are no longer susceptible), or those immunized.

INCIDENCE AND ATTACK RATES

A segment of a population may occasionally be at risk of illness or exposure to a disease or injury for a limited time period. The limited time period often has much to do with the gathering of a group of people at one location for a special occasion, or may be due to exposure at work. Thus, the time span of the outbreak is for only a short period of time and limited to a specific group of people. When these circumstances occur, it makes calculation of incidence quite simple. Incidence and risk of exposure often remain the same even if the time period is shortened some, or if the time period is a bit longer. The limited period of exposure and risk and the limited group of people at risk are what make attack rates unique. **Attack rates** are cumulative incidence rates and are used in epidemics. The term *infection rate* is sometimes used with attack rate. The infection rate shows the incidence of ill persons with signs and symptoms of the disease and also includes the unapparent cases of infection. The number of persons ill from a specific disease in a limited time period in a specific group makes up an attack.[4,5,6,7,14]

Attack rates are most commonly used in food poisoning situations (Figure 5.3) or chemical exposures in a group of workers. The classic case scenario for the use of attack rates is when a food poisoning event occurs at a church or school picnic. Often these potluck feasts include potato salads and other cream-based salads (which are great mediums for bacteria growth) prepared at home and brought by participants. Food sanitation preparation measures vary and are not easily controlled. As a result some participants may come down with one of several bacteria-caused food poison illnesses. An investigation of an outbreak includes the various food sources, who prepared what food, cases of ill people versus well people, who ate what, when, and how much. From the results of the investigation, attack rates are calculated.[4,5,6,7,14]

The epidemiological concept is to determine whether there is an association between the risk of exposure (eating the food) at a specific event and the specific illness. There are three attack rate formulas: (1) crude attack rate, (2) general attack rate, (3) food-specific

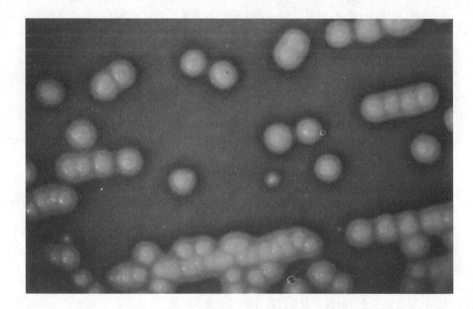

FIGURE 5.3   Above is *Clostridium botulinum*, toxin-forming anaerobic bacteria, responsible for a serious form of food poisoning. A small amount of the toxin quickly causes death. (Picture courtesy of Centers for Disease Control and Prevention, Atlanta, Georgia)

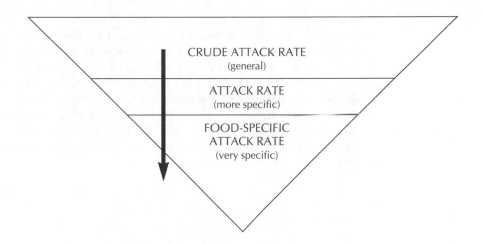

FIGURE 5.4   Attack rates are calculated from the more general crude attack rate down to attack rates to the food-specific attack rates.

attack rate. Attack rates are determined from the broad perspective (crude attack rate) downward to a more narrow focus (attack rate), and then finally a very specific assessment is conducted (food-specific attack rate). See Figure 5.4.

$$\text{Crude attack rate } = \frac{\text{Number of persons ill with the disease}}{\text{Number of persons attending the event}} \times 100$$

$$\text{Attack rate } = \frac{\text{Number of persons ill (new cases) within the time period}}{\text{Number of persons/population at risk within the time period}} \times 100$$

$$\text{Food-specific attack rate } = \frac{\begin{array}{c}\text{Number of persons who ate}\\ \text{a specific food and became ill}\end{array}}{\begin{array}{c}\text{Total number of persons}\\ \text{who ate a specific food}\end{array}} \times 100$$

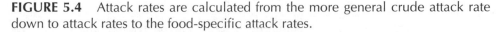

Secondary Attack Rate

Secondary attack rates are used in infectious disease investigations in which a limited time period exists and involves a pathogen with a short incubation period. The secondary attack rate is often used when the cases of an illness occur in the same household or work group, and when a primary case of the disease is present in a period of time before others in the group get the disease. When others in the group come down with the disease, and are secondary caused from the primary infection, they are secondary cases. The persons who come down with the disease after being infected from the primary case are determined by use of the secondary attack rate. The numbers of persons who had contact or exposure to the primary infectious person or the primary source of infection within the incubation period of the pathogen, are used in calculating the rate. This assessment uses the total number of exposed cases. The number of cases per number of persons exposed minus the index case are multiplied by 100. Stated another way, it is the number of infected persons per number of susceptible and exposed persons multiplied by 100.[4,5,6,7,14]

The numerator in the secondary attack rate includes the number of cases of the disease that occurred within the same group or household following the onset of the primary or first case and who are infected by the primary case. The number of infected persons is used in the numerator. The number of susceptible and exposed persons is used in the denominator. The denominator excludes individuals who have previously had the disease and now are immune, or who have had immunizations; susceptible people are the only ones used in the denominator.[4,5,6,7,14]

$$\text{Secondary attack rate} = \frac{\text{Number of exposed persons developing the disease within incubation period}}{\text{Total number of persons exposed to the primary case}} \times 100$$

$$\frac{\text{Number of cases among contacts of primary cases during the period}}{\text{Total number of contacts}} \times 100$$

Occupational Health and Safety's (OSHA) Approach to Incidence Rates

When dealing with the occupationally related health and safety events a rate of occurrence is used. This rate of occurrence is referred to in the occupational health and safety field as an *incidence rate*, this causes some confusion and should not be mixed up with epidemiological incidence rates.

Occupational health and safety incidence rates are based on the exposure of 100 full-time workers using 200,000 employee-hours as the equivalent (100 employees working 40 hours per week for 50 weeks per year.) The occupational health and safety incidence rate is computed for each category of days lost or cases of occurrence, depending what number is placed in the numerator of the formula. The denominator should be the total number of hours worked by all employees during the same time period as that covered by the number of occurrences or cases. To calculate the incidence rate for occupational health and safety for total recordable cases at the end of the year, multiply the number of cases/occurrences by 200,000 and divide that by the number of hours worked by all workers for the year. Here are the Occupational Safety and Health Incidence rate formulas:

$$\text{Incidence rate (total recordable cases)} = \frac{\text{Number of injuries and illness} \times 200,000}{\text{Total hours worked by all employees during the time period}} \times 100$$

$$\text{Incidence rate (work days lost)} = \frac{\text{Number of lost workdays}}{\text{Number of hours worked by all employees during the time period}} \times 100$$

PREVALENCE

The companion to incidence is prevalence. As a measure of morbidity, **prevalence** is the number of cases of disease, infected persons, or condition, present at a particular time, in relation to the size of the population from which it is drawn, for example, the number of cases of measles within a population as of the first of July. Prevalence of chronic diseases such as arthritis are high when compared to its incidence. Incidence includes the number of new cases and prevalence does not. Prevalence equals incidence multiplied by the average case duration.[2]

Several factors affect prevalence in a population (see Table 5.1). Some of these factors include

- As a new disease develops in a population, as new cases arise incidence goes up. As incidence goes up prevalence goes up.

- The duration of the disease affects prevalence. When a disease has a long duration, prevalence remains higher longer.

- Intervention and treatment have effects on prevalence. As treatment reduces cases, duration of the disease and numbers of cases go down, prevalence goes down. Immunization prevents new cases and reduces prevalence. Prolongation of life can increase duration and can add to the prevalence of chronic disease.

- Prolongation of a nondiseased and healthy population can reduce prevalence of acute disease and as healthy individuals become more hardy, life duration increases and so does life expectancy.[2]

Prevalence Rates

Prevalence means *all*. The prevalence rate assesses the total number of people in a group or population who have a disease at a specific time. The **prevalence rate** is equal to the incidence rate multiplied by the average duration of the disease. Prevalence is controlled by two elements, (1) the number of individuals who have been diseased in the past, and (2) the length or duration of the illness. Prevalence will vary in direct relation to both duration and incidence. Successful intervention and treatment will prolong life and will have an effect on

TABLE 5.1 Comparative factors affecting prevalence rates

Rates Are Increased by	*Rates Are Decreased by*
Immigration of ill cases	Immigration of healthy persons
Emigration of healthy persons	Emigration of ill cases
Immigration of susceptible cases or those with potential of becoming cases	Improved cure rate of cases
	Increased death rates from the diseases
Prolongation of life of cases without cure (increase of duration of disease)	Decrease in occurrence of new cases
	Shorter duration of disease
Increase in occurrence of new cases (increase in incidence)	Death

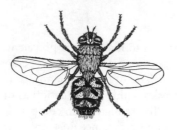

FIGURE 5.5   The cluster fly is a common housefly known to spread disease from garbage and feces to unprotected food. (Picture courtesy of Centers for Disease Control and Prevention, Atlanta, Georgia)

reducing prevalence. The decrease in incidence and shortening of the duration of a disease decreases prevalence. When duration decreases significantly, prevalence can decrease despite an increase in incidence (see Table 5.1).

Prevalence rates and the information they provide have been found useful in planning community and public health services and medical services, and are used in projecting medical care and need for hospital beds. Some epidemiologists become confused in ascertaining the correct denominator. The epidemiologist needs to determine who the total population is (see prevalence formulas).[3,4,5,6,7,10,11,12]

Two additional prevalence concepts need to be addressed. First is **lifetime prevalence**, which is the total number of individuals that have had a condition, problem, or disease throughout their life, or at least for a major part of it. Lifetime prevalence is considered a form of period prevalence (see Period Prevalence, next page). Another concept is *annual prevalence*. Annual prevalence is the total persons with a condition, problem, and disease at any given time throughout a given year. Cases of disease that started before the start date of the prevalence count but extend into the study period, are included in annual prevalence rates. Those cases that started prior to the end of the study period, extended throughout the year and/or had not yet recovered before the study period ended, are also counted. Health care administrators, public health professionals or epidemiologists want to know if cases of an epidemic are new and are of concern or if they are old. In some cases period prevalence data may be of limited value as it includes both point prevalence and incidence. Clearer information is available through incidence rates than point prevalence rates, as they are more specific in their information. Incidence is difficult to measure where prevalence is measured by a single study or survey. More than one approach to the prevalence rate has been suggested but the information used remains the same regardless of minor modifications or approaches.[3,4,5,6,7,10,11,12] Prevalence rate formulas are

$$\text{Prevalence rate 1} = \frac{\text{Number of existing cases of the disease}}{\text{Total population}} \text{ At a point in time} \times 1{,}000$$

$$\text{Prevalence rate 2} = \frac{\text{Total number of cases of the disease at a given time}}{\text{Total population at risk at a given time}} \times 1{,}000$$

Period Prevalence

Period prevalence is more complex than crude prevalence or point prevalence. **Period prevalence** includes the total individuals who have had the disease of concern at any time during the specified time period. But it is more than that. Period prevalence starts at a point in time and stops at a point in time. All persons with the disease that have carried over from the previous time period or have become ill at the end of the time period are included. New cases (incidence) occurring within the time period are included, *recurrences* during a succeeding time period (usually one year) are included. The epidemiologist should define any unclear issues and so state them. For example, if the epidemiologist decides to include all recurrences from the previous six months in period prevalence, he or she should make a statement in the tables and narrative of the report.

Another way that period prevalence has been expressed is to include point prevalence (see Point Prevalence, page 155) at the beginning of the time period plus all new cases that occur within the time period. However it is done, period prevalence requires the establishment of a specific time period for the study of a specific disease. Period prevalence is a complex measure. It is established from prevalence at a point in time, plus incidence (new cases), and recurrences during a succeeding time period such as one year. Persons not at risk of acquiring a new case of the disease are not included in the numerator. Below is the formula for period prevalence rate.[3,4,5,6,7,11,12]

$$\text{Period prevalence rate} = \frac{\substack{\text{Number of existing} \\ \text{cases of the disease}}}{\text{Average study population}} \ \text{Within a time period} \times 1{,}000$$

Disease Recurrence in Period Prevalence

The epidemiologist, when dealing with period prevalence and point prevalence, often has to define parameters which affect the study and the calculating of rates. Some parameters are defined by the nature of the disease or occurrence. Some epidemiologists struggle in dealing with defining recurrent cases. The nature of the disease helps to define some parameters. For example, the chance of a recurrence of a case of measles is small. On the other hand gonorrhea could be a recurrence or a current case. If the nature of the disease lends itself to recurrence, then the epidemiologist would make a statement to this effect and would count it as a new case in period prevalence. If the nature of the disease is to not recur, or if immunizations are prevalent within the population or the case, then the recurrent case would not be a new case.

Another factor to consider in recurrences is time. If a significant amount of time had passed from the end of the course of disease to the onset of the recurrent case, then it could be counted as a new case. The epidemiologist must identify and define the unusual factors surrounding the recurrence of a case in period prevalence and it must be consistent with the nature and course of the disease under study. According to Mausner, recurrent cases such as found in case 7 and case 15 in Figure 5.6 are to be excluded from the numerator. Persons not at risk of acquiring a new case of the disease are not to be included in the numerator. Cases of recurrences within the study period are counted only once in the numerator and

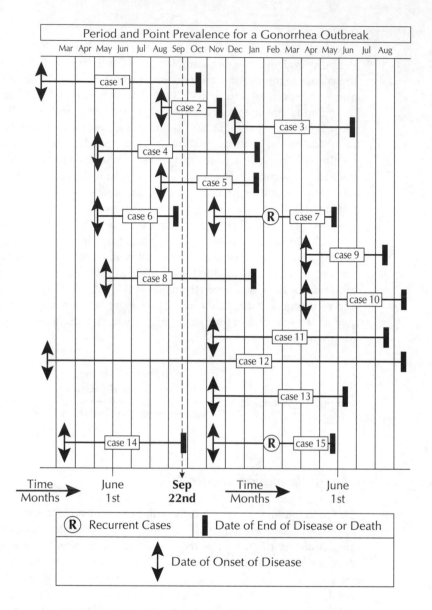

FIGURE 5.6   Graph of period and point prevalence.

once in the denominator; counted as an individual not as cases.[5] However, the nature of the disease, and its ability to recur has to be taken into account as well as immunity to a disease, both naturally acquired and through vaccinations. If a disease such as gonorrhea can recur over and over, the risk remains and new cases are not based on the individual. If natural immunity does not occur, each new case must be accounted for in the rate formula, both as a new case and as being within the population at risk.

Pingpong Gonorrhea (Recurring Diseases)

College Students Reinfect Each Other with Gonorrhea

Period prevalence and point prevalence are often difficult to determine when recurring diseases are involved. The epidemiologist can become confused as to when to count a case as a *new* case or as a *recurring* case. Generally, each case occurrence is counted as a new case, even if it is a recurring case of the disease.

One area in which diseases recur is venereal diseases (VD, now called sexually transmitted diseases or STDs). In many colleges and universities, sexual activity is higher than average. One college senior in particular had a common VD problem, but with a twist. He contracted gonorrhea four times in one winter, even though he insisted that he had only one girlfriend. How did either one of them get the disease in the first place? The attending physician speculated that a marijuana bash they attended developed into a love-in. "I think I was always having relations with my girlfriend but I can't be sure—you get a bit fogged up," was his reply. The girl stated that, even at the parties, "I always stayed loyal to Jim—I think." Because the two did not have simultaneous treatment, Jim would show up at the clinic with gonorrhea symptoms and get treated, and a few days later his girlfriend would present herself at the clinic for treatment. Jim would then show up again, sometime later, with the disease. This process repeated itself for several clinic visits before the doctors finally caught on. Epidemiologists called this the case of "ping-pong gonorrhea." In the process of getting cured, each partner was reinfected by the other in turn.

(*Source:* Time, *Vol. 9, No. 9, September 1, 1967, p. 32*)

Point Prevalence

Point prevalence is the number of cases of individuals with a disease, condition or illness at a single specific point in time—the number of existing cases at a point in time. Point prevalence measures the presence of a disease or condition on a single short-time point, theoretically stopping the clock for a minute, hour or a day and counting the existing cases of the disease. The point prevalence rate is presented below.

$$\text{Point prevalence rate} = \frac{\text{Number of existing cases of the disease}}{\text{Total study population}} \text{ At a point in time} \times 1,000$$

Understanding Point and Period Prevalence

Gonorrhea is a common sexually transmitted disease. Symptoms of the disease appear in about a week after exposure. Women are frequently symptomless carriers of the pathogen for weeks or months with symptoms appearing in 7 to 21 days and are often identified through tracking sexual contacts. In men the incubation period is from 2 to 14 days. Symptoms in men include a tingling sensation in the urethra followed by dysuria and a purulent discharge from the penis. Symptomless infections have been identified in homosexual men and rectal gonorrhea is found in both sexes.[1,13]

From the point and period prevalence grid in Figure 5.6, several morbidity rate factors can be identified.

- Total cases, 13 persons and 15 cases of gonorrhea.

- Total population of the study was 300 seniors from Central City High School. The total population of the three grades in the high school was 1,100 students.

- Point prevalence on Sept. 22nd includes 7 cases which are used in the numerator (cases include—cases: 1,2,4,5,8,12,14,15).

- Period prevalence, includes all cases from June 1st through May 31st, with recurrences treated as new cases since recurrent cases are like new cases, due to the nature of the disease gonorrhea. 15 cases are used in the numerator.

- Incidence for November includes all new cases in that time period over the population at risk. Four cases are new in November. Recurrences are treated as new cases.

EPIDEMICS: TWO TYPES—COMMON SOURCE AND PROPAGATED

The type and amount of disease spread in a population determines if an epidemic is at hand. Diseases that persist at a moderate and steady level in a community are referred to as being *endemic*. When a disease level rises above an endemic amount, and a significant number of cases appear, an epidemic has begun. A few dozen cases might constitute an epidemic of measles, whereas only two or three cases of rabies (Figure 5.7) might be considered an epidemic of this deadly disease, due to the potential for death or serious illness.

As mentioned in Chapter 1, there are two major types of epidemics, (1) common source and (2) propagated or progressive. The differences between these two types of epidemics are based on the differences in distribution of the disease in a population and time of onset, based on an epidemic curve. An **epidemic curve** is developed by the epidemiologist who uses a graph to plot the distribution of individual cases of disease by time of onset. For example, using a bar graph to plot the epidemic curve, and only one case occurs the first day, but 5 cases the next and 15 the third day, and 20 the fourth day and 10 the fifth day, five bars would be used, and length of each would be plotted according to the numbers of cases each day of onset. The same would hold true for cases that occur by the hour or the week. Date of onset is determined by identification of the index case, the incubation period, type of pathogen, primary source, primary case(s), and duration of the disease. (Plotting and construction of bar graphs and frequency polygons/ line graphs are covered in Chapter 7.) The bar graphs of the cholera outbreak

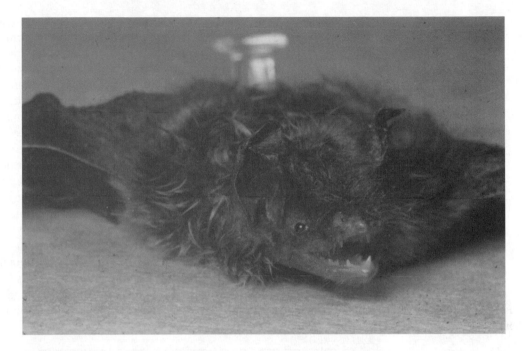

FIGURE 5.7 A rabid brown bat known to cause rabies epidemics. Droppings from brown bats have also been implicated in common source epidemics of histoplasmosis, caused by inhaling dust from bat droppings, which results in lesions on the lungs. Inapparent infections of this disease can occur in areas where people frequent caves with bat droppings. (Picture courtesy of Centers for Disease and Control and Prevention, Atlanta, Georgia)

investigated by Dr. John Snow in the 1850s shown in Case Study I, pages 419 to 441, are good examples of an epidemic curve.

Common Source Epidemic This is an epidemic in which the event or exposure of a disease to a group of persons comes from a single source that all persons in the group had a chance to encounter. When the group is exposed to the source of the epidemic almost simultaneously or only exposed for a brief time period, the cases that develop are usually within the common incubation period of the disease. One way to recognize a common source epidemic is through the rapid rise and fall of the epidemic curve. Examples of such diseases would be staphylococcal food poisoning as can occur in potato salad at a church picnic and with most persons eating the food. A second example would be Legionnaire's disease transmitted by the air conditioning system in a hotel while people attended a convention. Noncommunicable disease sources can also be the cause of common source epidemics. Chemicals, gases, injuries, and air pollution are but a few agent/noncommunicable disease causes.[4,5]

Propagated or Progressive Source Epidemic A propagated source epidemic is caused by either direct or indirect transmission of a communicable disease from one individual to another and can have multiple sources from which the disease can be transmitted. As explained in Chapter 2 under herd immunity, for such a disease to spread there have to be susceptible individuals. Propagated epidemics occur from person-to-person transmission. These epidemics can also involve several levels of progression of the transmission of the disease, including vectors and fomites. Because of the erratic nature of the transmission of the disease, the plotting of new cases does not produce a nice epidemic curve as seen in the common source epidemic. When a propagated epidemic is plotted, an upward trend from the onset is seen with increasing numbers of cases as the successive time periods pass. A resurgence of the epidemic curve may be seen over and over, as it reflects the time frame of the incubation periods and waves of recurring cases. Due to the multiple sources of a propagated epidemic susceptibles, they have a logarithmic increase in the chance of being exposed to the disease. Eventually the curves will show a continuing drop as the number of susceptible individuals dwindles. Propagated epidemics are also affected by *place* factors. Geographical distribution also differentiates the two different sources of epidemics. Common source epidemics are usually found in one place or in limited locations. Propagated epidemics spread laterally and also with circle shaped configurations as well and continue to spread from one generation of cases to successive generations. Propagated epidemics can occur not only in infectious diseases but can include occupational health related occurrences, environmental events, behaviorally caused diseases and conditions from chemicals and other agents.[4,5]

Figures 5.8 and 5.9 present two charts depicting examples of a propagated epidemic. Bar graph and line graph examples are used. The line graph shows multiple sources of the

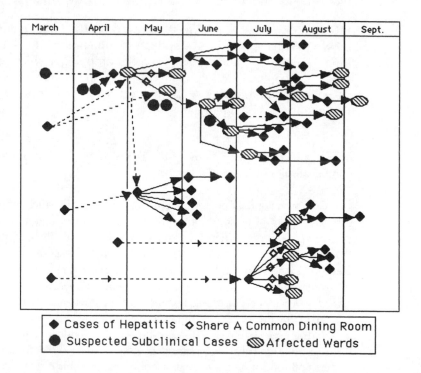

FIGURE 5.8   A line graph of an example of a propagated epidemic of infectious hepatitis in an institution for the mentally retarded. The line graph is a representation of probable hepatitis transmission among patients and employees and shows heavily infected wards. (Source: Adapted from Matthew, E.B., et al., "A Major Epidemic of Infectious Hepatitis in an Institution for the Mentally Retarded," *American Journal of Epidemiology*, Vol. 98, pp. 199–215, 1973)

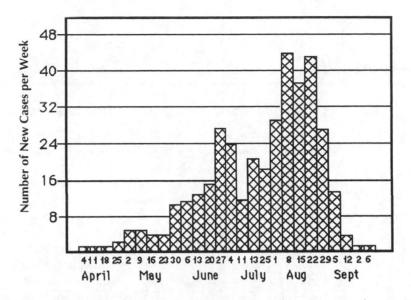

FIGURE 5.9   Example of a bar graph showing the epidemic curve of a propagated epidemic of infectious hepatitis in an institution for the mentally retarded. (Source: Adapted from Matthew, E.B., et al., "A Major Epidemic of Infectious Hepatitis in an Institution for the Mentally Retarded," *American Journal of Epidemiology*, Vol. 98, pp. 199–215, 1973)

disease and the time lag factors in a propagated epidemic. The bar graph represents the epidemic curve and the time lag and the second surge in the epidemic.

> In 1970, 375 apparent cases of infectious hepatitis occurred among 3600 patients in an institution for the retarded in Lynchburg Training School and Hospital, Lynchburg, Virginia. One employee had a case of hepatitis during the epidemic. The incubation period for infectious hepatitis is about 29 days. The route of transmission of the disease was from person to person by the fecal-oral route by direct contact or through fomites. The attack rate was 57% out of 473 in the study group. Attack rates were lower among those patients with the least levels of retardation as they had better personal hygiene. The epidemic produced two deaths. Long-term patients of 18 years or more and patients over age 40 years had lower attack rates. An index case was not identified early on in the outbreak.[16]

ODDS RATIO

Another ratio used in the assessment of morbidity data is that of **odds ratio**. The chance of exposure and risk of getting a disease can be determined by odds ratios. Various approaches to odds ratio have been used in epidemiology and are *prevalence odds ratio, cross-product ratio, exposure odds ratio, disease odds ratio*, and *risk odds ratio*.

Prevalence odds ratio is used in cross-sectional study analysis. Odds ratios are applied to prevalence studies instead of incidence studies.

Cross product/odds ratio can be best understood by the use of the 2 × 2, four-celled epidemiological grid as it compares the various arrangements of diseased states found using the grid.

NEWS FILE

Hantavirus (Emerging Infections)

Untreatable Hantavirus Remains a Threat to Public's Health

Of the confirmed cases of hantavirus since 1980, the Centers for Disease Control and Prevention report that almost half died. Fifty cases per year are predicted to occur throughout the United States. The hantavirus erupted in June, 1993 in the New Mexico/Arizona border region. It killed a young woman and her boyfriend, both of them athletes and runners who were in excellent health. Both were stricken and died of acute respiratory failure within hours of the disease attack. Hantavirus disease is transmitted by the droppings of the deer mouse, a common rodent found in most of the United States. The hantavirus is usually inhaled after becoming airborne in dust containing mouse urine or feces, and attacks the lungs (hantavirus pulmonary syndrome, HPS). The hantavirus causes hemorrhagic fever with renal syndrome (HFRS). The disease is called the Four Corners Disease because it was found in the Four Corners area on a Navajo reservation. However, it is not restricted to this place or the mouse host, as it has been found in rats in Baltimore, and 11 people in California have died of the disease.

Control measures include keeping rodent populations down and out of buildings, and avoiding contact with all rodents, dead or alive. If rodent droppings are found in a seldom-used house, air it out completely, clean up wearing face masks and rubber gloves, wet down the area with disinfectant, wipe up the droppings and place them in a double leak-proof plastic bag, and dispose of them along with all cleaning materials. Do not sweep, vacuum, or do anything to stir up dust and make the virus airborne.

(Sources: Reports from National Center for Infectious Diseases, Centers for Disease Control and Prevention, Division of Communicable Disease Control, Department of Health Services, State of California)

Cross-product ratio/odds ratio compares exposed/disease (**A**) and unexposed/no disease (**D**) with unexposed/diseased (**B**) and exposed and no disease (**C**) or a comparison of **AD/BC**.

Exposure odds ratio is the ratio of the odds of exposed in diseased subjects to the odds of being exposed in nondiseased subjects, or **A/B** compared to **C/D**.

In incidence and in rare cases or exotic diseases, **AD/BC** is used as an estimate of the risk ratio as well as the ratio of person-time incidence rates. Additionally forces of morbidity (see force of morbidity on page 138) can be used in determining the risk ratio in the exposed and unexposed.

In cohort studies and cross-sectional investigations, the *disease-odds (rate-odds) ratio* is used. The disease-odds ratio is the ratio of the odds of getting a disease among the exposed (**A/C**) compared to the odds of getting the disease among the unexposed (**B/D**). This process eliminates some options and reduces **AD/BC** and is equal to exposure-odds ratio.

Risk odds ratio is the ratio that determines the chances of getting a disease, if exposed, to the chance of getting the disease, if not exposed and is useful when applied to cross-

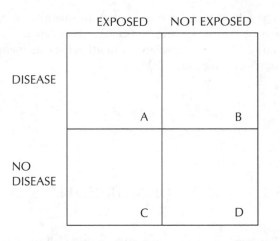

FIGURE 5.10 2×2, four-celled grid for assessing class-product ratio/odds ratio.

sectional, cohort studies and possibly to case control studies (see these terms). In determining odds ratio the epidemiology grid (Figure 5.10) is again used. In the case of odds ratio, however, the term *exposed* replaces *disease*. The term *not exposed* replaces *no disease*. The term *present* replaces *exposed*, and the term *absent* replaces *not exposed*. The proportion symbol of P_1, P_2, P_3, P_4 are used in the grid to replace A,B,C,D, respectively. Thus, we have Figure 5.11.

The ratio of incidence rates, which is actually relative risk, becomes the following formula:

$$\frac{P_1}{P_1 + P_2} \div \frac{P_3}{P_3 + P_4}$$

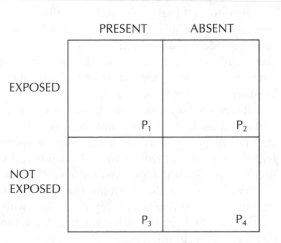

FIGURE 5.11 2×2, four-celled grid for odds ratio.

The following is the odds ratio as the quantities can be considered as the odds in favor of having the disease with the behavior or disease causing factor present and the factor absent. The odds ratio is obtained by multiplying diagonally in the 2 × 2 epidemiology grid, producing cross products.[3,4]

$$\frac{P_1}{P_2} \div \frac{P_3}{P_4}$$

FORMALIZED SOURCES OF MORBIDITY STATISTICS AND DATA

Five areas of morbidity statistics are generally used in epidemiology: (1) communicable disease reports, (2) clinical records and hospital medical records, (3) institutional and industrial records, (4) health and disease surveys, (5) ongoing observations of incidence of illness in a population.

Communicable Disease Reports and Sources of Data

Reports and publications developed and distributed by local public health departments, state departments of health and national federal agencies are the main sources of communicable disease data. The Centers for Disease Control and Prevention publishes *MMWR (Morbidity and Mortality Weekly Report)* which is the most common and widely distributed source of morbidity information in the United States. The National Center for Health Statistics of the U.S. Public Health Service produces several publications on a regular basis. *Advance Data* is a publication which is published on a regular basis, and covers the whole range of chronic and acute disease research.

Other special morbidity reports, life tables and research reports are regularly produced and distributed. Many states produce similar publications from their own centers of health statistics. For example, California produces *California Morbidity* and *Data Matters*. Such reports provide a means of notification for those who need to know about disease outbreaks that are of concern. In some cases the timely development and distribution of such reports have little value in preventing or controlling a current outbreak, especially in communicable diseases with short durations.

Reports of notifiable diseases, also referred to as reportable diseases, are also developed and distributed. Such reports provide a means of notification to those who need to know about disease outbreaks that are of concern to a population's health status or that pose a potential epidemic. The reports are useful in prevention, control or intervention of future outbreaks or disease occurrence and for research and study.[3,8,9]

The Centers for Disease Control and Prevention (CDC) maintains a standardized regular disease reporting system on all diseases with a major focus on notifiable diseases. Records are also kept on gunshot wounds, AIDS, abortions, congenital anomalies, and other factors affecting health status.

Disease reporting originates with the physician and laboratories who report to public health departments. The reporting of a notifiable disease or a life-threatening disease may also be reported directly to CDC. However, as far as a quick response to an epidemic is concerned, those who can intervene the quickest are those closest to the patient. Thus, local public health officials, local physicians, and hospitals are most likely to respond first and need to be notified and involved immediately. State health officials and CDC officials are often brought in to assist. However, the most immediate control and response is at the local level. Rabies, food-borne disease outbreaks, cholera, or any other disease of major concern that need control measures require prompt reporting and response in order for control and prevention of future epidemics. Control and prevention activities can contain the disease, as well as provide data and information about disease distribution, transmission, source, and the potential to infect groups in the future.

Disease reporting is legally vested in each individual state and territory of the United States and the list of notifiable diseases can vary from state to state. However, the Centers for Disease Control and Prevention's list of notifiable diseases remains the standard for reporting of disease outbreaks or occurrences for the nation. The list of CDC's notifiable diseases is presented in Chapter 2. The World Health Organization requires four diseases to be reported, cholera, plague, yellow fever, and AIDS. Smallpox was required to be reported in the past, but is no longer on the list.

Disease reporting still lacks consistency and completeness. Efforts are made to make the reporting process more effective and easier for the reporting sources. Physicians can now call by telephone, FAX or use an easily filled out postcard. Some physicians are hesitant to report diseases which may carry a stigma, such as AIDS and sexually transmitted diseases, for family members or certain persons of position. (When Liberace died of AIDS in 1987, the attending physician tried to report the death as being something other than AIDS. An investigation by the Riverside County California Coroner showed that he died of AIDS and this information was released to the public.)

Physicians are legally and ethically required to report the occurrence of all notifiable disease, including any that may have a stigma attached. Common diseases that are seen often by physicians and rare diseases that are difficult to recognize may be overlooked in the reporting process. The more rare or serious diseases such as rabies, cholera, plague, or Lyme disease are more likely to be reported. The reporting of common conditions may be important in pinpointing an epidemic but may not be reported. Measles, chickenpox, flu, streptococcal infections are commonly seen by practicing physicians and may be seen as having minimum reporting importance. When cases are reported by a multitude of physicians in separate private practices to a central public health department, an epidemic can be identified. The cumulative reporting effect can show an outbreak, whereas in the private practice, the physician may see only an occasional case. (See Notifiable Diseases in the United States in Chapter 2.)

The first contact or entry point to the health care system, most likely with the primary care physicians, are the first occasion exposure to a reporting source. Physicians are required to report cases of reportable diseases or unusual occurrences to local public health departments. The information is sent on to CDC and then on to the World Health Organization. However, newspaper or television reports from investigative reporters who check out stories from schools, colleges, universities, industries or government agencies may find an epidemic in the making long before it is officially reported to the public health department. (See Notifiable Disease Reporting System, Figure 2.7, in Chapter 2.)

Clinical Records and Hospital Medical Records

On the surface, clinic and hospital medical records seem to be a reliable source of disease data. However, this is not always true. Medical record data can be biased. Under the new prospective payment system using diagnosis related groups, physicians have a tendency to use a diagnosis that will provide the most income for the hospital. A primary diagnosis may be made a secondary diagnosis if it pays more.

Morbidity data from hospitals are not necessarily reflective of the level of disease of the community for a variety of reasons. Not all people go to the physician or clinic for health care when experiencing a disease, what is treated in the physician's office may not be reported nor may it show up in the hospital records. People will travel great distances to see a special physician and then may return to a different community in order to avoid a disease being reported, especially to the public. Health insurance policies limitations, access to care problems, availability of care problems, managed care's limited choices, lack of insurance, staff privileges of physicians at certain hospitals, and the effectiveness of the disease reporting system including tumor registry all affect reporting processes. Often there is no set or defined population for some general hospitals and a whole array of diseases are seen. In specialized hospitals such as children's hospitals or geriatric medical centers a certain set of diseases are commonly seen.

Given the limitations of hospital based data, morbidity information from hospitals provides opportunities for disease surveillance of specific disease or conditions. If certain diseases are serious and widespread enough to require hospitalization, then the data would be of value and rates could be developed. Hospitals do provide a select group of cases to study and provide a defined group or population on which to develop disease rates. Hospital studies are not reflective of the general population in the community. The defined and select population from a hospital based study does make the determination of the denominator for rates relatively easy.

Hospital studies provide a unique set of occurrences not often seen outside of the hospital setting. Nosocomial infections, iatrogenic illness or occurrences, adverse drug reactions, and other related hospital caused illness or diseases can and should be studied. Psychiatric treatment, alcohol and substance abuse, and other abuse studies can also be made in health care facilities using medical records. The medical records of private practice physicians or small clinics have been used very little by epidemiologists. In fact, these records may be a large yet untapped source of morbidity data. Accessing these medical records poses the greatest barrier. Physical access to records often has to be done by hand, as no database of primary care private practice is available or maintained. Financial constraints are also a barrier. No one is willing to fund a massive collection of data from the private physician's medical record.

Managed Care Organization's Records and Data

Managed care programs have increased at high rates over the last few years. The data available from the larger HMO, PPO, IPA health care organizations may allow an increase in study by epidemiologists. Larger HMOs, being prevention and cost containment oriented, routinely keep very good patient and medical records and databases. Information on morbidity and mortality not only affects the management of these organizations but also are excellent sources of epidemiologic data. The epidemiologist must recognize the limitations of the data and that the data do not represent the entire community. HMOs have contracts with large employers and the data used by them represent more of a middle class population than a cross-section of society. Some HMOs try to contract with only groups that are known to be more healthy. In managed care programs data collected is more for internal use in planning and financial management. Data gathered for medical or epidemiological reasons often has been collected more for use in administration of the insurance program than for disease prevention or control unless the disease related measures have some financial significance.

Morbidity Registry and Record Linkage

A disease registry is an organized system for identifying and recording information on all cases of an identified diagnosed disease. The terms *register* and *registry* are used interchangeably. To be more correct the term **register** refers to the actual report, or to the computer base of the data. A register is a file of data on diseases or of a certain disease or other health condition affecting the health status of a population or community. A **registry** is the system of collecting and registering disease-related data. Cancer and tumor registries are the most common register systems in recent times. Some states have made major efforts to computerize and develop centralized cancer tumor registry systems. In the mid 1980s Colorado, through the cooperation of the Colorado Department of Health and the Colorado Hospital Association developed such a system.

Registry

Diseases and conditions for which registries have been developed include, cancers, tuberculosis, psychiatric disorders, twins, blindness, physical handicaps, birth defects and rheumatic fever. Registries are expensive to develop, require the cooperation of many health care providers and entities, and need excellent management. A registry should be attempted only with a serious effort for success. Disease registry systems are only of value if the disease has a good prospect for intervention, control, prevention, and for research that can lead to these ends.

For a registry to exist and function registration must be done. **Registration** is the development of a register by creating a permanent record with demographic and identifying data, diagnosis, frequency of occurrence, survival, follow-up work or treatment and other information important and unique to a condition or disease. Cancer is a good example as it can be identified by type of tumor and location. Registration creates a databank from which studies and research can be conducted.

Record Linkage and Computerization

Record linkage systems seem like a new concept that is computer driven. Since the mid-1940s, there has been an effort to link individual birth certificates, death certificates, and marriage and divorce records. A more recent concern is to link cancer registries to hospital records to death certificates for those who have died from cancer. **Record linkage** is the connecting of data and information contained in two or more medical, morbidity, mortality records, and other vital event records.

In recent years, with the advances in computer technology, the linkage of morbidity, life, and mortality events occurs on a regular basis. Several major linkage systems have been developed and many are in the planning stages. Some hospitals have implemented computer systems that capture information from every activity within the hospital, which possibly could be shared with external organizations. Many projects are organization-specific and need to be linked to a central national system using standardized computer systems and software programs. The Oxford Record Linkage Project in England was established in 1962. More modern programs have been implemented in the United States. One of the more ambitious is the MUMPS program (Massachusetts General Hospital's Multi-Programming System) and many others are being developed and implemented in the United States and in many other countries.[2,5] Countries with a centralized, single health care system have made major advances with record linkage systems. Occupation, place of residence, and other data have been linked to medical records in these national health care systems.

Record linkage systems provide an excellent source of information on the courses of diseases, demographic data, use of health care services, fertility, genetic studies, maternal health issues, child health concerns, chronic disease tracking and development over time, family and genetic disease histories, and the natural history of specific diseases or morbidity-related events.[2,3,4,5]

Surveys of Disease and Health Status

The disjointed morbidity and health-related data collected from physicians and hospital medical records fall short of a complete picture on disease in a community, a state, or the nation. Moreover, these data do not present a comprehensive picture of health status or factors that influence, contribute to, or detract from a nation's overall health status. Surveys on specific diseases are conducted in both rural and urban localities. Medical care, control and prevention information is gathered to include stage of disease at diagnosis, sites and information about tumors in cancer cases, and basic information on a whole range of diseases.[3,4,5,6]

In order to gain further knowledge and information, local, state and national morbidity surveys are conducted. Some surveys are aimed at selected diseases or groups of related diseases. In 1956, The U.S. Congress established the ongoing National Health Survey (NHS), which was to provide an ongoing source of data and information about the health status of the United States population, and is to collect comprehensive information on morbidity. The NHS is a major source of nationwide information on common illnesses, injury, disability, functional deficits, and utilization of health care services. The NHS is carried out by the National Center for Health Statistics. Several national surveys are conducted on a continuing basis.

- **The Health Interview Survey**—interviews of noninstitutionalized individuals in households across the nation. Limitation of daily activities, acute disease, chronic conditions, physician visits and hospitalization are some of the items of the interview.
- **Health and Nutrition Examination Survey** (formerly the Health Examination Survey)—conducted to augment the information gathered in the Health Interview Survey. Individuals are sampled from general populations and are examined through health screenings and physical exams in three-year cycles.

- **National Hospital Discharge Survey**—used to collect data about the populations utilizing and discharged from hospitals.

- **National Notifiable Disease Surveillance System**—conducted by the Centers for Disease Control, this system is primarily used to provide weekly information on the occurrences of diseases defined as notifiable. Summary data are provided on an annual basis to health departments and epidemiologists across the nation. *Morbidity and Mortality Weekly Report* and the *Summary of Notifiable Disease in the United States* are the mediums for reporting the notifiable disease status. (See Notifiable Diseases in the United States and Notifiable Disease Reporting System, Figure 2.7, in Chapter 2.)

- **National Nursing Home Survey**—used to collect data about long-term care populations and health status of nursing home residents in the United States.

- **National Ambulatory Medical Care Survey**—a national probability sample survey conducted by the Division of Health Care Statistics, Centers for Disease Control and Prevention. Statistics are presented on patient, physician and visit characteristics for visits of a variety of diseases, acute and chronic.

- **National Family Growth Survey**—provides information about family planning activities and fertility conducted every 5 years, using individual interviews.

- **Survey Linked to Vital Records**—information is obtained from individuals, families, physicians or hospitals about death and birth information to augment birth and death certificate data as well as provide prenatal care and fertility information. Information on morbidity and hospitalization over the previous year is gathered.[3,4,5,6]

EXERCISES

Key Terms

Define and explain the following terms.

attack rate	point prevalence
attributable risk	population at risk
cumulative incidence rate	prevalence
epidemic curve	prevalence rate
force of morbidity	record linkage
gradient of risk	register
incidence	registration
incidence rate	registry
lifetime prevalence	relative risk
morbidity	risk
odds ratio	risk difference
period prevalence	risk factor
per-person incidence	risk marker
person-years	risk ratio

Study Questions

5.1   a. From the case on "Rubella Among the Amish," on page 140 list the factors that are to be included in the numerator of an incidence rate.

   b. What information is needed to complete the denominator part of the incidence rate? List them.

   c. Show the formula (without the denominator data, but a statement for it) for the incidence rate for the Amish rubella outbreak.

   d. Complete the rate formula and calculate the incidence rate using the following fictitious population data. Total Amish population for the 4 states was 79,600, with the children accounting for 29,500 of the total population. Assume the children are the susceptibles and are the population at risk.

5.2   From Figure 5.12 (Tuberculosis outbreak in Lincoln Senior Center).

   a. Determine the incidence rate for June 1st through May 31st.

   b. Determine the period prevalence rate for June 1st through May 31st.

   c. Determine point prevalence rate for April 8th.

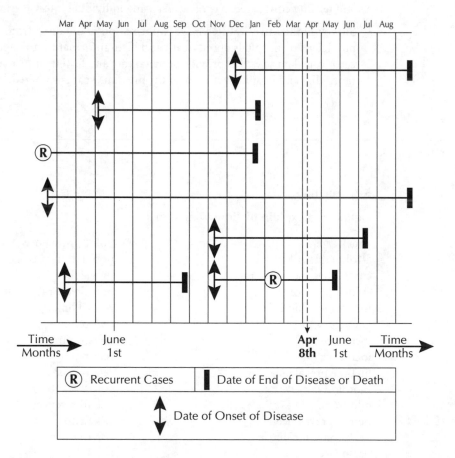

FIGURE 5.12   Tuberculosis outbreak in Lincoln Senior Center with 300 participants.

5.3 From the case example on the *E. coli 0157: H7* outbreak at the Little League barbecue, on pages 143–145.

    a. Set up the epidemiological grid used to determine relative risk for the two different cooks, I. R. Macho and R. M. Cooke.

    b. Calculate the relative risk for those eating hamburger patties cooked by I. R. Macho as compared to R. M. Cooke's. What is the relative risk of getting infected with *E. coli* from hamburgers cooked by I. R. Macho as compared to R. M. Cooke's? Use this information: Mr. Macho cooked 175 hamburgers and 103 people got sick from eating his hamburgers. Mr. Cooke cooked 145 hamburgers and 128 people did not get sick from eating his hamburgers.

    c. Outline in detail the public health standards for cooking hamburgers served to the public. (This information can be sought from the public health department, library, Internet, or textbooks on food services preparation and sanitation.)

5.4 Hillside Elementary School held an end of the school year pot-luck picnic for the 6th grade class. At the picnic, 135 6th graders and 315 parents attended. The menu was green salad, fruit salad, potato salad, rolls, soft drinks, lasagna, and brownies. Of the parents, 275 ate all of the food and 125 pupils ate all the foods. It was found that 45 students came down with staph food poisoning as did 65 parents. Of the people who got sick 90 ate the potato salad. Of the people who got sick 105 ate lasagna. 50 persons had drink only and ate no food.

    a. Calculate the crude attack rate.

    b. Calculate the attack rate.

    c. Calculate the food-specific attack rate for lasagna and for potato salad.

5.5 From the Hillside Elementary School picnic in Question 5.4, 35 people took leftover potato salad home and a total of 95 family members ate it the next day. 55 family members in 15 families came down with staph food poisoning after eating the leftover potato salad. They got ill either that same evening or the next day. 15 other family members got an upset stomach and were ill 3 days later. This is all the information available to you, the epidemiologist.

    a. Calculate the secondary attack rate for this food-poisoning outbreak.

5.6 Explain and discuss in detail the issues surrounding recurrence of cases in period prevalence.

5.7 Explain and discuss all facets of a propagated epidemic, including *time, place,* and *person* factors.

REFERENCES

1. Crowley, L.V. 1992. *Introduction to Human Disease*, 3rd edition. Boston: Jones and Bartlett Publishing Inc.
2. Timmreck, T.C. 1987. *Dictionary of Health Services Management*. Owings Mills, MD: National Health Publishing.
3. McMahon, B. 1970. *Epidemiology: Principles and Methods*. Boston: Little, Brown and Company.
4. Lilienfeld, A.M. and Lilienfeld, D.E. 1980. *Foundations of Epidemiology*. New York: Oxford University Press.
5. Mausner, J. and Bahn, A. 1983. *Epidemiology, An Introductory Text*, 2nd edition. Philadelphia: Saunders.

6. Kelsey, J.L., Thompson, W.D., and Evans, A.S. 1986. *Methods in Observational Epidemiology.* New York: Oxford University Press.

7. Slome, C., Brogan, D., Eyres, S., and Lednar, W. 1982. *Basic Epidemiological Methods and Biostatistics: A Workbook.* Monterey, CA: Wadsworth.

8. Sydenstricker, E. "Statistics of Morbidity," in Buck, C., Llopis, A., Najer, E., and Terris, M. 1988. *The Challenge of Epidemiology: Issues and Selected Readings.* New York: Pan American Health Organization.

9. Wilcox, K.R. 1991. "Outbreaks of Rubella Among the Amish," *Morbidity and Mortality Weekly Report. Centers for Disease Control and Prevention*, Vol. 40, No. 16, April 26, 1991, p. 264.

10. Fox, J.P., Hall, C.E., and Elveback, L.R. 1970. *Epidemiology: Man and Disease.* New York: Macmillan.

11. Morton, R.F., Hebel, J.R., and McCarter, R.J. 1990. *A Study in Epidemiology and Biostatistics.* Gaithersburg, MD: Aspen Publishing.

12. Hennekens, C.H., and Buring, J.E. 1987. *Epidemiology in Medicine.* Boston: Little, Brown and Company.

13. Berkow, R. (Editor). 1982. *The Merck Manual,* 14th edition. Rahway, NJ: Merck.

14. Rothman, K. J. 1986. *Modern Epidemiology.* Boston: Little, Brown and Company.

15. Cieslak, P.R., et al. 1997. "Hamburger-Associated *Escherichia coli 0157: H7* infection in Las Vegas: A hidden epidemic," *American Journal of Public Health*, Vol. 87, No. 2, pp. 176–180.

16. Matthew, E.G., et al. 1973. "A Major Epidemic of Infectious Hepatitis in an Institution for the Mentally Retarded," *American Journal of Epidemiology*, Vol. 98, pp. 199–215.

6

Epidemiology Vital Statistics and Health Status Indicators

CHAPTER OBJECTIVES

This chapter on vital statistics and health status indicators

- presents an overview of vital statistics and their use in epidemiology;
- defines *vital statistics* and related epidemiological terms;
- reviews the census and its role in developing vital statistics information and data;
- reviews the Standard Metropolitan Statistical Area (SMSA) concept and how it applies to epidemiology and vital statistics;
- reviews vital events and the vital events registration process;
- reviews major vital events such as births, deaths, marriages, and divorces, and the epidemiological implications;
- presents sources of epidemiological and vital statistics data;
- presents exercises that assist in review of the concepts and principles of the chapter.

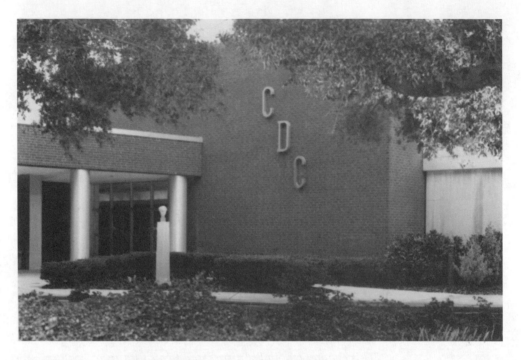

FIGURE 6.1   Centers for Disease Control and Prevention (CDC) produce a variety of statistical reports useful to epidemiologists across the United States. (Picture courtesy of Centers for Disease Control and Prevention, Atlanta, Georgia)

INTRODUCTION

Demographic information and vital statistics data useful to epidemiology, public health, and community health services are available from numerous sources. Of the multitude of sources of data, some are more useful than others to the epidemiologist. Applicability of data also has to be considered. Federal and state sources of demographic and vital statistics data have limited value at the county or city level, while city, county, and regional sources of data are useful for the state. Local and state data are important sources of information for the several national centers that compile and distribute data such as the U.S. Public Health Service, Centers for Disease Control and Prevention (see Figure 6.1), and National Center for Health Statistics. Data has to be collected and distributed using a routine, standardized method and a reliable system. Comparison of data from other countries is difficult due to the lack of standardized collection and publication and a general lack of information.

Vital Statistics

Vital statistics, also called **vital events**, refer to the process of collecting data and applying basic statistical methods to the data in order to identify vital health facts in a given community, population, or region. Morbidity, mortality, life expectancy, births, deaths, marriages, divorces, demographics, and census data are all part of vital statistics. Vital statistics includes population data combined with information pertinent to health status, disease, injury, and death events. In summary vital statistics consists of all population data plus health (disease) related data. The information gained from the collection, analysis, and distribution of data is important for planning and predicting population shifts and changes. Morbidity and mortality information are fundamental to and are useful in planning health services.

Some health insurance companies, health maintenance organizations, and medical clinics gather and compile vital events data. These organizations mostly gather data for internal use to assess financial viability and economic related trends which can be affected by general vital events. Only a few major insurance companies distribute vital statistics reports for general use. The data of insurance companies are limited in their usefulness as the data do not represent general populations. Vital statistics from such sources represent only the clientele/population of the insurance company or HMO. The most useful and reliable data comes from standardized data collection, compilation, publication, and distribution systems of governments. Vital statistics have been and continue to be a government function and responsibility. The U.S. federal government has several data collection systems. The most complex, thorough and oldest of these data collection systems is the U.S. census.

CENSUS OF THE POPULATION

The earliest government **censuses** were conducted in Egypt, Palestine, Babylonia, Rome, and China. The New Testament records census taking in Luke (2:1–3). Taxation apparently was also a reason for census taking. The shortcomings of asking people to go to their city of birth to be taxed are obvious. It is more effective and reliable to have paid government workers to take a census than to ask people to come to be taxed and counted. Rome in the height of its administration and rule also took a regular count of all citizens and slaves.

In the 1860s it was estimated that only about 17 percent of the world's population had been counted. Based on United Nation reports, Weeks suggested that in 1974 only 55% of the world's population had been enumerated. In underdeveloped nations censuses are not taken as often as in developed nations, mostly due to cost. In the United States a census is required by Congress to be taken every 10 years at the beginning of the decade, to determine seats in the House of Representatives.[1,2]

In the United States a census has been conducted every ten years since 1790. Since the seats in U.S. House of Representatives are apportioned on the size and distribution of populations, a census has been mandated by law. Currently the census has an even wider reaching importance. Federal dollars for various health, social, and economic programs are distributed to individual states based on their census. An inaccurate census means unfair distribution of funds.

In 1902, the U.S. Census Bureau became a government agency. *Census* in Latin means "to estimate or assess." In the United States this has meant a ten-year periodic counting of the total population. In 1976 President Gerald Ford, being concerned for the rapid social change taking place within the U.S., passed a bill authorizing a census to be taken midpoint between the regular ten-year census. This census cannot be used for reapportionment.

Grouping and Categories of Groups

In 1970, 1980, and 1990 the census suffered under enumeration of ethnic minorities and each time caused great controversy. Ethnic identity was expanded in the 1980 census to include 15 categories.

The **ethnic and racial categories** include

white	black	Japanese	Chinese
Filipino	Korean	Vietnamese	Asian
Indian	Hawaiian	Guamanian	Samoan
Eskimo	Aleut	American Indian (Tribe should be listed)	

Spanish/Hispanic origin or descent may have several categories:

1. Mexican-American, Mexican, Chicano
2. Puerto Rican
3. Cuban
4. other Spanish

People are often categorized in a rather arbitrary manner that does not present a complete and factual picture. Epidemiologists have much to learn in reporting ethnic and racial background in reports and documents. It is still common today to see many government reports presenting data with only three categories: white, black, others. When there exists so much diversity in health status due to culture, beliefs, genetic makeup, health practices, and behaviors in these highly diverse groups, it is a wonderment how a demographer, or epidemiologist would, in good conscience, make such limited categories. A greater effort must be made to develop reports that accurately represent all nationalities and their differences. The "other," category should be used very conservatively or not all. It does take more time and effort to include more categories of races and ethnic make-up. Reporting systems are not adequately geared to handle the additional categories, but efforts along this line need to be initiated at all levels of government and in private research as well. There is much to be learned in the future when all of the different tribes of Native Americans are treated separately and blacks will be categorized by their group or tribe of origin, instead of naively thinking all Native Americans, blacks, and Asians are alike.

A similar problem exists in the reporting of religion related health occurrences and statistics. The reporting of only three or four categories—Catholic, Protestant, Jewish, and other—presents a problem of reporting misinformation due to the narrow reporting practices. How devout one is in their religion and how strictly one adheres to the practices and beliefs of that religion can be extremely influential on health status. Mormons (members of the Church of Jesus Christ of Latter Day Saints) and Seventh Day Adventists have strong health codes within their religious beliefs. The effect of the health codes will only be significant if the members devoutly participate in the health codes and should be ascertained in any study. If the members do not closely follow the health codes they would be more similar to members of the general of society and religion would have little effect on health statistics. Religions that rely solely on faith healing, such as The Church of Christ, Scientist would also have a much different health status than those religions who use traditional medical care services.

Approaches to Counting the Population

Several approaches to counting a population can be done. Two approaches, based on location of the person at time of enumeration are suggested: *de jure population* and *de facto population*. A *de jure* population count is one of people who belong in a certain place regardless of whether they were in that location on the day of the census count; people are assigned according to the usual place of residence. *De facto* population count is when people are counted by their location at the time of enumeration; counts of people who are in a given place on the census day.[1,2]

When the census is conducted only a few questions are asked of all people and more detailed items are asked of samples of the population. Sample questions are changed each time the census is conducted in order to meet the social, health, and economic needs of the nation at the time. Some census takers visit every household and others receive mail-in questionnaires.[1,2] The Census Bureau conducts a census of population and housing every 10 years. The resulting series of bulletins shows the questions asked in the 1990 census and the answers that the American people gave. Each bulletin focuses on a question or group of questions appearing on the 1990 census questionnaires. Census questions asked include

- gender
- race
- marital status
- Hispanic origin
- type of housing and tenure
- number of rooms and bedrooms
- ancestry
- residence in 1985
- language spoken at home
- year moved in and year structure built
- place of birth, citizenship, and year of entry
- education
- employment status
- work experience in 1989
- complete plumbing and kitchen facilities
- telephone and vehicle availability
- home heating fuels

Questions Asked of All Persons

- household relationships
- sex
- race
- age
- marital status
- number of housing units at address
- plumbing facilities
- number of rooms
- tenure

- rented or owned
- value of home
- rent paid
- vacant, for rent, for sale period of vacancy

Questions Asked of Sample Population (sample of items)

Population related items

- state of birth
- citizenship/year of immigration
- language
- ancestry
- veteran status
- disability or handicapped
- all children ever born
- marital history
- employment status last week
- place of work
- transportation to work
- carpooling
- occupation
- income

Housing related items

- year house built
- year moved in
- source of water
- sewage disposal
- heating equipment and sources
- number of bedrooms
- number of bathrooms
- telephone
- number of automobiles

Assessment and Estimates Between Census Years

For planning of social services, health services, and public health programs, current demographic information about the general population may be needed. The 10-year census data may be dated and of little value, thus current data are needed. How does one go about getting accurate and current data between census years?

Several approaches to projecting **intercensal** counts are used. Reinterviewing is one approach. Reinterviewing is done by selecting a sample of households included in the census and then matching the people in the sample with persons enumerated in the census. Reinterviews are done in order to obtain a better and more accurate count. However, households missed in the regular census count may also be missed in a reinterviewed effort.

Case by case matching is another approach. Case by case matching compares lists of people in the census with lists from agencies and organizations and are matched in order to try to obtain accuracy.[1,2]

Intercensal cohort analysis is still another method. This method is based on the idea that some people of certain ages are more likely to be missed in the count than people in other age groups. By comparing the numbers of females ages 25 to 29 in 1990 with the numbers of females aged 15–19 in 1980, it can be determined whether or not fewer females in 1990 existed than would be expected.[1,2]

Another intercensal method is the *arithmetic method*. The arithmetic method takes the average annual increase between the last two censuses and is used to project the current population. Annual average increase is figured. The annual average increase is divided by the number of years and then added to the last census figure for the community under consideration, giving a fairly accurate projection of the current census.[3]

P_1 was population previous census.
P_2 is population recent census.
P_3 is to be the population next year.

Arithmetic method:

$$P_3 = [(P_2 - P_1) \div 10] + P_2$$

Still another method of census projection in intercensal years is used. The *geometric method* assumes that the population will increase on an average rate for the 10 intercensal years, rather than by the average number used in the arithmetic method. The rate of average growth is projected and then the average growth is used as a projection for each intercensal year. In all cases, migration has to be considered in both methods.[3]

Geometric method:

$$\frac{P_2}{10P_1} \quad \text{rate of growth}$$

$$P_3 \times P_2 + \left(P_2 = \frac{P_2}{10P_1} \right)$$

STANDARD METROPOLITAN STATISTICAL AREA (SMSA)

Communicable diseases and their spread know no boundaries and are no respecters of lines that establish cities, counties, and states. As cities have grown large, their influence has been extended far beyond the city limits that once drew the line between city and country, urban and rural, metropolitan or nonmetropolitan. Due to expanded transportation and the automobile, suburban and urban life have merged, both economically and in the ability to spread disease. The federal government recognized the merger of urban and suburban activity and felt it needed a unit that would encompass both for statistical reasons. Thus, in 1949 the Standard Metropolitan Statistical Area (SMSA) was developed. Each SMSA is made up of a major city with a population of 50,000 as its core and all those who live in the contiguous areas, focusing on the sharing of economic and health services in that area. **Standard Metropolitan Statistical Area (SMSA)**, as defined by the U.S. Bureau of Census, is any county or group of contiguous counties that contain at least one city of 50,000 inhabitants or more and any contiguous counties that are socially and economically integrated with the central city or cities. In New England, where counties are smaller, SMSAs are determined differently.[1,2,4]

SMSAs are used to assess the amount of urbanization and rural area in the United States. The loss of agriculture land to urbanization is tracked and determined by the SMSAs. As cities grow and urban sprawl reaches out into the agriculture areas new SMSAs are formed.[1,2,4]

The key source of data for planning for national health, social, economic, and related activities is the census; data gathered every decennial (ten years). Once the census data have been gathered and analyzed the information is bound in large volumes in the census bureau. Summaries of census data for the nation, each state, and for SMSAs are made available for use in various government agencies and organizations. The census bureau produces subject reports, published from the census information on health and human services, such as fertility, marriage, migration, ethnic groups, etc., which are of value to epidemiology, public health, health planning, and health services.[1,2,3]

SMSAs are used in a variety of ways from assessing public programs, funding of programs, and needs to determining what is rural and what is not. For example, a hospital on the edge of a metropolitan area, to be considered "rural," for special funding exceptions under Medicare, has to be 25 miles from any other hospital.[1,2,3]

VITAL EVENTS REGISTRATION

When you entered this world as a newborn, a certificate of birth was completed by one of your parents and a physician. When you have completed your stay on this earth and die, a death certificate will be filled out and signed by a physician. Somewhere in the middle of these two events was another major event or two. You possibly may have gotten married, and a marriage certificate was completed and registered with the county. Should you have the misfortune of ending the marriage, divorce papers are filed and the statistics are recorded by the county on the divorce.

All vital events are recorded and data of the events are put into charts and graphs. Vital statistics are the data which relate to the vital events of life, namely, birth, death, marriage, divorce, abortion, and succumbing to certain serious diseases. However, morbidity and mortality reporting are presented in separate chapters. The mechanisms of morbidity reporting, obtaining information and handling the data are done quite differently. The completeness of morbidity data is much less than that of mortality and births thus the reliability of the information obtained from these latter sources is much better.[1,2,3,4,5]

In countries where education levels are high, economic conditions are good and a high level of literacy exists, we find the most complete vital statistics registration systems. Less developed countries have less complete and less effective vital statistics systems. Even though the vital events produce statistics about births, and deaths, other demographic and public health information can also be obtained from the recording of the events and the records that the events create. Sex, age, race, religion, education, and occupation and information that may show the risks of these people can also be obtained from the recording of vital events.[1,2,3,4]

When vital statistics data are coupled with census data a more complete picture of a population emerges. Insights into health and social trends can be seen, with the information being used in planning and developing to meet health and human services needs.[1,7] (See Table 6.4 for selected vital events in California in 1990.)

Registration is the recording of births, deaths, marital status, abortion and notifiable diseases and the recording and tracking of persons with selected communicable diseases. Registration of certain other events that might produce data and research insights is also done, for example, the registration of twins. Research on twins, especially if separated at an early age, can provide valuable knowledge gained under no other circumstances, due to the identical genetic make-up of twins.[6]

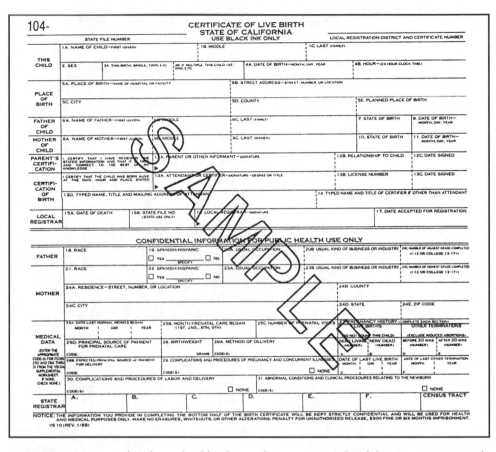

FIGURE 6.2 Sample of standard birth certificate—state of California. (Source: California Center for Health Statistics)

Birth certificates are needed for a variety of reasons such as entering public school, military service, obtaining a driver's license, social security card, acquiring citizenship, professional licenses, insurance, passports, right to vote, etc. Figure 6.2 is a sample birth certificate for the State of California. The National Center for Health Statistics sets forth a standard birth certificate, indicating the minimum information that should be on a birth certificate. Individual states then develop their own using the standard with some states adding additional information, but no state is to use less information than set forth in the standard certificate.[5,6,8]

BIRTH RATE AND CRUDE BIRTH RATE

Birth rates of a total population usually are crude rates and crude rate refers to the total population (see Table 6.1). When using crude rates (birth or death) it is important to consider further assessment with the use of specific rates and age distributions as the characteristics of a population can vary, causing crude rates to vary and be inaccurate. Age is a variable that

TABLE 6.1   Trends in the numbers of births and deaths in the United States for the years 1910 through 1990

Year	Live Births	Birth Rate[1]	Deaths[2]	Death Rate[1]
1910	2,777	30.1	N.A.	14.7
1920	2,950	27.7	N.A.	13.0
1930	2,618	21.3	N.A.	11.3
1935	2,377	18.7	1,393	10.9
1940	2,559	19.4	1,417	10.8
1945	2,858	20.4	1,402	10.6
1950	3,632	24.1	1,452	9.6
1955	4,097	25.0	1,529	9.3
1960	4,258	23.7	1,712	9.5
1965	3,760	19.5	1,828	9.4
1970	3,731	18.4	1,921	9.5
1975	3,144	14.6	1,893	8.8
1980	3,612	15.9	1,990	8.8
1981	3,629	15.8	1,978	8.6
1982	3,681	15.9	1,975	8.5
1983	3,639	15.5	2,019	8.6
1984	3,669	15.5	2,039	8.6
1985	3,761	15.8	2,086	8.7
1986	3,757	15.6	2,105	8.7
1987	3,829	15.7	2,127	8.7
1988	3,913	15.9	2,171	8.8
1989	4,021	16.2	2,155	8.7
1990	4,179	16.7	2,162	8.6

[1] Per 1,000 total population.
[2] Excludes fetal deaths.
(Sources: *Monthly Vital Statistics Reports, Vital and Health Statistics 1989*, National Center for Health Statistics, U.S. Department of Health and Human Services)

can cause any rate based on a total population to produce varying results in different age groups. **Crude birth rates** (and crude death rates, which are presented in Chapter 4) are most useful as they provide summary information as well as general statistics for large populations. **Crude rates** are useful in international comparisons as well as for general comparisons of vital events over time. Crude rates often use a mid-year (July 1st) average population as the denominator. The formula for the crude birth rate is presented below. Specific rates can be used for specific population groups and circumstances. The denominator of a specific rate would be that of the population group under study rather than the total population.[1,2,3,5]

$$\text{Crude birth rate} = \frac{\text{Number of live births to residents in an area in a calendar year}}{\text{Average population in the area in the same year (midyear population)}} \times 1,000$$

MORTALITY AND DEATH CERTIFICATES IN VITAL STATISTICS

Death certificates are also important documents for the families of the deceased and are presented in Chapter 4. The first and obvious need of a death certificate is to meet any legal concerns. Death is taken seriously and laws protect against wrongful death possibilities by tracking and registering deaths in a secure manner. Many novels and movies are made based on the premise of the disposition of a body of a dead person. A death must be registered and if any foul play is suspected it is investigated including an autopsy being performed. Death certificates are also needed for making claims for benefits from retirement pensions and life insurance. Mortality rates and related relevant data (as discussed in Chapter 4) are generated from the death certificate registration process. The National Center for Health Statistics sets forth a standard death certificate, and a standard certificate of fetal death indicating the minimum information that should be on the certificates. Individual states then develop their own using the standard. Some states add additional information to the certificate but no state is to use less information than set forth in the standard death certificate.[2,3,5,6,8]

The detailed filling out of the certificate, in addition to the cause of death being listed on the death certificate, includes the listing of the "underlying cause of death." There is a designated space on the death certificate for other important conditions that contributed to the death. Diagnostic terminology must be that of International Classification of Disease (ICD or ICD-9-CM). (See Chapter 4 for details of the death certificate.)[2,3,5]

Fetal Deaths and Fetal Death Certificates in Vital Statistics

The fetal death certificate (Figure 4.7) provides some information not available elsewhere, produces data on the loss of life that could have been and information on medical services used for the treatment of fetal death situations. **Fetal deaths** include all deaths regardless of age or length of gestation period. In the United States, an embryo after 20 weeks of gestation is considered a fetus and thus counted as a fetal death. The various parties of the debates on abortion attempt to set the time an embryo becomes a fetus at different times, but vital statistics uses the 20 weeks of gestation as the standard.

A standardized vital statistics registration system has been established in the United States. This system outlines the flow of reporting activities of birth certificates, death certificates, and fetal death certificates. The flow of information and paperwork is from the local level, including those persons with closest and most direct contact, i.e., the physician, coroner, funeral directors, and hospital personnel to the local public health department, to the state office of vital statistics to the National Center For Health Statistics. Figure 4.5, on page 106, shows how the registration system works.

THE ROLE OF THE MEDICAL EXAMINER AND CORONER

When a death has any suspicion of homicide, suicide, foul play, or is due to an accident, the attending or family physician cannot sign the death certificate. Local officials, usually the medical examiner or coroner and possibly the police, are notified. An autopsy is usually required and is performed by a medical examiner, who is usually a board certified physician usually in forensic pathology. Medical examiners can be public officials, work under contract, or can be employees of a coroner's office. Each state seems to have different approaches to the public position of coroner and/or medical examiner. A medical examiner may be the one to pronounce a person dead and is the one who will sign the death certificate. A **coroner** is an elected official and may or may not be a physician, let alone a forensic pathologist. In some states the coroner, being an elected official, may be a farmer or a school teacher, yet may have the authority to pronounce a person dead and sign death certificates. The ultimate decision about whether or not to do an autopsy rests with the medical examiner or coroner. Autopsy reports are a source of non-random data which contribute significantly to the understanding of the natural history of disease.

Reportable Deaths to Coroner

Most state governments have set forth laws governing the circumstance, manner, and cause under which a death must be reported to a coroner. The following is an example of a usual list of reportable deaths to the coroner.

1. Unattended deaths
2. Deceased not attended by a physician in the 20 days prior to death
3. Physician unable to state cause of death
4. Known or suspected homicide
5. Known or suspected suicide
6. Involving any crime
7. Related to self-induced or criminal abortion
8. Associated with a rape or crime against nature
9. Following an accident or injury
10. Drowning, fire, hanging, gunshot, stabbing, cutting, starvation, exposure, alcoholism, drug addiction, strangulation, or suffocation
11. Accidental poisoning
12. Known or suspected contagious disease constituting a public hazard
13. All deaths in operating rooms, and all deaths where a patient has not fully recovered from an anesthetic
14. Occupational diseases or occupational hazards
15. Deaths in prison or while under sentence
16. Deaths of all unidentified persons

    (List taken from Code, State of California, Section 27491 and Health and Safety code Section 10250 and Coroner, County of San Bernardino material)

Some coroners are political appointees with a staff of physicians and investigators. Realizing the limitations of the coroner as an elected official, and lack of scientific background, the role has become more investigative and more of a public official than that of dealing with the state of death. Medical examiners and coroners both may have the responsibility to investigate the cause of death. In some counties the coroner has the role to "determine to be dead" but a physician has the responsibility to "pronounce" a person dead. In some counties the medical examiner's office is located within the public health department. Other large counties may have a separate office or the office may be affiliated with a county hospital.

MARRIAGE AND DIVORCE STATISTICS

The family in modern society has changed in structure in the last 30 years. Marriage has become less popular and has decreased while cohabitation has increased, with marriage rates down and divorce rates very high. Marital status affects family structure, socioeconomic status, mental health, access to medical care, and a variety of other health status related factors. An estimated 2.45 million couples married in 1990 which was a 1% increase from 1988 and 1989. In 1960 40% of all women married, but by 1990, only 11% of women were marrying. In the 20 years between the years 1970 and 1990 the percentage of 30- to 34-year-olds who never married had risen from 6% to 16% for females and 9 to 27% for males. In 1960, about 92% of all females were married prior to reaching their 30th birthday. Tables 6.2 and 6.3 present the marital status of the population of the United States by age and sex for 1990. Figure 6.3 presents the marriage and divorce rates in the United States for a 30-year span of time.

For the epidemiologist to gain an understanding of daily occurrences of key vital events, a graph similar to Figure 6.4 and a table like Table 6.4 can be developed for a city, county, state, or country. This graph allows for the comparison of the vital events as well as presenting the events of most concern. Similar graphs could be developed for the list of notifiable diseases or other risk factors of interest to epidemiologists and public health.

TABLE 6.2   Marital status in the United States—Females by age and sex for 1990

		Percent Distribution by Marital Status				
Age	Total Number ('000s)	Single, Never Married	Married, Spouse Present	Married, Spouse Absent	Widowed	Divorced
Female						
18–19	3,683	90.3%	8.2%	1.1%	N.A.	0.4%
20–24	9,117	62.8	31.1	3.2	0.1%	2.8
25–29	10,685	31.1	56.6	4.8	0.4	7.1
30–34	11,094	16.4	67.0	5.3	0.8	10.5
35–39	10,047	10.4	69.7	4.6	1.4	13.8
40–44	8,817	8.0	69.1	4.8	2.3	15.8
45–54	13,012	5.0	70.7	4.6	5.3	14.4
55–64	11,230	3.9	66.1	2.9	17.2	9.9
65–74	9,966	4.6	51.1	2.1	36.1	6.2
75–84	5,792	5.2	27.7	1.4	62.0	3.6
85+	1,475	6.2	10.1	0.5	79.8	3.4
Total 18+	94,977	18.9	56.0	3.7	12.1	9.3

(Source: *Marital Status and Living Arrangments, March, 1990*. U.S. Bureau of the Census, 1991)

TABLE 6.3   Marital status in the United States—Males by age and sex for 1990

		Percent Distribution by Marital Status				
Age	*Total Number ('000s)*	*Single, Never Married*	*Married, Spouse Present*	*Married, Spouse Absent*	*Widowed*	*Divorced*
		Male				
18–19	3,639	96.8%	2.8%	0.3%	N.A.	N.A.
20–24	8,811	79.3	18.4	1.3	N.A.	1.1%
25–29	10,515	45.2	47.4	2.7	0.1%	4.7
30–34	10,947	27.0	61.2	3.8	0.2	7.9
35–39	9,844	14.7	70.0	4.0	0.4	10.9
40–44	8,487	10.5	74.0	3.6	0.5	11.3
45–54	12,292	6.3	77.8	3.6	1.2	11.1
55–64	10,002	5.8	79.5	3.3	3.3	8.1
65–74	8,013	4.7	78.2	2.0	9.2	6.0
75–84	3,562	3.3	71.2	2.6	19.5	3.3
85+	758	3.5	46.9	4.2	43.4	2.0
Total 18+	86,872	25.8	61.3	3.0	2.7	7.2

(Source: *Marital Status and Living Arrangments, March, 1990.* U.S. Bureau of the Census, 1991)

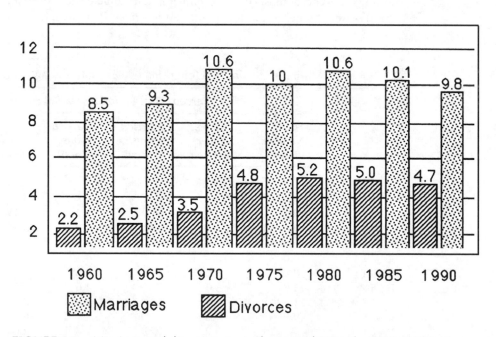

FIGURE 6.3   Marriage and divorce rates in the United States for 1960–1990. Rates are per 1,000 population. (Source: National Center for Health Statistics, *Annual Report—Vital Statistics of the United States, 1991.* Public Health Service,. U.S. Department of Health and Human Services)

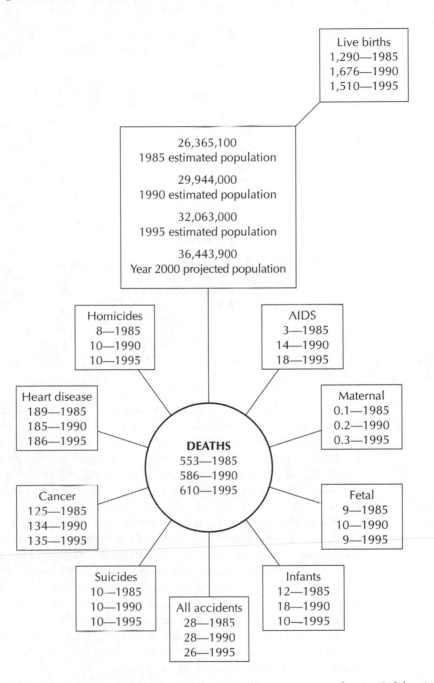

FIGURE 6.4 A day in California. Vital events for an average day in California for the years 1985 through 1995. (Source: Special thanks to Phillip Coon, Health Information and Evaluation Section, Department of Health, County of Riverside, California, and California Center for Health Statistics, 1997)

TABLE 6.4   Selected vital event totals for the year 1990 for the state of California, used to determine information in Figure 6.4

Totals—Selected Vital Events 1990	
Live Births	611,666
Homicides	3,703
Heart Disease	67,425
Cancer	48,896
Suicides	3,735
All Accidents	10,170
Infant Deaths	4,828
Fetal Deaths	3,989
Maternal Deaths	55

(Source: Health Information and Evaluation Section, Department of Health, County of Riverside, California, 1992, and *Data Matters*, California Center for Health Statistics, 1992)

COMPUTER USED IN VITAL STATISTICS AND EPIDEMIOLOGY

The first computer ever developed was a mechanical counting machine developed to assist in counting the census in England in the late 1800s. Mechanical adding machines evolved over time to become highly compact, powerful, electronic data processing devices. What is a bit surprising is that the development of software to assist local public health departments and vital statistics departments in processing and analyzing the data has been slow in its development even though computers were originally developed to help with vital statistics work.

Spreadsheet software programs for both desktop and mainframe computers have been coming forth on regular basis, including those programs that not only analyze the data but produce one-, two-, and three-dimensional graphic displays of the data. Large network and systems of computers, interfaced with central processing areas make access to data readily available to the epidemiologist. The use of computers to process the data and findings of epidemiological studies is discussed in Chapter 7 and the use of computers and networks to collect morbidity data was discussed briefly in Chapter 5. Computer network reporting systems used by federal agencies are mentioned below under the various sources of data. Introductory literature addressing the specific use of computers in vital statistics data analysis and graphic presentation of the findings is needed.

SELECTED SOURCES OF DATA FOR EPIDEMIOLOGICAL AND VITAL STATISTICS INFORMATION

Information in documents from government and nongovernment sources have data that is gathered and reported in various approaches and manners. Thus, the data may vary with respect to source, method of collection, definitions, reporting structure, and time periods. Populations covered by various data collection systems may not be the same, and understanding these differences is critical to interpreting the data. Most data on morbidity and utilization of health resources cover the civilian, noninstitutionalized population. Government reports often exclude certain populations in their reports and the epidemiologist needs to take this into account. Populations excluded from most general studies are military personnel, persons who are younger, institutionalized people of any age, nursing home populations, persons who are older.

All data collection systems have limitations and are subject to error. Records may be incomplete or contain inaccurate information. Some tables and data openly state their limitations. Some studies are limited to only certain populations, or segments of the population. However, the federal government has advanced its survey and data collection to a high level with sampling errors kept to a minimum and large population bases used and in some cases, such as vital statistics, complete counts completed.

The main data gathering activities and sources are from the Department of Health and Human Services, Public Health Service, Centers for Disease Control and Prevention, and National Center for Health Statistics, and additional sources.

National Vital Statistics System
(National Center for Health Statistics)

Through the National Vital Statistics System, the National Center for Health Statistics collects and publishes data on births, deaths, fetal deaths, marriages, and divorces in the United States. Information is received from the registration office of all states, New York City, the District of Columbia, Puerto Rico, U.S. Virgin Islands, and Guam. Some states send their information through the Cooperative Health Statistics System, using computers to report their data to the National Center for Health Statistics called the Vital Statistics Cooperative Program. After 1985 all 50 states participated in the cooperative program.

Studies have shown that 99.3% of all births in the United States are registered. No comparable information is available for deaths, but it is generally believed that death registration is at least as complete as birth registration. Provisional death rates by cause, age, race, and sex are estimated from the Current Mortality Sample. The Current Mortality Sample is a 10% systematic sample of death certificates received each month in the vital statistics office in the states and territories and New York City. All death certificates received during the 1-month period are sampled regardless of the month or year in which the death occurred.

National Survey of Family Growth
(National Center for Health Statistics)

Data from the National Survey of Family Growth are based on samples of women ages 15–44 years in the civilian, noninstitutionalized population living in the United States. The first and second cycles excluded women who had never been married, except those with offspring in the household. The third and fourth cycles include all women ages 15–44, regardless of whether they have ever been married.

The purpose of the survey is to provide national data on the demographic and social factors associated with childbearing, adoption, and maternal and child health. These factors include sexual activity, marriage, unmarried cohabitation, divorce and remarriage, contraception and sterilization, infertility, breastfeeding, pregnancy loss, low birthweight and use of medical care for family planning, infertility, and prenatal care. Interviews are conducted in person by female interviewers using a standardized, printed questionnaire.

National Health Interview Survey (National Center for Health Statistics)

The National Health Interview Survey is a continuing nationwide sample survey in which data are collected through personal household interviews. Information is obtained on personal and demographic characteristics, illnesses, injuries, impairments, chronic conditions, utilization of health resources, and other health topics. The household questionnaire is revised each year. For most health topics data are collected over a calendar year, using a continuous sampling of the civilian noninstitutionalized population in the United States. The survey is designed so that the sample scheduled each week is representative of the target population and the weekly samples are additive over time. The response rate for the survey has been between 95–98% over the years. The expected sample of 49,000 will yield a probability sample of about 127,000 persons. In 1989 a sample of about 117,000 was done.

National Health and Nutrition Examination Survey (National Center for Health Statistics)

The first National Health Examination Survey was conducted in 1960–1962. The focus was on the total prevalence of certain chronic disease as well as the distributions of various physical and physiological measures including blood pressure and serum cholesterol levels. Forty-two primary sampling units in 1,900 geographical units were surveyed. In 1971 a nutrition surveillance component was added and the survey name was changed to the National Health and Nutrition Examination Survey (NHANES).

The first NHANES was conducted from 1971 through 1974, with the purpose of measuring and monitoring indicators of the nutritional status of the American people through various tests and measures, including clinical assessments by physicians. Subsamples of adults on overall health care needs and behavior, with detailed data collected on cardiovascular, respiratory, arthritic, and hearing conditions. NHANES target population was the civilian, noninstitutionalized population ages 1 through 74. Reservations of Native Americans were excluded. Household surveys of 96% of 28,043 people selected by a sampling process were examined.

National Health and Nutrition Examination Survey II was conducted from 1976–1980. Areas of focus were diabetes, kidney and liver functions, allergy, and speech pathology. NHANES target population was the civilian, noninstitutionalized population ages 6 months through 74 years, with 20,322 persons examined. In NHANES three geographically and ethnically distinct populations were studied, Mexican Americans in Texas, New Mexico, Arizona, Colorado, California; Cuban Americans living in Dade County, Florida; and Puerto Ricans living in parts of New York.

National Master Facility Inventory
(National Center for Health Statistics)

The National Master Facility Inventory is a comprehensive field of inpatient health facilities in the United States. The three broad categories of facilities are hospitals, nursing and related care homes, and other custodial or remedial care facilities. To be in the survey a hospital has to have at least 6 beds and a nursing facility has to have 3 beds. The survey is kept current by periodic addition of names and addresses obtained from state licensing agencies for newly established inpatient facilities.

Annual surveys of hospitals and periodic surveys of nursing homes and other facilities are conducted to update the data. From 1968 through 1975, the hospital survey was conducted in conjunction with the American Hospital Association Annual Survey of Hospitals. Nursing homes and related facilities were surveyed off and on from 1963 through 1982. In 1986 nursing homes and related care homes and facilities for the mentally retarded were covered and called the Inventory of Long-Term Care Places.

National Hospital Discharge Survey
(National Center for Health Statistics)

The National Hospital Discharge Survey is a continuing nationwide sample survey of short-stay hospitals in the United States. Prior to 1988 the scope of the survey was patients discharged from hospitals, excluding military and veterans administration hospitals. To be included in the survey a hospital has to have 6 or more beds and 30 days or less length of stay. In 1988 all general and children's hospitals were included with no regard for length of stay.

Information and data from all discharges from hospitals are included in the survey, excluding discharges of newborn infants and all discharges from federal hospitals.

The original sample was selected in 1964 from a list of hospitals from the National Master Facility Inventory. Hospitals were randomly selected according to number of beds and geographic region. Systematic random sample of discharges were from the daily listing sheet. In 1988 the survey was redesigned. Hospitals with the most beds and/or discharges annually were selected with certainty. The remaining sample was selected using a three-stage sampling design. The basic unit of estimation from the survey is the sample patient abstract which is arrayed by primary diagnoses, sex, age group, and date of discharge. In 1989, 408 hospitals participated in the survey.

National Nursing Home Survey
(National Center for Health Statistics)

The National Center for Health Statistics has conducted three National Nursing Home Surveys in 1973, 1977, and 1985–86. In the first survey data were collected on nursing homes, chronic disease and geriatric hospitals, nursing home units and chronic disease wards of general and mental hospitals. The second survey focused on nursing homes and geriatric hospitals. The third survey concentrated on nursing and personal care homes. The third survey was of 1,220 nursing homes selected from 20,479 units. Information was collected through a personal interview with the administrator. Accountants were asked to complete a questionnaire on expenditures or provide a financial statement. Resident data were provided by a nurse familiar with the care provided. Additionally, a sample of registered nurses completed a questionnaire. Health and discharge data were gotten from the medical record. Additional data about the residents were obtained in telephone interviews with next of kin. Data were obtained from 1,097 facilities, 2,763 registered nurses, 5,243 current residents, and 6,023 discharges.

National Ambulatory Medical Care (National Center for Health Statistics)

The National Ambulatory Medical Care Survey is a continuing national survey of ambulatory care medical encounters. The survey covers physician-patient encounters in the offices of non-federally employed physicians classified by the American Medical Association or American Osteopathic Association as office-based, patient-care physicians. Excluded are hospital-based outpatient treatments and nontreating specialties such as pathology, radiology, and anesthesiology. A sample of about 71,594 patient visits was used.

AIDS Surveillance (Center for Infectious Disease, Centers for Disease Control and Prevention)

Acquired immunodeficiency syndrome (AIDS) surveillance is conducted by health departments in each state, territory, and the District of Columbia. Although surveillance activities range from passive to active, most areas employ multifaceted active surveillance programs, which include four major reporting sources of AIDS information: hospitals, and hospital-based physicians, physicians in nonhospital practice, public and private clinics, and medical record systems (death certificates, tumor registries, hospital discharge abstracts, and communicable disease reports). Using a standard confidential case report form, the health departments collect information without personal identifiers, which is coded and computerized either at the Centers for Disease Control and Prevention (CDC) or at health departments from which it is transmitted to CDC.

AIDS surveillance data are used to detect epidemiologic trends, to identify unusual cases requiring follow-up, and for publication in the HIV/AIDS Surveillance Report. Studies to determine the completeness of reporting of AIDS cases meeting the national surveillance definition suggest reporting at greater than or equal to 90%.

National Notifiable Diseases Surveillance System (Centers for Disease Control and Prevention)

The Epidemiology Program Office (EPO) of the Centers for Disease Control and Prevention (CDC) in partnership with the Council of State and Territorial Epidemiologists (CSTE), operates the National Notifiable Diseases Surveillance System. The purpose of this system is primarily to provide weekly provisional information on the occurrence of diseases defined as notifiable by CSTE. The system also provides summary data on an annual basis. State epidemiologists report cases of notifiable diseases to EPO, which tabulates and publishes these data in the *Morbidity and Mortality Weekly Report (MMWR)* and the *Summary of Notifiable Diseases, United States.*

Notifiable disease reports are received from 52 areas in the United States and 5 territories. Completeness of reporting varies because not all cases receive medical care and not all treated conditions are reported. Although State laws and regulations mandate disease reporting, any reporting to CDC is voluntary. Some diseases not considered notifiable and reportable by CDC may be reportable by some local and state authorities. Under-reporting of some diseases continues to be a problem.

Abortion Surveillance (Center for Health Promotion and Education, Centers for Disease Control and Prevention)

The Centers for Disease Control and Prevention (CDC) acquire abortion statistics from the states where they occur, usually from three different sources—central health agencies, hospitals and other medical facilities, and the National Center for Health Statistics. Most central health agencies have developed direct reporting systems. Epidemiologic surveillance of abortion was initiated in eight states in 1969, and now statewide abortion data are reported by all states. The total number of abortions reported to CDC is about 16% less than the total estimated by the Guttmacher Institute.

Alan Guttmacher Institute Abortion Survey (The Alan Guttmacher Institute, Planned Parenthood Federation of America)

The Alan Guttmacher Institute conducts an annual survey of abortion providers. Data are collected from hospitals, nonhospital clinics, and physicians identified as providers of abortion services. The survey included 3,092 health care providers. The purpose was to assess the completeness of the provider and abortion counts. Supplemental surveys are conducted of a sample of obstetrician-gynecologists and a sample of hospitals not in the original survey, identified by the American Hospital Association as providing abortion services.

U.S. Immunization Survey (Division of Immunizations, Centers for Disease Control and Prevention)

This system is the result of a contractual agreement between the Centers for Disease Control and Prevention (CDC) and the U.S. Bureau of Census. Estimates from the immunization survey are based on data obtained during the third week of September in certain years for a subsample of households which are interviewed by the current population survey.

The reporting contains demographic variables and vaccine history along with disease history when relevant to vaccine history. The system is used to estimate the immunization level of the nation's child population against the vaccine-preventable diseases. From time to time, immunization level data on the adult population are collected.

Starting in 1979, the questionnaire was modified to solicit information regarding the source of immunization as given by the interviewee. This change was made to measure the percent of responses for which a family immunization record was the source of the information. In this last survey 37,500 households were surveyed.

National Occupational Hazard Survey
(National Institute for Occupational Safety and Health)

The National Occupational Hazard Survey was conducted by the National Institute for Occupational Safety and Health (NIOSH) to obtain data on employee exposure to particular chemicals and physical agents in various industries. A sample of 4,636 urban workplaces that fall within the scope of Occupational Health and Safety Act were selected by the U.S. Department of Labor, Bureau of Labor Statistics for the survey that was conducted from 1972 to 1974. Information solicited profiled the size of facility, medical and industrial hygiene programs, and a "walk through" of the worksite. Also, employees, who were potentially exposed to the same chemicals and physical agents were listed by job title. All materials and physical agents each employee group encountered, regardless of toxicity; hazardous nature; conditions of use; and the presence, absence, or effectiveness of any exposure control measures were examined. For each potential exposure listed within an occupational group the surveyor also recorded the duration, intensity, form, and the control utilized, and whether it functioned.

National Occupation Exposure Survey
(National Institute for Occupational Safety and Health)

During 1981–83, the National Institute for Occupational Safety and Health (NIOSH) conducted a second national survey of worksites. The second survey, National Occupational Exposure Survey information was collected essentially identical to the previous one mentioned above.

National Survey of Drinking
(National Institute on Alcohol Abuse and Alcoholism)

Data on trends in alcohol consumption were drawn from national surveys funded by the National Institute on Alcohol Abuse and Alcoholism and the National Institute on Drug Abuse. The 1979 survey was based on self-reported consumption and was designed to represent adults 18 years of age and over, living in households in the United States. 1,772 interviews were conducted.

National Household Surveys on Drug Abuse
(National Institute on Drug Abuse)

The National Household Surveys on Drug Abuse are done to show trends in use of marijuana, cigarettes, and alcohol among youths 12–17 years of age and young adults 18–25 years of age. The 1988 survey is the ninth in a series since that began in 1971 under the auspices of the National Commission on Marijuana and Drug Abuse. Since 1974, the survey has been sponsored by the National Institute on Drug Abuse.

The survey covers the population 12 years of age and older in the United States. Youths, young adults, blacks, and Hispanics are over sampled. The most recent survey (1988) is based on home personal interviews of 8,814 Americans 12 years of age and older.

The Drug Abuse Warning Network
(National Institute on Drug Abuse)

The Drug Abuse Warning Network (DAWN) is a large-scale ongoing drug abuse data collection system based on information from a nonrandom sample of emergency room and medical examiner reports. DAWN collects information only about those drug occurrences which have resulted in a medical crisis or death. The major objectives of the DAWN data system include the monitoring of drug abuse patterns and trends, identification of substances associated with drug abuse episodes, and the assessment of drug-related consequences and other health hazards. Data come from 21 metropolitan area emergency rooms throughout the United States. Medical examiner data are collected from 27 metropolitan areas.

Surveys of Mental Health Organizations
(National Institute of Mental Health)

Several inventories of mental health organizations are conducted. The Inventories of Mental Health Organizations are the primary source of information for the National Institute of Mental Health. Questionnaires are mailed every other year to mental health organizations in the United States. The purpose of these surveys is to determine the socio-demographic, clinical, and treatment characteristics of patients served by mental health facilities.

Surveillance, Epidemiology and End Results Program
(National Cancer Institute)

In the Surveillance, Epidemiology and End Results Program (SEER) the National Cancer Institute contracts with 11 population-based registries throughout the United States and Puerto Rico to provide data on all residents diagnosed with cancer during the year and to provide current follow-up information on all previously diagnosed patients.

Data are submitted to the institute twice a year. Patients included are those diagnosed between 1973 and 1986 and are included in survival calculations using the actuarial method. Population estimates used to calculate incidence rates are obtained from the U.S. Bureau of the Census. Life tables used to determine normal life expectancy when calculating relative survival rates were obtained from the National Center for Health Statistics. Separate life tables are used for each race-sex-specific group included in the SEER program.

Estimate of National Health Expenditures Survey
(Health Care Financing Administration)

Estimates of National Health Expenditures for Health (National Health Accounts) are compiled annually by type of expenditure and source of funds. Health expenditure estimates presented go back to 1960 with extensive revisions. Revisions include the addition of new categories of service, such as home health. New categories of sources of funds are also included, such as nonpatient revenues as well as changes in concepts, data sources, and methodology in dealing with data and its sources.

An array of sources are used. The American Hospital Association data on hospital finances are the primary source for estimates relating to hospital care. Salaries of facility-paid physicians and other health care providers are included in the survey process as components of hospital care. Expenditures for services of private health professionals (physicians, dentists, chiropractors, etc.) are estimated from Internal Revenue Service (IRS) data. U.S. Bureau of Census Services Annual Survey and the quinquennial Census of Service Industries have been used to augment IRS data. Expenditures for drugs and other medical nondurable goods and vision products and durable products purchased in retail outlets are based on estimates of personal consumption expenditures prepared by the U.S. Department of Commerce's Bureau of Economic Analysis and on industry data on prescription drug transactions. Durable goods provided by health care providers are excluded under this category.

Nursing homes and homes for the mentally retarded expenditures cover care rendered. Spending estimates are based upon revenue data from the National Nursing Home Survey. Sources used to estimate state and local government spending for health are the U.S. Bureau of Census' Government Finances report and Social Security Administration reports on State-operated Workers' Compensation programs. Overall sources of funding estimates come from a multiplicity of sources including private professional health care provider associations.

Medicare Statistical System
(Health Care Financing Administration)

The Medicare Statistical System provides data from examining the program's effectiveness and for tracking the eligibility of enrollees and the benefits they use, the certification status of institutional providers and the payments made. Records are maintained on about 33 million enrollees and 24,000 participating institutional providers, with about 420 million bills for services processed annually.

The four major areas, accessed through computer files are the health insurance master file, the service provider file, the hospital insurance claims file, and the supplementary medical insurance payment records file. The files contain specific detailed information ranging from basic demographic information to types of supplies and services used to facility statistics to amounts paid out by type of provider.

Data from the Medicare statistical system provide information about enrollee use of benefits from a point in time or over an extended period. Reports are produced on enrollment, characteristics of participating providers, reimbursements and services used.

Medicaid Data System
(Health Care Financing Administration)

The majority of Medicaid data are compiled from forms submitted annually by State Medicaid Agencies to the Health Care Financing Administration (HCFA) for Federal fiscal years (ending Sept. 30th).

Data and counts are based on eligibility and only count each person once, in the year they enroll. Some states handle data differently and report an individual in several categories, making the sum of all basis-of-eligibility cells greater than the "total recipients" numbers.

Expenditure data include payment for all claims adjudicated or paid during the fiscal year of the report. This differs from summing payments for services rendered in the same reporting period. Some states fail to send in all forms, which leaves data missing. For errors in data HCFA estimates values that appear to be more reasonable.

U.S. Census of Population
(Bureau of the Census, Department of Commerce)

The census has been taken every ten years in the U.S. since 1790. In the 1980 census, data were collected on sex, race, age and marital status from 100 percent of the enumerated population. More detailed information such as income, education, housing, occupation and industry were collected from a 20% sample. Places of 2,500 or less population received 50% coverage and places of 2,000 population took one out of 6 households to survey.

Current Population Survey
(Bureau of the Census, Department of Commerce)

The Current Population Survey (CPS) is a household sample survey of the civilian, non-institutionalized population conducted monthly by the U.S. Bureau of the Census. The survey is conducted to provide estimates of employment, unemployment, and other characteristics of the general labor force, the population as a whole, and various other subgroups of the population. The last sample was from 729 sample areas in all states and District Columbia. In 1989, 55,800 households were interviewed.

Population Estimates
(Bureau of the Census, Department of Commerce)

National estimates are derived by use of decennial census data as benchmarks and from data available from various agencies as follows: births and deaths (Public Health Service); immigrants (Immigration and Naturalization Service); the Armed Forces (Department of Defense); net movement between Puerto Rico and the U.S. mainland (Puerto Rico Planning Board); and Federal employees abroad (Office of Personnel Management and Department of Defense). State estimates are based on similar data and also on a variety of data series including school statistics from state departments of education and parochial school systems.

Current estimates are generally consistent with official decennial census figures and do not reflect the amount of estimated decennial census under enumeration.

Consumer Price Index
(Bureau of Labor Statistics Department of Labor)

The Consumer Price Index (CPI) is a monthly measure of the average change in the prices paid by urban consumers for a fixed market basket of goods and services. This index represents the buying/spending habits of 80% of the population in the United States.

In calculating the index, price changes for various items in each location were averaged together with weights that represent their importance in the spending of all urban consumers. Local data were then combined to obtain a U.S. city average.

The 1987 revision of the CPI reflected spending patterns based on the Survey of Consumer Expenditure from 1982 to 1984, the 1980 Census of Population, and the ongoing Point-of-Purchase Survey. Using this improved sample, prices for goods and services required to calculate the index are collected in 85 urban areas throughout the United States and from about 21,000 retail and service establishments. Data on rents are collected from 40,000 tenants and 20,000 owner-occupied housing units. Food, fuels, and a few other items are priced monthly in all 85 locations.

The 1987 revision changed the treatment of health insurance in the cost-weight definitions for medical care items. Three new indexes have been created by separating previously combined items, for example, eye care from other professional services and inpatient and outpatient treatment from other hospital and medical services.

Employment and Earnings
(Bureau of the Census, Department of Commerce)

The Division of Monthly Industry Employment Statistics and the Division of Employment and Unemployment Analysis of the Bureau of Labor Statistics (BLS) publish data on employment and earnings. The data are collected by the Bureau of the Census, State Employment Security Agencies, and State Departments of Labor in cooperation with the BLS. The major source of data is the Current Population Survey.

National Aerometric Surveillance Network
(Environmental Protection Agency)

The Environmental Protection Agency (EPA), through extensive monitoring of activities conducted by federal, state and local air pollution control agencies, collects data on the six pollutants for which National Ambient Air Quality Standards have been set. These pollution control agencies submit data quarterly to EPA's National Aerometric Data Bank (NADB). About 3,400 total stations report air pollution data.

Demographic Yearbook
(Statistics Office, United Nations)

The *Demographic Yearbook* is a comprehensive collection of international demographic statistics. Questionnaires are sent annually and monthly to more than 220 national statistical services and government offices. To insure comparability, rates, ratios, and percentages have been calculated in the Statistical Office of the United Nations.

Lack of international comparability between estimates arises from differences in concepts, definitions, and time of data collection. The comparability of population data is affected by several factors including (1) the definitions of the total population, (2) the definitions used to classify the population into its urban and rural components, (3) difficulties relating to age reporting, (4) the extent of over- or under-numeration, and (5) the quality of population estimates. The completeness of vital statistics data vary from one country to another. Differences in statistical definitions of vital events may also influence comparability.

World Health Statistics Annual (Statistics Office, United Nations)

The *World Health Statistics Annual* is an annual volume of information on vital statistics and causes of death, designed for use by the medical and public health professions. Each volume is the result of a joint effort of the United Nations and the World Health Organization (WHO).

Information published on late fetal and infant mortality is based on official national data available through WHO. Selected life-tables are calculated from a uniform methodology used on national mortality data of WHO. International comparability of estimates are affected by the same limitations as mentioned under the *Demographic Yearbook*.

PRIVATE PROFESSIONAL ASSOCIATIONS AS SOURCES OF DATA

American Association of Colleges of Osteopathic Medicine

This association compiles data on various aspects of osteopathic medical education.

American Dental Association (ADA)

The ADA conducts annual surveys of predoctoral dental educational institutions, reports information from dental schools on student characteristics, financial management, and curricula.

American Hospital Association (AHA)

The AHA conducts an annual Survey of Hospitals—all hospitals in the United States. Overall 6,322 hospitals report data.

American Medical Association (AMA)—Surveys:

Physician Masterfile: Since 1906 the AMA has maintained a master file on almost every physician in the United States. A census of physicians is conducted every 4 years. Masterfile data are obtained for 2,100 organizations and institutions. Data are collected and processed on an ongoing basis for over 550,000 physician records.

Association of American Medical Colleges

Information is collected on student enrollment in medical schools, through the annual Liaison Committee on Medical Education questionnaire: the fall enrollment questionnaire.

Other data sources are the institutional profile system, the premedical students questionnaire, the minority student opportunities in medicine questionnaire, the faculty roster system, data from the Medical College Admission Test, and one-time survey developed for special projects.

National League of Nursing

The annual survey of Schools of Nursing is conducted each October. Questionnaires are sent to all graduate nursing programs for RN and LPN programs. Enrollments, admissions and graduates data are recorded.

Public Health Foundation—Association of State and Territorial Health Officials Reporting System

The Association of State and Territorial Health Officials Reporting System is operated by the Public Health Foundation as a statistical system that provides comprehensive information about the public health programs of state and local health departments. An annual survey of the official state health agency in each state or territory is conducted. The survey includes extensive detail on the agencies' expenditures and funding sources, and the services and activities in two program areas: personal health and environmental health. Supplementary data on clients, services, and selected health outcomes are collected in the areas of maternal and child health, handicapped children's services, dental health, and tuberculosis control. Special studies are done on public health topics of high national priority.

InterStudy; National Health Maintenance Organization Census

InterStudy conducts a census of all HMOs in the United States.

EXERCISES

Key Terms

Define and explain the following terms.

birth rate	intercensal
census	registration
coroner	Standard Metropolitan Statistical Area
crude birth rate	(SMSA)
crude rates	vital events
ethnic and racial categories	vital statistics
fetal death	

Study Questions

6.1 Calculate the current intercensal population for your county for last year, the current year and for the next 2 years using

a. the arithmetic method.
b. the geometric method.

(Hint: Contact your local Department of Health / Vital Statistics Office, County Planning Office to obtain census statistics. Appropriate reference books in libraries have population statistics about counties, as do some on-line computerized databases that may be accessed by personal computers or in libraries.

6.2 You are faced with a case of a 71-year-old female born on May 12th, who has just died today in the emergency room of COPD. She was brought to the emergency room due to automobile accident that injured her head and ribs. The Hispanic patient smoked 2.5 packs of cigarettes a day and weighed 365 lbs. On the Certificate of Death (Figure 4.6) which boxes can you fill in from the information given above? List the box number and the information you would place in each box. (Some personal investigation and use of ICD-9-CM may be needed.)

6.3 Anne T. Emm, a 15-year-old female has just given birth to a 4 lb, 6 oz, 18-inches-long baby. The baby has been born with cleft lip. She was born in Cornfield View Hospital, Cornfield County, Hays, Kansas. The father's name is Leo L. Ianhearted. The father's name is to be listed on the birth certificate. The parents are not married. Dr. Spock is the attending physician. The birth was to be normal, but the baby had to be taken by C-section due to fetal distress after 40 hours of labor. You name the child. On the certificate of birth, which boxes can you fill out in the birth certificate from the information given above? List the box number from the birth certificate and the information you would place in each box.

6.4 Research the annual vital events data for a city, county, or a nation (the United States), and develop a graphic presentation of the vital events which occur each day for the chosen population as found in Figure 6.4.

6.5 List all vital statistics, health statistics and demographic data that is available on

a. a birth certificate;
b. a death certificate.

6.6 List all of the various ethnic and racial categories used in the U.S. Census. Explain and discuss the importance of using all of the various race and ethnic categories in research and reporting the findings of epidemiological studies.

6.7 Using the information found Figure 4.5, draw a diagram and label it in detail, including appropriate official personnel, the flow of the filing and registration process for

a. a birth certificate;
b. a death certificate.

6.8 Using a computer spreadsheet, computer graphics, and the information in Table 6.1 on page 180, develop a chart of bar graphs comparing the live birth rate to the death rate for all years listed from 1910 through 1990.

REFERENCES

1. Weeks, J.R. 1981. *Populations*. Belmont, CA: Wadsworth.
2. Mausner, J.S. 1985. *Epidemiology: An Introductory Text*. Philadelphia: Saunders.
3. Grant, M. 1987. *Handbook of Community Health*, 4th edition. Philadelphia: Lea & Febiger.
4. Timmreck, T.C. 1987. *Dictionary of Health Services Management*, 2nd edition. Owings Mills, MD: National Health Publishing.
5. Fox, P.J., Hall, C.E., and Elveback, L.R. 1970. *Epidemiology, Man and Disease*. New York: Macmillan.
6. MacMahon, B., and Pugh, T.F. 1970. *Epidemiology*. Boston: Little, Brown and Company.
7. Timmreck, T.C. 1991. *Handbook of Planning and Program Development for Health and Social Services*. San Bernardino, CA: Health Management Development Associates.
8. National Center for Health Statistics. 1991. *Health in the United States 1990*. Hyattville, MD: U.S. Department of Health and Human Services, Public Health Service, Centers for Disease Control and Prevention, National Center for Health Statistics.

7

Descriptive Statistics in Epidemiology

CHAPTER OBJECTIVES

This chapter on descriptive statistics as used in epidemiology

■ reviews the role of descriptive statistics in epidemiology;

■ presents the basic concepts and principles of descriptive statistics;

■ presents concepts such as different kinds of data, percentages, central tendency, and measures of dispersion;

■ presents the formation and use of tables and the different approaches commonly used;

■ presents the formation and use of graphs, charts, and figures and the different approaches commonly used;

■ presents examples of the different approaches to and use of charts and graphs in the practice of epidemiology and in epidemiological reports;

■ reviews the concepts of the chapter through exercises and defining related terms.

INTRODUCTION

Epidemiology is a scientific methodology used to study epidemics and the findings, and results of epidemiological studies are used by public health and the practice of medicine to control disease outbreaks and prevent future occurrences of disease. The general purpose for and existence of epidemiology is to support the activities of public health programs. In its infancy epidemiology studied epidemics in relation to time, place and person, a construct that is still valuable and used today. Additionally, epidemiology has had a strong biological and medical science foundation, which is also still important today. Even though the understanding of illness, disability, and causes of death have changed over time due to chronic disease, behaviorally implicated and lifestyle related disease, the disease model is still viable and useful for the study and practice of epidemiology. The basic foundation of and premise on which epidemiology has functioned in the past remains today.

COMPUTERS IN EPIDEMIOLOGICAL DESCRIPTIVE STATISTICS

Due to technology, the biomedical foundations of epidemiology have evolved to a highly complex science as have the statistics used in support of the analysis of epidemiological findings. Computers provide the ability to develop databases on a whole range of diseases, both communicable and chronic, and have changed the face of epidemiology data collection and analysis. Using computers for compiling and analyzing data has made the assessment of data both easier and more complex at the same time. Easier, because the computer does the calculations that used to be done by hand or machine; complex, because of the numerous possibilities, approaches and arrangements of data analysis, that computers provide. Due to the intricate and complex analysis that computers provide, the scientist now has the ability to do many more statistical analyses and can use many more types of statistical approaches, all of which can generate a whole range of different tables, graphs, and charts, providing an easy-to-study pictorial representation of the data.

The foundational activities of epidemiology are based on logical thinking, common sense and deductive reasoning. As science and the field of statistics has advanced in recent years, so have the approaches to epidemiologic studies and the computerized analysis. Because of the advances in statistics and the use of statistics in medical science research, and the close relationship of epidemiology to these fields, epidemiology seems to have become mixed up in and confused with the field of biostatistics. Unfortunately, epidemiology has become more of a mathematical and statistical exercise in search of not only the numerator and denominator of rates and ratios, but the p value of empirical studies basic to biostatistics. The merging of epidemiology and biostatistics has caused epidemiology to begin to be lost to biostatistics and causes epidemiology's identity to become clouded. Many new textbooks address epidemiology in terms of statistical analysis and biostatistics and say little about basic epidemiology.

This introductory textbook takes the position that epidemiology and biostatistics are two separate fields of study. Biostatistics do provide advanced analysis and probability assessment, as used in clinical trials, prospective studies and pure empirical research. The true foundation of epidemiology, founded on retrospective studies, descriptive statistics, and the tables used in the presentation of data, will be retained as the foundation of epidemiology in this text. The focus of epidemiology is on basic public health activities, disease control and prevention and will remain the emphasis. Thus, this text will take the student through descriptive statistics and tabular presentations up to the edge of inferential statistics or biostatistics but will not go into a study of biostatistics nor get lost in search of the p value. The development of a plethora of multivariate statistical approaches combining an ever increasing number of variables, will be left to traditional empirical research, the scientific method as used in basic scientific research design and inferential statistics. The student wishing advanced inferential statistical analysis should consult a text on basic statistics or biostatistics.[1,2,3,4,5,6]

Empirical research methods are the research approaches which use prospective studies and an experimental research design. **Inferential statistics** are the statistical methods, using mathematical formulas which are applied to parametric data, rely on the reasoning that uses probability statistics, approaches and formulas, and have a final statement about the levels of probability about the findings. **Biostatistics** is the application of mathematical statistics and techniques to research information and data collected related to medicine, biomedical science, health and social problems, using inferential statistics as the basis for analysis of the data which includes a statement about p values, the results, and analysis.

DESCRIPTIVE STATISTICS BASICS

Descriptive statistics are used in epidemiology to develop rates, ratios, and proportions (percentages) of morbidity and mortality statistics for use in public health and vital statistics. Moreover, descriptive statistics are used for the understanding, prevention, and control of diseases in populations. The student of and professional in epidemiology must not lose sight of the fact that all activities of the epidemiologist are applied and are for studying and controlling epidemics and disease outbreaks affecting populations and the health status of cities, counties, and states, as well as the nation as a whole. The student of epidemiology and the professional must not get lost in the process of conducting pure research and lose sight of the fact that epidemiological research is a tool used to understand the cause of, prevention of, and control of the spread of disease, disability, injury, disorders, conditions, and death. Fascination with the research process must not give way to the original applied intent and purpose of epidemiology, epidemiology research, and the use of descriptive statistics.[1]

Descriptive statistics describe the frequency and distribution of morbidity and mortality and all the characteristics and causes associated with disease, conditions, disorders, disability, and death. Chapters 4 and 5 provide in-depth detail about the rates, ratios, and proportions used in the analysis of morbidity, mortality, and vital statistics.

Descriptive statistics provide data, information, and insights into the characteristics which are present in a group or population suffering an outbreak of a disease and the absence of disease in unaffected groups or populations. Descriptive statistics assist the epidemiologist in answering traditional epidemiological questions such as: Are there any characteristics present in the affected population that are not present in people who do not have the disease? For example, why are breast cancer rates lower in women who have had children and did breast feeding as compared with women who have had no children?

Descriptive statistics also rely on and refer to many variables associated with morbidity and mortality. The following is a list of variables useful in epidemiological descriptive statistics.

- age
- gender
- season
- marital status
- ethnicity
- income
- race
- occupation
- dates (year)
- geographical location
- education
- religion

Of the many variables used in descriptive statistics, age is the one variable that must be considered first and most often. *Age* will provide the epidemiologist with more information about a population and the variability of research findings than any other single variable.

The main use of descriptive statistics in epidemiology is to show the relationship and association between disease, conditions, and death and the implication caused by the above-mentioned variables. The cause-effect association between morbidity or mortality and certain variables or factors in life provide the epidemiologist opportunities to develop disease prevention and control programs. The underlying aim is the reduction of death in groups or populations and the society as a whole. The end goal is to understand the relationship of the causes of disease and death so interventions can occur, resulting in an improved overall health status of the population.

Mausner and Bahn suggest that descriptive epidemiology encompasses "person, place, and time," as foundational concepts that are used to describe the events and activities that surround or may affect disease outbreaks. Descriptive statistics are not to be confused with the descriptive aspects of person, place, and time, which are covered in Chapter 8.

Descriptive statistics are the mathematical aspects of epidemiology. Inferential statistics embrace the basic concepts of calculus and algebra. Descriptive statistics use basic math skills and stop where inferential statistics begin. Rate, ratios, and proportions are the common sources of descriptive statistics. The use of rates and ratios, covered in detail in Chapters 4 and 5, include many of the formulas and their applications to descriptive statistics in epidemiology. See Table 7.1 for a comparison of descriptive and inferential statistics.

TABLE 7.1　Descriptive versus inferential statistics

Descriptive Statistics	*Inferential Statistics*
Qualitative	Quantitative
Nonparametric	Parametric
Observational	Analytical
Rate, ratio, proportion	Probability, levels of chance/significance

AIDS/HIV
(Epidemics, Prevalence, Prevention, and Control)

AIDS Cases Continue to Grow in Young Adults

AIDS (Acquired Immune Deficiency Syndrome) cases in the United States continue to climb, yet deaths from HIV infection-related illness have decreased. Twenty-eight different diseases are used to define full-blown AIDS.

Teenage sexual activity and premarital sex has greatly increased in recent years, even in the face of the AIDS epidemic. The Centers for Disease Control and Prevention report that 25.6% of 15-year-old girls and 75.3% of unmarried 19-year-old girls have had sexual intercourse. Overall, an average of 51.5% of girls report having sex by their late teens, nearly double the 28.6% from 1970. Having several sex partners as a teen can haunt both males and females later, even if they end up married or monogamous, as they never really know if they were infected. With each new partner there is the chance of being exposed to HIV.

Blacks of both sexes have the highest premarital sex and cases of AIDS, followed by Hispanics, whites and Asians, who have the least. In a 1994 CDC report, one out of every 92 young American men, ages 27–39 are infected with the AIDS virus. The CDC warns that AIDS is threatening young adults more each year and in 1993, AIDS became their number one killer. AIDS started as a major problem in large cities and has now spread to smaller cities. In a CDC report in 1996, it was reported that the AIDS virus was responsible for a third of all deaths among black men ages 25 to 44 and a fifth of all deaths among black women. The death rate from AIDS for young black men in 1994 was 177.9 per 100,000, four times the rate for white males. The rate of AIDS for young black women was reported at 51.2 per 100,000 in 1994. This rate rose 28 percent from the 1993 rate of 40.1.

The AIDS epidemic has spread to all corners of America. Two rare types of HIV have been seen; in France an exotic hard-to-diagnose strain was reported in 1994 and a case was found in the United States. A second rare type of HIV, Group O, was recently discovered.

Tests for HIV/AIDS have improved, but not all strains show up in the current tests. Blood banks are experimentally testing a new saliva test that is simple, painless, and effective. Blood tests are currently the only way HIV/AIDS testing can be done. Vaccines for AIDS continue to be a major focus of research on prevention and control of this epidemic disease. One vaccine for use on infants failed, but an oral AIDS vaccine is being tested experimentally on humans in San Francisco that is claimed to be safe with the further advantage that the body responds by making both antibodies and infection-fighting cells.

(Source: Centers for Disease Control and Prevention)

TYPES AND SOURCES OF DATA FOR DESCRIPTIVE STATISTICS

Four types of data scales are generally used in descriptive statistics: (1) nominal, (2) ordinal, (3) interval, and (4) ratio.

Nominal

Nominal scales are used to classify observations using categories that lack order and cannot be numerically arranged. If numbers are used, the numbers are not for calculation but serve only as labels. Categories are age, sex, race, religion, occupation, etc. Nominal scales place each observation into a separate category. For example, when asking about race in an epidemiology survey, the epidemiologist would place the subjects into a range of different categories such as white, black, Hispanic, Native American, Asian, Puerto Rican. Categories do not have to be numbered and if numbers are used they are only used as labels for identifying categories.

Ordinal

Ordinal scales are used to put order to the categories. Categories are set up so that one is higher than others and other categories are lower, and numbers can be used to label these various categories. Numbering different levels within the scales puts order to the categories. The typical use of ordinal scales is the five-point scale that categorizes information from lower to higher with order in the categories. This is sometimes referred to as a Likert scale. Much more information is provided by the ordinal scale process. Quantity and quality are given to categories by placing them in an ordered scale. For example, if in a public health survey, potential participants are asked if they would go to an immunization clinic if provided in the neighborhood, a five-point ordinal scale could be used for this and other questions (categories). A sample 5-point scale question could be developed as presented below.

Example: (From a health clinic survey questionnaire).

Question 3. If an immunization clinic was held in your neighborhood would you take your children to the clinic for their immunizations? (Check the box that applies most to your intention.)

1 _____	2 _____	3 _____	4 _____	5 _____
Not likely to attend	Will consider attending	May attend	Most likely will attend	Will attend for certain

Interval

The **interval scale** divides categories with equal distance between categories or units of measure. The interval scale has no zero point. Interval scales provide more information than nominal and ordinal data. The number structure in interval data has value assigned to it and the distance between numbers or the number differences provides measurement. Meaning is given to the numbers as the difference between the numbers are equal and useful in data analysis. An example of an interval scale is Intelligence Quotient or IQ (see Figure 7.1). An average IQ is 100. A 0 on the IQ test does not mean the subject is lacking intelligence but that the test has too high a useful range to measure such a low level of intelligence. Lower numbers in the IQ scale (under 100) mean low IQ. Numbers that are high on the IQ scale

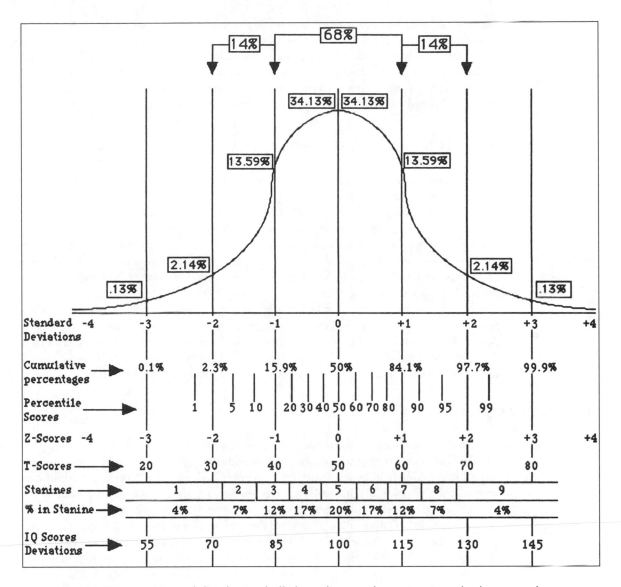

FIGURE 7.1 Normal distribution bell-shaped curve plus various standard score scales shown in relationship to the bell-shaped curve. (Source: The Pyschological Corporation/Harcourt Brace Jovanovich: San Diego, CA. Adapted and used with permission.)

mean above average IQ. The key to the IQ interval scale is the 100 average so comparison can be made. Weight of a person is also an example of no zero point.

Ratio Scale

The **ratio scale** has much the same characteristics as the interval scale plus the zero point. A tire gauge, thermometer, weight measuring scale, speedometer, numbers of participants attending an immunization clinic, numbers participating in a survey are some examples of uses of ratio scales. The ratio scale relies on an equal distance between all numbers and a consistent value of all numbers and the distance between them in the scale; the distance between 7 and 8 is the same as the distance as between 77 and 78, 50 is half the amount of 100, 30 is twice the amount of 15, etc. Ratio scales are used in time assessments, elapsed time, scores of exams, etc. Ratio scales are basic to most descriptive and inferential statistical analysis, and are at the least, a starting point for most analysis.

PARAMETRIC AND NONPARAMETRIC DATA

Data are categorized in several ways; one way is to place data in one of two different categories: parametric and nonparametric.

Parametric data are used only with interval and ratio scales. Inferences with parametric data are made about the information of a group or population parameters. The following are some assumptions about parametric data: random sampling is used to gather the data, the distribution of the scores fall within a possibility of a normal distribution, and when the data come from more than one group, variances of the different populations from which the data were gathered were drawn equally.

Nonparametric data are used with nominal and ordinal scales of measurement. Nonparametric data are not used to make inferences about values or information of a group or population. It is assumed that the information used in nonparametric data are drawn from the group or population at random. This tells you where the center line falls on the normal distribution curve, and the proportions of the scores that lie around the mean.

Measures of Dispersion

Some measures of dispersion are also used in descriptive statistics.

The **range** uses the highest score in a list of numbers minus the lowest score. This score is used in descriptive statistics. Ordering of scores is basic to range scores, so it is not used with nominal scales. If ordinal scales are used numbers have to be assigned to categories.

The **deviation from the mean** is how far a score is located either to the right (higher) or to the left (lower) of the mean. Standard deviation refers to how the groups of numbers pile up under/within the bell curve. (More correctly, the standard deviation is the average distance that values fall from the mean.) One standard deviation (referred to as one standard deviation from the mean and when the distribution is a normal one and has the bell curve shape) is when 34.13% of the numbers fall (are grouped together) to the left of the mean or when 34.13% of the numbers fall (grouped together) to the right of the mean (see Figure 7.1). The second standard deviation (or 2 standard deviations from the mean) adds 13.59% to the 34.13% to the left and to the right of the mean. The third standard deviation adds another 2.14%, and the fourth standard deviation takes on the last .13% which is added to the previous numbers, all of which fall in the tail of the bell-shaped curve. These percentages will change and vary as the shape of the distribution changes. If the distribution is flat or mostly flat, then the percentages do not remain as shown in Figure 7.1.

The **sum of squares** tells how much and how far the normal distribution is spread out (see normal distribution in Figure 7.1). It is the sum of the squared deviations about the mean. A low number means the scores are piled up in the middle, around the mean. A high score means the numbers are spread out, which makes the bell curve flattened. With a large sample size, the sum of squares would be large and still be a tall narrow bell curve. The sum of squares is needed for and aids in the calculation of the standard deviation.

The **variance** is the average of the squared deviations around the mean. Variance takes into account how many numbers there are. If there is a high sum of squares number and a large amount of numbers, this causes the sum of the squares numbers to be high and the variance numbers to be low, all which shows that it is a tall narrow distribution curve. Low numbers make a tall narrow distribution and high numbers make a flat distribution.

The **standard deviation** is found mathematically by taking the square root of the variance. This tells you where the center line, (the mean) falls on the normal distribution curve.

CENTRAL TENDENCY

Using the Normal Distribution Curve

The normal distribution curve is the foundation of the bell-shaped curve, and shows the placement of the mean, mode, and median. Below is a detailed presentation of the standard distribution, with various transformed scores presented in relationship to the bell-shaped curve. **Central tendency** refers to the ways of designating the center of data. The most common measures are mean, mode, and median.[8]

Mean, Mode, and Median

Three standard measures of central tendency are used in descriptive statistics: mean, mode, and median. The most common is the average (arithmetic average) which takes on a new name and is called the mean.

The **mean** is the sum of all of the scores added and then divided by the total number of scores. The mean is mathematically responsive to each score in the group of scores. The problem with the mean is that it is sensitive to extreme scores. One high score or one or two low scores will cause the mean to be less representative of the typical average, as the arithmetic average will be offset toward the high or low scores. This form of central tendency is used with interval and ratio scale.

The **mode** is the number or score that occurs most often; the number with the highest frequency. This score is easy to identify and is of value in descriptive statistics. This form of central tendency is used with nominal, ordinal, interval, and ratio scales.

The **median** is the number or score that divides a list of numbers in half. The median is the balance point of the list of scores and is used with ordinal, interval, and ratio scales. If the middle number is a whole number it is used. If the middle lands between two numbers, the distance between the two is split in half. For example, if the middle is between 44 and 45 the median is 44.5. This form of central tendency is used with ordinal, interval, and ratio scales.

Percentile Rankings and Z Scores

Percentile ranking transforms an individual score to the percent of observations that fall below the score given. The reference point is all other scores in the group. The score is assessed in relation to all other scores. The given score, the one you might receive on a licensing exam for example, is viewed in relationship to whether your score is higher or lower than all others in the battery of scores. If you are given a score that places you in the 70th percentile ranking on an exam, that means that 69% of the people did not do as well as you and that 29% did better than you.[8]

The **Z-score** is a measure of relative standing in a data set. It is a single figure that indicates whether a score is higher or lower than the average for a population. A Z-score is found by subtracting the population mean from the sample mean, and then dividing by the standard deviation of the population (you divide by the standard error with small sample sizes less than 30). A Z-score of +3.0 indicates that the score is 3 standard deviations above the mean and usually considered a good score.[8]

SKEWNESS OF STANDARD DISTRIBUTION BELL CURVE

The shape of the standard distribution bell curve often departs from the "normal," distribution because groups of scores do not always pile up in the middle but at one end or the other, or at least a bit offset one way or the other from the normal distribution. Most sets of numbers do not pile up in a neat normally distributed pile with most scores in the middle and with half of the scores nicely distributed on the positive and negative side of the mean. The normal distribution is mostly an ideal that is used as a standard to be compared to.[8]

Standard distributions are skewed either to the left or right, or positively or negatively skewed. The shape of the distribution is determined by how scores pile up in the distribution. The skewness of the distribution is used to determine how to label the shape that results. Several shapes of skewness have been identified.[8]

Positive Skewed Distributions

Positive skewed distributions are distributions that are skewed to the right. This is backward of what seems logical. As the scores pile up left of the mean, this makes the distribution skewed to the right. The skewness is located in the tail. The side of the tail that is the flattest determines the direction of the skewness. The median is found at the top of the curve. In a skewed distribution, the mean is often found on the tail (skewed) side of the median. The positive skewed distribution shows that the scores piled up below the mean. If this was an exam for certification of environmental specialists, for example, it would mean that the test was too difficult, with few persons achieving high scores. Figure 7.2 is a positive skewed distribution.[8]

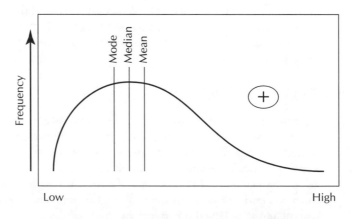

FIGURE 7.2 A positive skewed distribution.

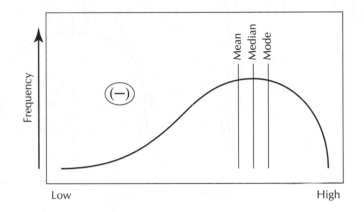

FIGURE 7.3   A negative skewed distribution.

Negative Skewed Distributions

Negative skewed distributions are distributions that are skewed to the left. The negative skewed distribution shows that the scores piled up above the mean. If this was an exam for certification of environmental specialists, for example, it would mean that the test was too easy with few persons achieving low scores below the mean. Figure 7.3 is a negative skewed distribution.[8]

Kurtosis: The Shapes of Distributions

In addition to the "normal distribution," or the "normal bell curve," that is seen in Figure 7.1, two other general distributions are seen. A whole array of possible distributions are possible from almost a straight point to an almost flat curve. But, examples of two common but unusual shaped distributions are those with a certain extent of peakedness and certain extent of flatness of the shape of the distribution. Peakedness is described by the term "leptokurtic," and the flatter distribution is called "platykurtic." Figure 7.4 is an example of leptokurtic distribution and Figure 7.5 is an example of a platykurtic distribution.[8]

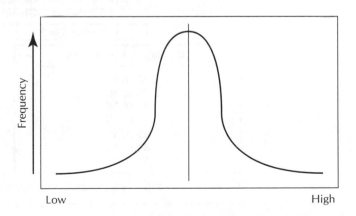

FIGURE 7.4   A leptokurtic distribution (note the peaked distribution and the long tails as representatives of the way the data is distributed).

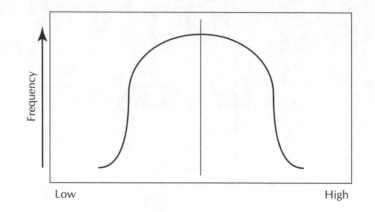

Low   High

FIGURE 7.5   A platykurtic distribution (note the wider and flattened distribution with limited tails which is representative of the distribution of the data).

TABLES AND THE PRESENTATION OF DATA IN EPIDEMIOLOGY

Tables are the best way to provide a pictorial representation of data. Tables assist in the analysis and understanding of data. The epidemiologist should construct and present tables that show the frequency of scores providing pictorial view of the findings of epidemiologic studies. Scores, numbers, or the frequency of numbers are first presented in frequency tables or frequency distribution tables. Examples of frequency tables are presented in Figure 7.6 and Figure 7.7.

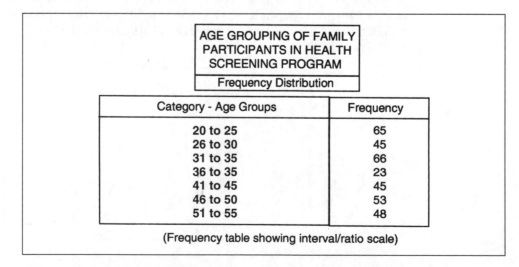

AGE GROUPING OF FAMILY PARTICIPANTS IN HEALTH SCREENING PROGRAM	
Frequency Distribution	
Category - Age Groups	Frequency
20 to 25	65
26 to 30	45
31 to 35	66
36 to 35	23
41 to 45	45
46 to 50	53
51 to 55	48

(Frequency table showing interval/ratio scale)

FIGURE 7.6   Example of frequency contingency table—interval/ratio scale.

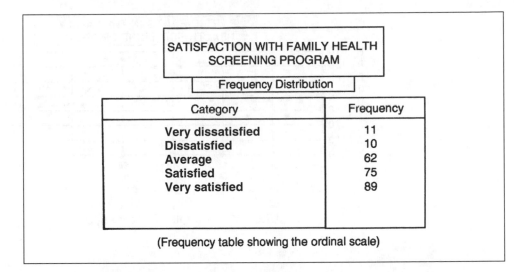

FIGURE 7.7   Example of contingency table—ordinal scale.

GRAPHS AND CHARTS IN THE PRESENTATION OF DESCRIPTIVE STATISTICS DATA

Several types of graphic presentations are commonly used in epidemiology, vital statistics, and presentation of health status indicator data reports. Following are several forms of graphs and charts, some which are computer generated. A variety of graphic approaches is used to present epidemiology data and statistics.

Some graphic and charting approaches are standardized and others are not. In government generated reports, graphs are fairly standardized in their presentation, while others appear to rely on either the creativity of the person creating the graph or are limited by the software producing computer generated approaches.

Several descriptive statistics graphic presentations commonly produced by computer spreadsheet programs are area graph, scattergram graph, pie chart, column graph, bar graph, line graph, and a whole range of three-dimensional graphs and charts. Figures 7.8 through 7.13 are examples of computer generated graphs and charts.

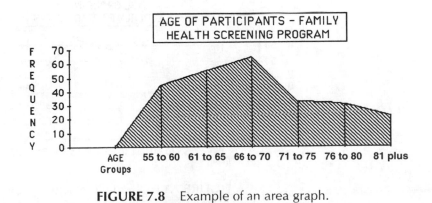

FIGURE 7.8   Example of an area graph.

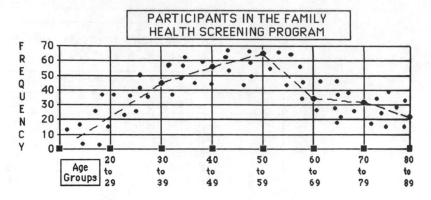

FIGURE 7.9   Example of a scattergram graph.

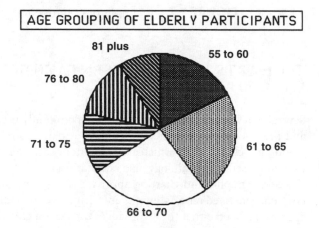

FIGURE 7.10   Example of a pie chart.

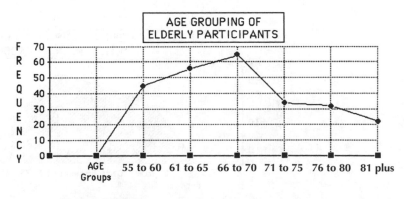

FIGURE 7.11   Example of a line graph.

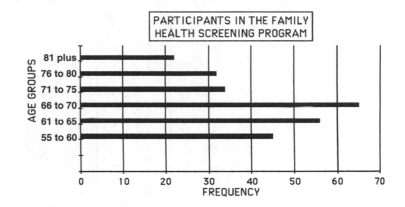

FIGURE 7.12   One example of a bar graph (computer generated).

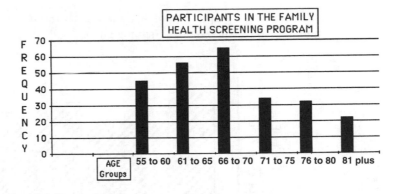

FIGURE 7.13   One example of a column graph (computer generated).

The preceding graphs and charts are computer generated. Program charts and graphs can come in a variety of shapes and arrangements, depending on the computer software. Traditional descriptive statistics are usually presented in forms similar to the computer generated charts shown. Additional representations of charts and graphs are presented in Figures 7.14 through 7.18. These charts are representative of the four types of scales mentioned previously. Nominal and ordinal data are presented in the bar charts of Figures 7.15 and 7.16. Bar charts are often presented in a vertical fashion (called columns in the computer generated charts). Fundamental to the construction of bar charts are two basic rules. First the bar width should always be the same for each bar. If bars are not the same width, the size gives a visual presentation of being different, implying that the data are different, i.e., wider bars would mean bigger or more numbers or narrower bars would give the idea of being smaller in size or less in number. Height of the bars should be the only variable to present visual differences in the data (see Figures 7.14, 7.15, and 7.16). Secondly, the space between the bars should be the same for each bar and all bars and spaces should be consistently spaced, but be close enough to each other to get a good visual comparison and not be spaced wide distances apart.

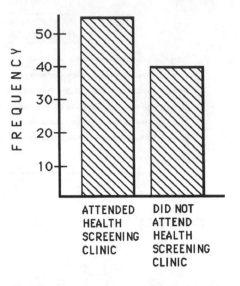

FIGURE 7.14   Bar graph—nominal data: elderly members of a senior citizen center attending an on-site health screening clinic.

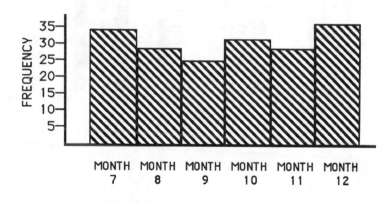

FIGURE 7.15   Histogram—ratio scale. Numbers of immunizations per month administered to elderly in nursing homes.

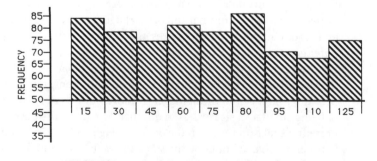

FIGURE 7.16   Histogram—interval scale.

Interval and ratio scales data are shown in a bar graph in Figure 7.15. Interval and ratio scales are shown through a **histogram**. The bottom line (*x*-axis or abscissa) uses the numbers of the data. The numbers have numerical meaning rather than serving as labels. The *frequency* at which the data occur is presented on the *y*-axis. Figures 7.15 and 7.16 are charts using interval scale data and ratio scales data presented as a histogram.

The histogram as shown in Figure 7.16 is a bar chart type presentation of interval scale data. In a histogram, each bar is butted up against the next. In a **bar graph** a space is provided between each bar and each interval between the bars must be equal. If a 1/2-inch-wide bar (interval) is used for one bar in the bar chart then all intervals and bars must be 1/2-inch wide in the entire chart.

The data of the histogram can also be presented in a line graph type chart called a "frequency polygon." The **frequency polygon** presents the same information as the histogram but uses a line graph instead of bars. Figure 7.17 shows a frequency polygon overlaid on a histogram demonstrating that both are the same numerically and different pictorially. The frequency polygon, Figure 7.18, uses the same data as the histogram (interval scale).

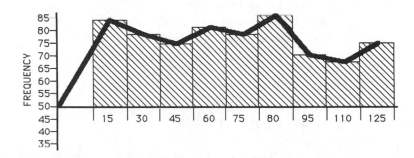

FIGURE 7.17 Combined frequency polygon and histogram. An example of a frequency polygon (line graph) overlaid upon a histogram, showing the commonality of both charts (uses interval scale data).

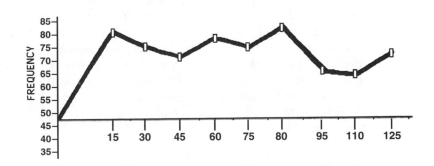

FIGURE 7.18 Frequency polygon (line graph—using interval scale data).

RATES, RATIOS, AND PROPORTIONS IN EPIDEMIOLOGY

Rates (comparing mortality, morbidity, and related health status occurrences to population groups of 100 or 1,000 or 10,000) are commonly used in epidemiology descriptive statistics and may serve the epidemiologist in presenting data. Ratios are also a common form of epidemiology descriptive statistics and are used throughout epidemiology. Rates and ratios, their use, function, and epidemiological formulas are presented in detail in Chapters 4, 5, and 6. Rates, ratios, and percentages (proportions) are commonly used in public health planning reports, administrative decisions, and in planning public health services.

Proportions (percentages) are very useful descriptive statistics. Percentages can provide a clear picture of data if presented correctly or can mislead if presented incorrectly. Percentages should always be compared to the total numbers from which they come. For example, to show how many elderly persons participated in a flu immunization program, the epidemiologist could say 88% of the elderly were immunized. However, this percentage is meaningless when presented alone. Do we mean 88% of 10 or 88% of 1200 citizens? Thus, when showing percents, the epidemiologist should always present the total number of the participants or the N. (N stands for total number or subjects.) The letter N is used in statistics to show the total number of the study population or the total of any sub-group being compared in a study or compared statistically. The best way to show percentages is to state N, along with the percent, for example, "670 out of 750 persons or 89.3% of the participants in a health screening program needed flu immunizations."

SAMPLES OF TABLES AND CHARTS USED IN EPIDEMIOLOGICAL REPORTS

Most epidemiological reports and publications use fairly standard approaches in presenting epidemiology descriptive statistics.

Tables

Tables of various types are used to present basic and advanced epidemiological data. Tables use the fundamentals of various sources of data mentioned above, however tables do not necessarily express the types of data. It is implied that the epidemiologist understands the basics of the four types of data presented above. Some tables use a combination of the different data scales. Figures 7.19 through 7.21 are sample tables from *Morbidity and Mortality Weekly Reports*, representative of common practical use of various epidemiological tables. Tables are not graphs or charts but the arrangement of numbers (data) in a fashion that is easy to review, study, and assess. The examples that follow are presented for study and as examples for reference in order to better understand the tabulation of data.

Reporting Area	All Causes, By Age (Years)						P&I† Total
	All Ages	≥65	45-64	25-44	1-24	<1	
NEW ENGLAND	611	427	96	63	15	10	43
Boston, Mass.	195	117	42	26	3	7	21
Bridgeport, Conn.	51	35	11	4	1	-	5
Cambridge, Mass.	27	18	7	1	1	-	-
Fall River, Mass.	22	17	3	1	1	-	-
Hartford, Conn.	45	35	5	4	1	-	2
Lowell, Mass.	24	21	1	1	1	-	-
Lynn, Mass.	21	18	2	1	-	-	1
New Bedford, Mass.	22	18	1	3	-	-	1
New Haven, Conn.	47	33	2	8	3	1	3
Providence, R.I.	29	23	3	2	1	-	1
Somerville, Mass.	4	4	-	-	-	-	-
Springfield, Mass.	43	29	9	5	-	-	4
Waterbury, Conn.	25	14	5	5	1	-	3
Worcester, Mass.	56	45	5	2	2	2	2
MID. ATLANTIC	1,191	772	252	106	23	38	63
Albany, N.Y.	46	29	14	2	1	-	3
Allentown, Pa.	24	20	2	2	-	-	1
Buffalo, N.Y.	100	70	20	6	1	3	4
Camden, N.J.	38	21	11	1	1	4	2
Elizabeth, N.J.	26	14	9	3	-	-	1
Erie, Pa.§	30	21	7	2	-	-	-
Jersey City, N.J.	52	35	8	8	U	1	2
New York City, N.Y.	U	U	U	U	U	U	U
Newark, N.J.	85	35	23	18	3	6	3
Paterson, N.J.	29	12	6	3	-	8	1
Philadelphia, Pa.	323	199	83	24	7	10	9
Pittsburgh, Pa.§	47	31	9	4	-	3	3
Reading, Pa.	47	29	9	7	2	-	9
Rochester, N.Y.	109	78	22	8	1	-	8
Schenectady, N.Y.	28	22	4	1	1	-	3
Scranton, Pa.§	38	35	1	1	1	-	1
Syracuse, N.Y.	75	51	12	6	4	2	1
Trenton, N.J.	34	21	6	6	1	-	7
Utica, N.Y.	27	22	3	1	-	1	2
Yonkers, N.Y.	33	27	3	3	-	-	3
E.N. CENTRAL	2,035	1,323	392	188	92	40	81
Akron, Ohio	61	48	10	2	1	-	6
Canton, Ohio	34	26	8	-	-	-	2
Chicago, Ill.	337	145	60	69	57	6	8
Cincinnati, Ohio	112	70	29	6	5	2	12
Cleveland, Ohio	165	96	41	20	1	7	3
Columbus, Ohio	199	135	34	19	8	3	3
Dayton, Ohio	112	87	16	5	2	2	7
Detroit, Mich.	196	121	48	19	7	1	2
Evansville, Ind.	42	30	7	4	-	1	1
Fort Wayne, Ind.	59	40	13	4	-	2	5
Gary, Ind.	18	6	2	7	2	1	1
Grand Rapids, Mich.	63	42	11	7	1	2	3
Indianapolis, Ind.	169	126	30	8	2	3	3
Madison, Wis.	53	35	12	4	1	1	2
Milwaukee, Wis.	122	102	14	5	-	1	10
Peoria, Ill.	48	36	9	-	-	3	1
Rockford, Ill.	48	34	10	1	2	1	3
South Bend, Ind.	44	33	5	3	1	2	4
Toledo, Ohio	91	62	22	3	2	2	3
Youngstown, Ohio	62	49	11	2	-	-	2
W.N. CENTRAL	770	535	132	63	20	20	25
Des Moines, Iowa	70	54	11	4	-	1	2
Duluth, Minn.	26	24	2	-	-	-	-
Kansas City, Kans.	30	20	5	1	3	1	-
Kansas City, Mo.	121	91	21	7	2	-	4
Lincoln, Nebr.	28	18	6	4	-	-	-
Minneapolis, Minn.	184	131	31	16	2	4	11
Omaha, Nebr.	72	45	13	7	3	4	4
St. Louis, Mo.	111	63	23	10	8	7	-
St. Paul, Minn.	62	42	9	7	1	3	2
Wichita, Kans.	66	47	11	7	1	-	1
S. ATLANTIC	1,268	777	252	162	49	27	52
Atlanta, Ga.	148	86	36	21	4	1	3
Baltimore, Md.	183	106	38	27	5	7	9
Charlotte, N.C.	99	62	20	11	4	2	5
Jacksonville, Fla.	118	83	20	11	3	-	9
Miami, Fla.	110	56	24	19	7	4	-
Norfolk, Va.	65	39	8	10	5	3	5
Richmond, Va.	65	39	20	1	4	1	3
Savannah, Ga.	46	23	12	7	1	3	3
St. Petersburg, Fla.	76	63	3	6	2	2	2
Tampa, Fla.	140	97	25	14	4	-	10
Washington, D.C.	200	109	43	34	10	4	3
Wilmington, Del.	18	14	3	1	-	-	-
E.S. CENTRAL	716	446	163	59	24	24	31
Birmingham, Ala.	113	72	19	14	2	6	5
Chattanooga, Tenn.	56	38	13	3	2	-	6
Knoxville, Tenn.	98	68	22	4	2	2	7
Louisville, Ky.	100	57	24	11	3	5	5
Memphis, Tenn.	151	100	29	12	7	3	-
Mobile, Ala.	44	22	13	3	4	2	2
Montgomery, Ala.	27	15	6	2	2	2	1
Nashville, Tenn.	127	74	37	10	2	4	5
W.S. CENTRAL	1,292	802	246	137	63	42	58
Austin, Tex.	38	18	9	5	4	2	3
Baton Rouge, La.	49	34	10	1	2	2	2
Corpus Christi, Tex.	37	21	12	2	1	1	-
Dallas, Tex.	197	121	33	28	7	8	2
El Paso, Tex.	72	46	12	7	5	2	5
Ft. Worth, Tex.	90	51	23	11	2	2	2
Houston, Tex.	303	177	53	48	16	9	25
Little Rock, Ark.	55	44	5	2	3	-	3
New Orleans, La.	96	51	25	13	6	1	-
San Antonio, Tex.	173	113	30	12	13	5	5
Shreveport, La.	64	47	9	-	3	5	7
Tulsa, Okla.	118	79	25	8	1	5	4
MOUNTAIN	620	394	128	64	16	18	42
Albuquerque, N.M.	75	58	9	5	3	-	6
Colo. Springs, Colo.	46	24	10	8	3	1	2
Denver, Colo.	110	62	22	19	1	6	12
Las Vegas, Nev.	94	61	24	6	1	2	4
Ogden, Utah	19	13	3	3	-	-	3
Phoenix, Ariz.	140	86	31	13	4	6	3
Pueblo, Colo.	24	13	8	3	-	-	3
Salt Lake City, Utah	34	20	7	3	1	3	4
Tucson, Ariz.	78	57	14	4	3	-	5
PACIFIC	1,859	1,189	312	230	65	57	122
Berkeley, Calif.	30	19	3	1	-	7	1
Fresno, Calif.	63	43	9	3	3	5	17
Glendale, Calif.	43	33	7	2	1	-	1
Honolulu, Hawaii	76	53	9	11	2	1	13
Long Beach, Calif.	94	57	20	11	3	2	16
Los Angeles, Calif.	503	303	77	91	24	5	14
Oakland, Calif.	U	U	U	U	U	U	U
Pasadena, Calif.	28	21	4	2	1	-	3
Portland, Oreg.	131	101	19	2	3	6	3
Sacramento, Calif.	141	88	29	16	3	5	11
San Diego, Calif.	154	93	19	25	10	5	17
San Francisco, Calif.	151	78	28	39	6	-	1
San Jose, Calif.	167	104	41	12	2	8	17
Seattle, Wash.	131	86	22	11	4	8	3
Spokane, Wash.	53	43	6	2	1	1	2
Tacoma, Wash.	94	67	19	2	2	4	3
TOTAL	10,362¶	6,665	1,973	1,072	367	276	517

*Mortality data in this table are voluntarily reported from 121 cities in the United States, most of which have populations of 100,000 or more. A death is reported by the place of its occurrence and by the week that the death certificate was filed. Fetal deaths are not included.
†Pneumonia and influenza.
§Because of changes in reporting methods in these 3 Pennsylvania cities, these numbers are partial counts for the current week. Complete counts will be available in 4 to 6 weeks.
¶Total includes unknown ages.
U: Unavailable.

FIGURE 7.19   Example of epidemiological data table on deaths in selected United States cities. (Source: *Morbidity and Mortality Weekly Reports*, Vol. 40, No. 40, October 11, 1991, p. 690)

Percentage distribution of live births, by trimester that prenatal care began, race of infant, and marital status of mother — United States, 1980 and 1988

Race of infant/ Marital status of mother/Year	No. births	Trimester of pregnancy prenatal care began			No prenatal care
		1st	2nd	3rd	
White					
Married					
1980	2,578,669	82.6	14.3	2.5	0.7
1988	2,506,466	84.1	12.5	2.5	0.9
Unmarried					
1980	320,063	52.9	33.7	9.5	3.9
1988	539,696	57.1	30.2	8.5	4.2
All					
1980	2,898,732	79.3	16.4	3.2	1.0
1988	3,046,162	79.4	15.6	3.5	1.5
Black					
Married					
1980	263,879	72.3	22.0	4.2	1.5
1988	245,311	74.0	20.2	4.1	1.7
Unmarried					
1980	325,737	54.9	33.8	7.6	3.7
1988	426,665	53.5	32.6	8.4	5.5
All					
1980	589,616	62.7	28.5	6.1	2.7
1988	671,976	61.1	28.0	6.8	4.1
All races*					
Married					
1980	2,946,511	81.3	15.2	2.7	0.8
1988	2,904,211	82.9	13.4	2.7	1.0
Unmarried					
1980	665,747	53.8	33.7	8.7	3.8
1988	1,005,299	55.4	31.3	8.5	4.7
All					
1980	3,612,258	76.3	18.6	3.8	1.3
1988	3,909,510	75.9	18.0	4.2	1.9

***Includes races other than white and black.**

FIGURE 7.20   Example of epidemiological data table on distribution of live births and selected measures. (Source: *Morbidity and Mortality Weekly Reports*, Vol. 40, No. 23, June 14, 1991, p. 383)

Estimated number and percentage* of drivers† with a blood alcohol concentration ≥0.01% involved in fatal crashes, by year and age group—United States, 1982–1989

Year	Age group (yrs)							
	15–17		18–20		21–24		≥25	
	No.	(%)	No.	(%)	No.	(%)	No.	(%)
1982	910	(31.5)	3,468	(48.3)	4,645	(51.5)	12,168	(34.2)
1983	826	(29.1)	3,141	(46.8)	4,270	(50.6)	11,723	(33.1)
1984	799	(26.8)	3,128	(44.3)	4,392	(49.0)	11,741	(31.5)
1985	734	(24.0)	2,653	(40.2)	4,156	(45.9)	11,451	(30.2)
1986	910	(25.4)	2,850	(41.4)	4,313	(47.2)	12,008	(30.5)
1987	853	(23.6)	2,509	(38.1)	4,004	(45.5)	12,457	(30.3)
1988	776	(22.4)	2,562	(36.9)	3,935	(46.0)	12,624	(30.1)
1989	592	(18.9)	2,269	(34.8)	3,476	(45.0)	12,278	(29.5)

*Percentage of involved drivers in each age group who were alcohol-impaired.
†Regardless of whether driver was killed.
Source: Fatal Accident Reporting System, National Highway Traffic Safety Administration.

FIGURE 7.21   Example of epidemiological data table on traffic fatalities involving alcohol. (Source: *Morbidity and Mortality Weekly Reports*, Vol. 40, No. 40, October 11, 1991, p. 179)

Graphs and Charts

Graphs and charts of various types are used to present basic and advanced data. Most graphs and charts use the fundamentals of various sources of data previously discussed. Some graphs and charts use a combination of the different data scales. Figures 7.22 through 7.26 are samples of graphs and charts from *Morbidity and Mortality Weekly Reports*, presented as samples of possible approaches to chart and graph development available to develop epidemiological reports.

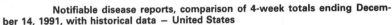

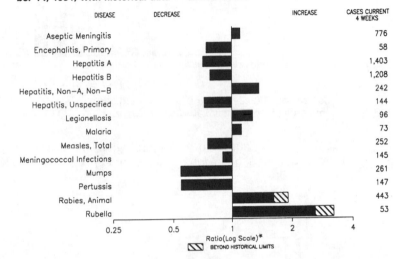

FIGURE 7.22   Example of epidemiological bar graph on notifiable diseases in the United States. (Source: *Morbidity and Mortality Weekly Reports*, Vol. 40, No. 50, December 20, 1991, p. 872)

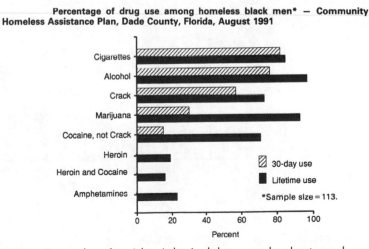

FIGURE 7.23   Example of epidemiological bar graph chart on homeless men and drug use. (Source: *Morbidity and Mortality Weekly Reports*, Vol. 40, No. 50, December 20, 1991, p. 867)

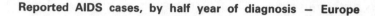

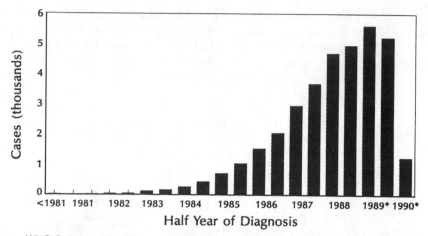

Source: WHO Collaborating Centre on AIDS, Paris.
*Reporting incomplete for 1989 and 1990.

FIGURE 7.24 Example of epidemiological bar graph chart on AIDS diagnosis. (Source: *Morbidity and Mortality Weekly Reports*, Vol. 39, No. 47, November 30, 1991, p. 850)

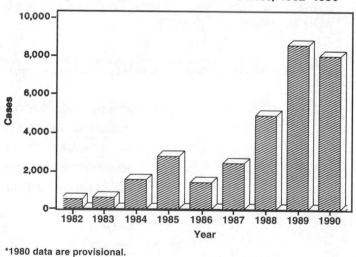

*1980 data are provisional.

FIGURE 7.25 Example of epidemiological two-dimension bar graph chart on Lyme disease. (Source: *Morbidity and Mortality Weekly Reports*, Vol. 40, No. 15, June 28, 1991, p. 418)

Cases of dracunculiasis detected during national surveys—Nigeria.

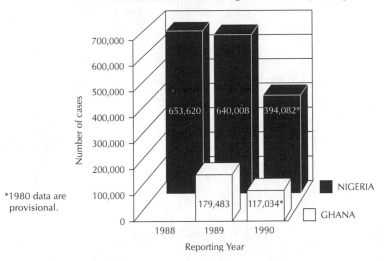

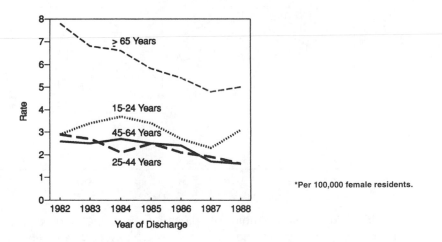

FIGURE 7.26 Example of epidemiological three-dimension bar graph chart on cases of Dracunculiasis (a parasitic nematode—worm). (Source: *Morbidity and Mortality Weekly Reports*, Vol. 40, No. 15, April 19, 1991, p. 246)

Line Graphs

Line graphs of various types are used to present basic and advanced epidemiological data. **Line graphs** use the fundamentals of various sources of data mentioned above. Some tables use a combination of different data scales. Figures 7.27 through 7.29 are some samples of various types of line graphs from *Morbidity and Mortality Weekly Reports*, presented as examples for possible use in developing epidemiological reports.

FIGURE 7.27 Example of epidemiological line graph chart on traumatic spinal cord injury for women. (Source: *Morbidity and Mortality Weekly Reports*, Vol. 40,. No. 50, December 20, 1991, p. 872)

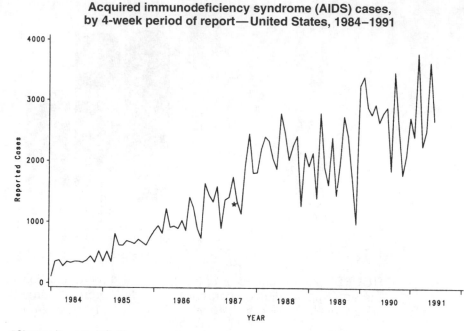

Acquired immunodeficiency syndrome (AIDS) cases, by 4-week period of report—United States, 1984–1991

*Change in case definition.

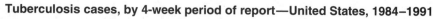

Tuberculosis cases, by 4-week period of report—United States, 1984–1991

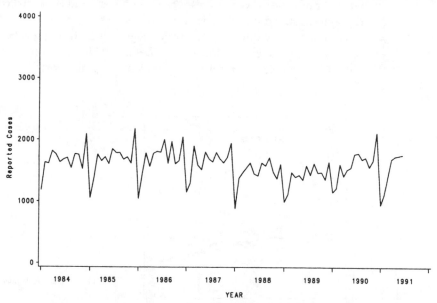

FIGURE 7.28   Two examples of epidemiological line graph charts, one on AIDS and one on tuberculosis cases. (Source: *Morbidity and Mortality Weekly Reports*, Vol. 40, No. 30, August 2, 1991, p. 529)

Acquired immunodeficiency syndrome (AIDS) cases, United States, 1985–1989

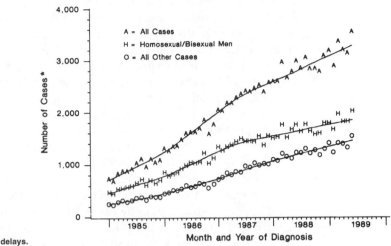

*Adjusted for reporting delays.

FIGURE 7.29 Example of epidemiological line graph on the incidence of AIDS. (Source: *Morbidity and Mortality Weekly Reports*, Vol. 39, No. RR-16, November 30, 1990, p. 3)

EXERCISES

Key Terms

Define and explain the following terms.

bar graph	interval scale	percentile ranking
biostatistics	line graph	proportion
central tendency	mean	range
descriptive statistics	median	ratio scale
deviation from the mean	mode	standard deviation
empirical research	nominal scale	sum of squares
frequency polygon	nonparametric data	tabular presentation
histogram	ordinal scale	variance
inferential statistics	parametric data	z-score

Study Questions

7.1 Based on the sample tables presented and from the *MMWR* examples in this chapter, make a table for the case situation presented below. Arrange the following data in a table. Read the following account and use the information to construct the table using a computer spreadsheet.

Table Data

Smoking and tobacco use for females was 31.7% for any tobacco use, 31.3% for cigarette use, 12.5% for frequent cigarette use and 1.4% for smokeless tobacco use. Smoking and tobacco use for males was 40.4% for any tobacco use, 33.2% for cigarette use, 13.0% for frequent cigarette use and 19.1% for smokeless tobacco use.

Smoking and tobacco use for 9th graders was 32.1% for any tobacco use, 29.5% for cigarette use, 9.9% for frequent cigarette use and 7.8% for smokeless tobacco use. Smoking and tobacco use for 10th graders was 33.9% for any tobacco use, 30.0% for cigarette use, 10.8% for frequent cigarette use and 10.9% for smokeless tobacco use. Smoking and tobacco use for 11th graders was 36.7% for any tobacco use, 32.8% for cigarette use, 12.6% for frequent cigarette use and 9.5% for smokeless tobacco use. Smoking and tobacco use for 12th graders was 41.2% for any tobacco use, 36.7% for cigarette use, 17.7% for frequent cigarette use and 11.9% for smokeless tobacco use.

Smoking and tobacco use for whites was 41.2% for any tobacco use, 36.4% for cigarette use, 15.9% for frequent cigarette use and 12.6% for smokeless tobacco use. Smoking and tobacco use for blacks was 16.8% for any tobacco use, 16.1% for cigarette use, 2.3% for frequent cigarette use and 1.9% for smokeless tobacco use. Smoking and tobacco use for Hispanics was 32.0% for any tobacco use, 30.8% for cigarette use, 7.4% for frequent cigarette use and 5.7% for smokeless tobacco use.

Show totals, and means as appropriate and where useful.

Provide discussion and explanations as to why the statistics for blacks differ from whites and Hispanics based on the data in your table.

7.2   Using a computer spreadsheet and graphics, construct a line graph by charting the following data. On the *y*-axis place the numbers of cases in 10,000 increments up to 50,000, starting with 0 at the bottom. On the *x*-axis place the year of diagnosis ranging from 1981, including each year through 1990. Draw three lines on the chart; one line for homosexual/bisexual men, one line for intravenous (IV)-drug users and one line for the totals of both of the other lines.

Line Graph Data

In 1980 there were 0 cases reported for homosexual/bisexual men, and 0 cases for IV-drug users. In 1982, 50 cases of AIDS were reported for homosexual/bisexual men and 25 cases for IV-drug users. In 1983, 500 cases of AIDS were reported for homosexual/bisexual men and 100 cases for IV-drug users. In 1984, 2,000 cases of AIDS were reported for homosexual/bisexual men and 500 cases for IV-drug users. In 1985, 6,500 cases of AIDS were reported for homosexual/bisexual men and 1,500 cases for IV-drug users. In 1986, 11,000 cases of AIDS were reported for homosexual/bisexual men and 3,200 cases for IV-drug users.

In 1987, 16,500 cases of AIDS were reported for homosexual/bisexual men and 4,500 cases for IV-drug users. In 1988, 20,000 cases of AIDS were reported for homosexual/bisexual men and 7,500 cases for IV-drug users.

In 1989, 23,000 cases of AIDS were reported for homosexual/bisexual men and 9,500 cases for IV-drug users. In 1990, 25,000 cases of AIDS were reported for homosexual/bisexual men and 10,000 cases for IV-drug users.

7.3   Using a computer spreadsheet and graphics, complete a bar chart for the following information and data. Homicide followed by suicide was studied in Kentucky from 1985 through 1990 and the following information was found.

Bar Chart Data

The clustering of the homicide followed by suicide cases was presented in MMWR for Sept. 27, 1991. On the y-axis construct a scale ranging from 0 to 20 at 5 point increments. On the x-axis use the following data: In 1985 there was a clustering of 11 homicide/suicides. In 1986 there was a clustering of 6 homicide/suicides. In 1987 there was a clustering of 13 homicide/suicides. In 1988 there was a clustering of 8 homicide/suicides. In 1989 there was a clustering of 17 homicide/suicides. In 1990 there was a clustering of 12 homicide/suicides.

7.4 List and explain the basic four types and sources of data scales used in descriptive statistics.

7.5 Draw a normal distribution bell curve. By placing an X on the bottom line (the one that makes the tails of the distribution) indicate with the X and a written label where the following fall.
   a. 9th stanine,
   b. 40th percentile,
   c. a Z-score of 0,
   d. a standard deviation of a −2,
   e. an IQ score of 115.

7.6 Draw a negative skewed distribution, label it with correct positive and negative directions, and indicate where the median and the mean would likely fall.

7.7 Explain and discuss the difference between the tabulation of data and the graphing of data. Provide an example of tabulated data and graphed data. The data for the example of tabulated and graphed data can come from an example in the chapter or from data you provide.

REFERENCES

1. Kuller, L.H. 1991. "Epidemiology Is the Study of 'Epidemics' and Their Prevention," *American Journal of Epidemiology*, Vol. 134, No. 10, pp. 1051–1058.
2. Kelsey, J.L., Thompson, W.D., and Evans, A.S. 1986. *Methods in Observational Epidemiology*. New York: Oxford University Press.
3. Slome, C., Brogan, D., Eyres, S., and Lednar, W. 1982. *Basic Epidemiological Methods and Biostatistics: A Workbook*. Monterey, CA: Wadsworth.
4. Morton, R.F., Hebel, J.R., and McCarter, R.J. 1990. *A Study Guide to Epidemiology and Biostatistics*. Gaithersburg, MD: Aspen Publishing.
5. Hennekens, C.H., and Buring, J.E. 1987. *Epidemiology in Medicine*. Boston: Little, Brown and Company.
6. Rothman, K.J. 1986. *Modern Epidemiology*. Boston: Little, Brown and Company.
7. Mausner, J.S., and Kramer, S. 1985. *Epidemiology: An Introductory Text*. Philadelphia: Saunders.
8. Thorndike, R.L., and Hagen, E.P. 1977. *Measurement and Evaluation in Psychology and Education*, 4th edition. New York: Wiley.

8

Research Methods, Study Design, and Analytic Studies

CHAPTER OBJECTIVES

This chapter on research methods, study design, and analytic studies

- reviews observational epidemiology and research design used in epidemiology;
- reviews the rationale for choosing certain research designs in epidemiological studies;
- distinguishes between different research design approaches;
- reviews the different epidemiological research study approaches;
- reviews the importance of controls or control groups in epidemiological research;
- presents the importance of and approaches to sampling in research methods;
- presents study questions that develop the use of the chapter materials;
- presents and defines key terms used in the chapter.

INTRODUCTION

Several types of research studies and designs are used in epidemiology. Research possibilities range from studies of mortality and morbidity to survey research to experimental designs. Research in epidemiology has been classified into two general categories: observational epidemiology and experimental trials. In epidemiological research on ill or diseased persons, groups or populations are compared with well persons and groups. In research design, the diseased persons are referred to as "cases," and the well persons or groups are referred to as "controls." (Concepts related to case are presented in Chapter 1.) Basic to all research is the development of hypotheses, which are developed for the overall study (statement of the problem) and are also developed for each facet or question in the study. (Hypothesis development is covered in detail in Chapter 10.)

Computers in Research Design

The epidemiologist should be familiar with how data are used by a chosen computer software program prior to developing a questionnaire or designing a research study. Analysis of the data is a task that is easier completed if the data are readily accepted into and processed by the computer program or spreadsheet.

OBSERVATIONAL EPIDEMIOLOGY STUDIES

Observational epidemiology and related research restricts the epidemiologist from being able to control any of the conditions of the research and is the most common and traditional type of research found in epidemiology. Observational studies usually include retrospective studies, cohort studies, cross-sectional studies, longitudinal and other prospective studies. **Observational study** uses the ability to categorize groups by occurrence of disease, conditions, injury, death, etc. Study groups are selected prior to any investigations, as they are set by those who have the disease and those who do not. The groups are predetermined by variables beyond the control of the epidemiologist. Past experience, lifestyle, personal behaviors, training, immunization levels, exposure to risk factors and environmental factors all influence the state of health and susceptibility to illness of individuals in groups, which are beyond the control of the epidemiologist/investigator. These limitations are what makes the approach observational; little or no control can be exercised over the study population by the epidemiologist.[1,2]

Some terms relating to research activities need to be defined. **Subjects** are the individual participants in research. A subject can be a white rat, a laboratory rabbit, or a person who is selected for participation in a research project. Another term common to research activities is **variable** which is any factor or influence upon the research activities or outcomes. Any event, attribute, interaction, or phenomenon that can vary or have different values is also referred to as a variable. (See dependent and independent variable concepts presented later in this chapter.)

Some factors of a research project may be influenced or changed before research activities occur. Any factor or attribute influencing research variables prior to the activity occurring is referred to as an **antecedent** or may be called an **antecedent variable**. Precursors, prior influencing factors or activities that are required to take place beforehand or which already occurred and influence research processes or outcomes, are also antecedents. Another term that has been applied to a variety of research approaches is that of *quasi* as in quasi-experimental study. **Quasi** means "done in the manner of, like unto it, or using the basic concept of." Thus, a quasi research design includes the basic foundations of good research design present but the study falls short of meeting the strict letter of the law of the design. A quasi-experiment is one in which the researcher falls short of meeting all the parameters of the experimental research design, but much of the study methodology is in place. It could also mean that the epidemiologist lacks the ability to control all variables within the study. Quasi research designs are modifications of the standard or traditional approach to a given research design but are used anyway, keeping all factors of a good design in place as much as possible.

Experimental studies are not true epidemiological studies, at least in the traditional sense but are clinical or planned research designs. In experimental research designs the researcher sets or specifies the conditions of the study or experiment. The researcher controls or establishes the cause-effect relations or associations, or controls characteristics or variables which can then be compared statistically. Controls, sampling methods, and established probability statistical assessments are used. Inferential statistics are used most often in the analysis of clinical or experimental design studies. **Community trials** (use nonrandom data), and **clinical trials** (use randomly assigned data) are the two most-used design approaches using the experimental design approach in epidemiology. Another term for these types of research designs is *analytical studies*.[1,2]

Clinical trials and experimental designs are useful in establishing sound cause-effect relations (association) of an agent or factor to a disease, condition, or death. However, observational studies, since they provide many more insights into the effects of diseases or conditions on groups or populations, are more useful to epidemiology as epidemiology must deal with population groups. Experimental designs are limited as they deal with individuals or smaller treatment or experimental groups and have limited inference value to large populations.[1,2]

DESCRIPTIVE VS. ANALYTICAL EPIDEMIOLOGICAL STUDIES

Two other ways epidemiological studies are classified are as *descriptive* and *analytical*. Descriptive studies are used when little is known about a disease. Analytical studies are used when insights or information about the various aspects of a disease are available.

Descriptive studies provide insights, data, and information on the course or patterns of diseases, conditions, injuries, disability, and death in groups or populations. The information is usually based on routinely collected data with the usual demographic characteristics of age, sex, race, marital status, education, socioeconomic class, occupation, geographical area, and time periods.[1,3] (See Chapter 7 on descriptive statistics.)

Analytical studies are used to test cause-effect relationships and rely on the development of new data. The key to analytical studies is to assure that the studies are properly designed so the findings are reliable and valid. If designs are properly done, the findings allow more definitive conclusions about cause-effect relationships. Planned analytical research is much the same as clinical trials and experimental designs.[1,3]

THE STUDY DESIGNS

The basic design of an experimental design research effort is to establish an experimental or treatment group and to identify a second group that gets no experimentation or no treatment and is used for comparison. The group receiving no treatment is called the *control group* or *controls*. The control group is to reflect the characteristics of the treatment group as closely as possible. If the research lends itself to it, individuals are assigned at random to both the control group and the experimental group. Additionally, the conditions, processes, procedures, environment, exposures to outside influences, etc., for both the treatment group and the control group should be kept exactly the same. The only factor that should be different is that the treatment is given to the experimental group and withheld from the control group. Most all experimental research designs have the basic design as the foundation of the research structure and approach. A variety of arrangements have been used, but the fundamental aspects of the basic design should be present. The types of approaches used include randomized controlled trials (control groups), multiple treatment groups, blind studies and nonrandomized treatment and control groups.[6,7,8,13,14]

Proper sampling techniques, as presented in this chapter, should be used in experimental designs just as in any research. Effective sampling approaches must be used in both the control and experimental groups. In some clinical trials sampling is not planned due to the nature of the research and subjects, such as in certain drug experiments or surgical techniques.

Two basic constructs used in experimental design research are dependent variables and independent variables. **Dependent variables** are those factors or conditions that occur and exist in both treatment and control groups. Dependent variables cause no change in the experimental group. When an intervention, treatment or change occurs in the treatment group it must be identified. The **independent variable** is the factor causing change in the treatment group and is withheld from the control group. The treatment or change agent is the independent variable. When the experimental group is exposed to a treatment such as a vaccine, drug, or other intervention and change occurs, the factor that caused the change is referred to as the independent variable.[6,7,8,13,14]

In experimental design research, a cause-effect relationship is easily observed. When no change occurs in the subjects and a treatment is then introduced (independent variable) and change occurs, a cause-effect phenomenon is observed. Change occurs in the treatment group and no change occurs in the control group. Thus, a deduction is made that the treatment (the independent variable) is what caused the change. Inferential statistics are used to demonstrate that a cause-effect relationship did not occur by chance and are used to show what level of probability occurred by cause and not by chance. The level of confidence is the effectiveness of the treatment in the subjects and the degree of change due to the action of the independent variable. For example, if an immunization was given to a set of patients who were then exposed to a disease and they did not get the disease after taking an experimental vaccine, it would be said that the experimental drug prevented the disease at the 95% confidence level (or whatever level it might be), and only 5% could be attributed to chance. Probability statistics are used to demonstrate levels of confidence. Another way of expressing levels of confidence is to state them as levels of significance. The research findings stated in terms of probability of effectiveness are usually stated at the 1.0, .1, or .01 level of significance.[6,7,8,13,14,15,16]

Later in this chapter is a brief description of the research designs for randomized controlled trials (control groups), multiple treatment groups, blind studies, and nonrandomized treatment and control groups. Study designs can be very complex when used in clinical settings, especially when studying treatment methods in laboratory animals or volunteer subjects. The type and amount of complex research designs are many and varied and no attempt is made to present them all. Entire textbooks have been devoted to research designs and should be sought if such a need arises.[6,7,8,13,14,15,16]

EXPERIMENTAL/ANALYTICAL DESIGN IN EPIDEMIOLOGY

Experimental design research is a common empirical research design and method. In epidemiology the basic experimental design approach has been given a variety of different labels. Some of the terms used include experimental epidemiology, therapeutic trials, experimental studies, prophylactic trials, randomized control trials, experimental trials. The term used frequently in epidemiology is *experimental epidemiology*. This author prefers to use the term *experimental design*, a term used more commonly in the general research field.

In a true sense of the definition epidemiology does not include experimental design research. Epidemiology studies the effect of epidemics, outbreaks in populations and groups. Experimental design research is used in basic empirical research on small populations. In the health care/medical field, experimental design is used in testing drugs, vaccines, treatment procedures, and patient treatment approaches, all of which are done on small sets, often on experimental animals or small experimental study groups. For the most part it is considered unethical to do such experiments on large populations due to the possible risks and potential bad outcomes. Thus, small groups of volunteers, sometimes people with a disease for which there is no cure, are used and informed of the hazards and risks. Sometimes people with little to lose are used. Sick individuals who may die anyway, prisoners, or other such populations may volunteer for a study.

One of the first experimental designs used in medical trials was done by Pasteur while trying to find a treatment or vaccine for rabies. The rabies experiments were first conducted on rabbits, rats, and mice. When a child bitten by a rabid dog was brought to Pasteur, he first refused to treat the child, as no human subjects had ever been treated for rabies. The parents persisted, the child would die anyway and the child was treated and cured. Later, another child was presented, but was in the latent phases of the disease. Pasteur, knowing the potential for a bad outcome, refused the treatment. The parents persisted and he treated the child and the child died. The death of the child was made a public concern and almost caused the research on vaccines to cease. In recent times, patients at the brink of death have volunteered to be placed on special heart-lung machines in the stages of being developed, or were exposed to experimental surgical procedures in order to further medicine and science. These important research activities helped to advance knowledge. Many were experimental design studies done on individuals or small groups of persons with specialized needs. These types of studies are not done on a large scale to large groups or populations, and thus fall short of being epidemiological studies.

Some control measures useful in public health and epidemiology are a direct result of biomedical experimental research designs. Most vaccines have been developed using experimental designs and clinical trials. Many outcomes of biomedical research have furthered the cause of public health and epidemiology, and in this sense experimental design is essential to the field of epidemiology. On the other hand, it is confusing to suggest that basic experimental designs/clinical trials on small groups in clinical settings, as used in biomedical sciences are epidemiological studies. There has been a trend in the last few years to call basic experimental design research analyzed using sophisticated inferential statistic approaches, epidemiological research. Many sources and references imply that these two separate fields are one, causing much confusion and diminishing the importance and significance of basic epidemiology methods. In order to provide a basic understanding of experimental design research and since it is a research design approach, some of the basics are presented.

In experimental design research one of the first things that is noted as being different is that the research process, procedures, inputs, and outcomes are under the direct control of the investigator. Experimental design resembles longitudinal and prospective study designs as the studies follow a subject over time (but usually only a short time period) and include follow-up assessments. The feature that stands out the most is that the investigator (I avoid calling this person an epidemiologist) manipulates the subject or provides some form of intervention, treatment, or change. In observational epidemiological studies no manipulation or change is done, only what has occurred is observed and studied.

Case Example: Experimental Design

One of the best examples of a study using an experimental design is Louis Pasteur's, demonstrating the effectiveness of his new vaccine against anthrax in the mid-1800s. The medical community issued a challenge to Pasteur to prove his vaccine, because there was much skepticism at that time about vaccines, germs, and the causes of disease. The Hippocratic theory of medicine still dominated medical practice.

Sixty sheep were donated for this politically charged experiment: 25 to be vaccinated, 25 to be used as a control group, and 10 merely to be observed. Twenty-five sheep were vaccinated and allowed to wait two weeks for the immunization process to occur. After two weeks, all 50 of the sheep were injected with a double dose of anthrax pathogens. The 10 sheep with no injections of bacteria or vaccine were kept separate. All 25 vaccinated sheep lived. All 25 unvaccinated sheep of the control/comparison group died, and all 10 sheep in the nontreatment control group lived.

OBSERVATIONAL STUDIES

Epidemiological studies are founded in observational studies. The most prominent observational studies are retrospective and case control studies.

Retrospective Studies and Case Control Studies

In order to define *retrospective*, we return to basic medical terminology. *Retro spicere* means "to look back," thus, retrospective studies are research activities that go back in time to study activities related to disease outbreaks that have already occurred. Slome, Brogan, Eyres, and Lednar suggest that the concept of retrospective study is interchangeable with case control study.[4] In a more strict definition, **retrospective studies** are research methodologies used to study and test hypotheses related to exposure or experiences in the past due to the etiology of a disease, condition, or disorder through which information about cause-effect relationships are derived from past characteristics of the population or group under study. Another term for this type of study is *ex post facto*. In an **ex post facto** study the epidemiologist does not manipulate the data but measures its effect after it has occurred. Retrospective studies are done ex post facto. Persons who are unaffected, (well persons/controls or case control) are compared to the affected (diseased) person's traits and experiences. Levels of severity, means of exposure, and other differences in individuals and populations are studied. *Case control study* is a phrase or term often used in epidemiology in place of retrospective study.[1,2,3,4]

Case control studies are retrospective studies as they are conducted after the onset of an outbreak and "look backward" to the possible causes of the outbreak. Case control studies begin with assessment of the persons or groups with a disease, condition, or disorder and identify a separate control group that has not been affected by the disease or condition. Case control refers to the way in which the study group is put together. Case control studies are also referred to as *case-comparison studies, case-referent studies*. The agent, risk factor, or causal element being studied is included in external causes as well as internal factors such as genetic makeup. The diseased and unexposed, nondiseased (well) are compared and examined with regard to the frequency of selected attributes and characteristics that each have, the level, severity, quantities, etc., are quantitatively analyzed with regard to the condition or disease.[1,2,3,4]

Retrospective studies are used to determine if the well group and the ill group differ in the proportion to those who have been exposed to a specific agent, risk factor, or pathogen. What makes the study retrospective is that the well and ill are compared with regard to the presence of some trait, characteristic, or factor resulting from past activities or experiences.

Since epidemiology classifies individuals in a study by either case (diseased) or control (non-diseased), groups for a retrospective study are to be selected and arranged using the same classification.

Case Example: A Retrospective Cohort Study—Infant Mortality Among Teenage Births at County Hospital

County Medical Center, that served the indigent populations of the central area of Metropolitan City in recent years observed a high rate of teenage births. The Committee for Quality Performance Improvement enlisted the aid of the hospital epidemiologist to determine death rates related to teen births. The epidemiologist obtained the support of the medical records department and set up a retrospective study to review all medical records and birth certificates for the past five years. The epidemiologist determined that she would ascertain perinatal, fetal, and infant mortality rates related to teenage births and set up the study design to identify a study group and a comparison group. The sampling method would be a blanket sample of all teenage births for the previous full five years, starting with January 1. The study group would consist of two cohort groups. The first cohort would consist of all teenage births of high-risk years (defined as all teen births within the hospital, consisting of mothers who had babies prior to their eighteenth birthday, all the way down to the very youngest mother, who was determined to be 12 years of age), all within the five-year period. The comparison/control group would be made up of all mothers past their eighteenth birthday, within the next 6 years. Each cohort would be placed in a category according to several variables: baby's birth weight, payment source, prenatal care history, method of delivery, race, sex of child, mother's marital status, mother's occupation, years of education, tobacco use, illicit drug use, and alcohol use. The epidemiologist planned to review all available records. Tick sheets and tabulation forms would be developed, the information entered into spreadsheets, proper descriptive statistics employed, and appropriate tables and graphs developed to present the findings, with a comprehensive report summarizing the findings presented to the committee.

CASE FILE

Data Collection in Case Control Studies

Collecting Occupational Job and Exposure Risk Data

When occupational data are collected for medical records or for survey research, responses are often limited to those given to general questions. But one group of researchers developed a procedure to acquire more detailed information in a standardized, efficient, and systematic manner in case control studies.

A computer-assisted generic work history is taken, which includes job elements that can aid in determining occupational health risk, exposure to risk, and some indication of health status. Information gathered in the interview includes chemicals and materials used, job activities, tools and equipment used, type of business, and job title. One research variable included was that each job after age 16 must have been held for six months or more. All responses are entered directly into the computer as the interview is conducted. The computer program searches for synonyms that will identify possible job-specific modules. Modules are detailed questionnaires on specific jobs, which ask further questions about the work environment, such as sources of exposure, the worker's exposure to hazardous agents, work in front of ventilation exhaust fans, work history, and chemicals handled.

When all the data have been collected, the work history and responses to the modules are sent to an industrial hygienist who reviews the information on a specialized software package called CAPI, or Computer-Assisted Personal Interview. The computer finds the job-specific module from the synonym file that links job titles and modules. If the word *repair* is used, for instance, all mechanic jobs will appear on the screen. Whereas generic work histories were not always useful, the module/synonym approach was found effective. Modules are optimal for jobs where level of exposure varies among similar persons having the same job. Modules were developed for 38 of the most frequently reported jobs, using more than 4,000 word synonyms, and sophisticated branching and skip patterns, so that the interviewer asks only the most important questions. Risk assignment is the last step, using industrial hygiene principles while avoiding misclassification of disease. Future occupational health epidemiologists will be able to utilize CAPI to enhance job risk, exposure, relative risk, and risk-ratio assessments for cancer and other occupational diseases.

(Source: Steward, P.A., "A Novel Approach to Data Collection in a Case-Control Study of Cancer and Occupational Exposures," International Journal of Epidemiology, Vol. 25, No. 4, 1996, pp. 744–752)

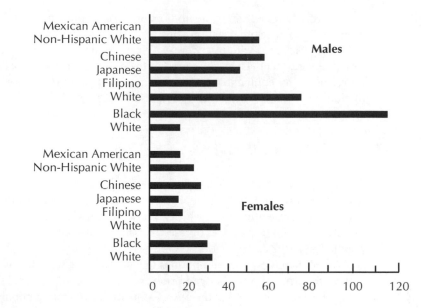

FIGURE 8.1 Retrospective study of lung and bronchus cancer incidence rates according to sex and race: Selected cancer registries, 1977–83. (Source: Centers for Disease Control and Prevention, *Health United States—1990*, Public Health, U.S. Department of Health and Human Services, March, 1991)

Selection of Cases for Retrospective Studies/Case Control Studies

In retrospective studies, cases usually have been sick and often have presented themselves for medical care or testing at a clinic, physician, or other health care provider. To establish a retrospective study, clear guidelines concerning the severity, extent, and stages of a disease must be set so that precise criteria about the cases can be established. The results of a retrospective study are important in establishing a cause-effect relationship (etiological relationship), more so than trying to generalize to a general population. For example, certain characteristics or behaviors may lead to certain types of cancer (see Figure 8.1). Once etiological relationships are established, then interventions can be made, and control and prevention measures can be planned and implemented.

Guidelines for Case Selection for Prospective and Cross-Sectional Studies

1. Cases should consist of all new cases (confirmed by diagnosis) having selected characteristics present during a specific time period in a specific population and a particular area.

2. Incidence is preferred over prevalence due to the duration of certain diseases.

3. Slanted or biased results must be avoided. The selection process should consider the effects of different sets of risk factors found in cases.[1,2,3,4]

Sources for cases can come from records from public health clinics, physician offices, health maintenance organizations, hospitals, and industrial and government sources. Medical records coupled with interviews with cases done in person are valuable sources of information and an effective approach. For the most part, records are the main source of data for retrospective epidemiology studies. The placement of past records (the data and information) into sets of cases becomes case control studies.[1,2,3,4]

Controls and Control Group Selection

To better assure that a retrospective study is valid and reliable, the cases used in the study need to be compared to normal or unaffected groups or persons that were the same as or equal to the population from which the cases came. Controls can come from the general population, from the relatives of cases, the same treatment center, HMO, hospital, or study population as the cases.

An epidemiological assumption is that controls are representative of the general population in terms of probability of exposure and that controls have the same possibility of being selected or exposed as the cases. Controls drawn from a population of the same area or populace of the cases should reflect the same sex, age groups, and other significant factors. Controls from a general population are assumed to be normal and healthy and to reflect the well population from the area. Sampling of controls from a general population for large studies is an expensive endeavor and thus not always realistic or possible. Regardless of where controls come from, every effort should be made to select them at random and have them be representative of the study group.

Randomized Control Groups

Also referred to as *randomized controlled trials*; once a large study group is established, the subjects are then assigned to the treatment group and the control group by random sampling/assignment techniques. (See *random assignment* on page 249.) Chance is the only determining factor that determines which group each subject is assigned to, thus allowing inferential statistical tests of probability to be applied and levels of significance to be determined. Cause-effect relationships can be shown in a clinical setting and randomized controlled trials are most common in these settings. The results of such studies in turn can be applied to public health, while disease, conditions, disorders, and disability can be reduced, controlled, and prevented when causal factors are identified.[6,7,8,13,14,15,16]

Multiple Treatment Groups

Using a modification of the basic research design presented above, subjects are assigned to three or four or more different study groups. Subjects can be assigned at random to the different treatment groups. For example if three groups are needed, i.e., treatment group A, treatment group B, and the control group, the subjects, are placed in equal numbers in each of the three groups using random assignment approaches. Treatment group A could be given drug A only to see its effects on the subjects. Treatment group B would be given drug

A and drug B together to study the effects of the combination of the two drugs on the subjects. The third group is the control group and is treated the same as the treatment groups but receives no drugs. As with the other research designs, inferential statistical tests of probability are applied and levels of significance determined. Cause-effect relationships can be shown and the results may be applied to public health and disease, control and prevention when causal factors are identified.[6,7,8,13,14,16]

Blind Studies

Also called *blind experiments* or *blind trials* these studies are used most with drug and pharmaceutical type research studies. As in basic design type studies, multiple study groups can be used. One group can receive drug A, one group can receive drug B, a third group could receive both drug A and B together, and a fourth group would serve as the control group. A multitude of arrangements can be made with the research subjects and treatment and control groups. The key to blind studies is to reduce bias and confounding variables. To reduce any outside influence, other than what the actual treatment does, the researcher or the subjects or both do not know to which group they have been assigned. A second researcher does random assignment to study groups and treatment is provided in a manner so that researchers or subjects do not know if they are given the treatment or if they are in the control group. Sometimes the subjects are kept "blind," from knowing which group they are assigned to. One way to keep subjects from figuring out which group they are in is for all to receive treatment, some by using fake treatments or placebos. Sometimes the researchers are kept blind so that the processes surrounding the experiment do not become an influencing factor, or researchers' biases will not influence study outcomes. Bias may creep in if the treatment subjects are treated differently, better and more warmly by the researcher than the control group. The researcher may unknowingly treat subjects differently as he or she may wish to see certain outcomes and thus may do things differently for the experimental group, resulting in a biased result.[6,7,8,13,14,16,17]

A **single blind study** occurs when the researcher knows the treatment structure, subject assignments, methods etc., but the subjects do not know. A **double blind study** takes place when neither the researcher nor the subjects know the treatments, subjects group assignments, and methods. A **triple blind study** is when not only are the treatment and research approaches kept a secret from researcher and subjects, but the analysis is also completed in a manner that is removed from the researcher.[6,7,8,13,14]

Nonrandomized Treatment and Control Groups

Several reasons exist for not using random assignment or random sampling. First, large research populations are not always available especially in clinical settings. Cost of research is expensive and funds may not be adequate for the research procedures, follow-up treatments and testing of both study and control groups that are large. Another restraint is the lack of subjects with the disease, condition, or a seen need to participate.

If a large population is to be treated with a preventive measure such as immunizations, the epidemiologist would not purposely leave half of the population, assigned at random as a control group and at risk of getting the disease due to not being protected by the immunization (as was done in the Tuskegee Syphilis Study, see Chapter 3). Randomization cannot be applied if an entire population is to be affected or subject to the treatment. If fluoride is added to the water supply of a city, there is no way to include or exclude certain individuals. If seat-belt laws are implemented, control groups are not selected and randomization is not used in the enforcement of the law.

If randomly selected control groups are available, a comparison group may be selected from individuals with traits similar to those of the subjects in the treatment group. A pretest/post-test approach will allow the treatment group to serve as its own controls. The changes from the pretest to the post-test results often show a statistically significant cause-effect relationship.[6,7,8,13,14]

Confounding Variables

Variables or factors known to be related to, associated with, or that can influence the state of the subjects being studied are **confounding variables**. Confounding variables can affect controls and may lead to biased or misguided association between disease and cause, the agent or risk factors. Any characteristic, trait, or other factor that can distort or slant the results of a study can be a confounding variable if not taken into account or considered. Some of the more important variables that can be confounding to cases or controls are age, sex, race, occupation, education, socioeconomic status. Any factor that distorts the outcome or effect of a study confounds the facts and objectivity of the results. Any factor that causes unequal distribution among the exposed and unexposed (cases and controls) can also distort or confound the outcome of a study.

Confounding of variables can be controlled by matching or by statistical control methods or approaches. **Matching** is the process of selecting controls so that they have similar effects or characteristics as the cases. Matching attempts to make the cases comparable with controls. Matching can include efforts to match ages closely (caliper matching), or to pair up individual cases with controls, one to one (pair matching). **Individual matching** compares separate individuals with a study subject who resembles the other individual. Frequency distributions of a matched characteristic should be the same or similar in cases and controls (**frequency matching**). The matching of cases and control groups in broad categories such as wide groupings of occupation, ages, or races is **category matching**.

Matching is an important part of research design, as is the control of confounding variables. Statistical control can be used to deal with confounding variables. The case groups and control groups can be controlled by **stratification**, which is used to remove the effect of confounding variables, and is accomplished by breaking the groups of cases and controls into sub-units or subsets.

Advantages of Retrospective Studies/Case Control Studies   Several advantages exist that encourage the use of retrospective and case control studies. The advantages are listed below. Retrospective studies and case control studies

1. are inexpensive to conduct;

2. make it easier to access a large number of subjects as the study uses records and the identification of cases which are then compared to controls with similar traits;

3. require fewer numbers than are required for prospective studies;

Retrospective and Outcome Studies

Epidemiological Outcome Studies in Hernia Repairs

In the managed care environment of the late 1990s, length of hospital stay, cost of treatment, and unnecessary readmissions are of utmost concern to physicians and health care administrators. Of more importance to the patient is a positive treatment outcome. Patients want successful treatment with no complications requiring further care, treatment, hospitalization, or loss of life.

A retrospective outcome case study on outpatient versus inpatient hernia repair was conducted through the outpatient department of St. Bernardine Medical Center of San Bernardino, California, There has been a national trend to do as many hernia repairs as possible on an outpatient basis, but after reviewing 149 records of all hernia repairs, it was found that it is not always best to do outpatient surgery on all types of hernia repair cases. The best candidates for outpatient surgery were those with inguinal hernias. The readmission rate is high for most forms of hernia repair other than inguinal. Infection rates, bleed rates, and readmissions were studied. The bleed rate was highest for outpatient surgery on all types of hernia repair including inguinal. Infection rates were the same for both inpatient and outpatient surgery. In England, a study of 30,675 records of England's National Health Service were retrospectively reviewed from 1976 to 1986, with 28,399 patients actually receiving the operation/hernia repair. Of all the cases, 6%, or 1,786, were done as day cases. In all, 425 had emergency readmissions within 30 days of the operation, with 17 of the day cases being readmitted. The causes of unplanned readmissions were complications of the operations, such as postoperative infection/ hemorrhage/hematoma (18%), deep vein thrombosis (8%), pulmonary embolism (7%), and other cardiovascular causes (7%), with 4% requiring a second emergency operation. In the year after the operation, there were 366 deaths following an elective procedure and 175 following emergency repairs. Retrospective epidemiological studies have proved to be extremely valuable for understanding health care treatment procedures, related morbidity, and mortality.

(Sources: Cantwell, Marie, an Outcomes Study: Outpatient Versus Inpatient Hernia Repairs, thesis for M.S. in Health Services Administration, California State University, San Bernardino, 1994; Primatesta, P., and Goldacre, M.J., "Inguinal Hernia Repair: Incidence of Elective and Emergency Surgery, Readmission and Mortality," International Journal of Epidemiology, Vol. 25, No. 4, 1996, pp. 835–839)

4. are useful in the study of etiological factors in unusual or rare diseases as fewer cases are needed;
5. allow results to be obtained quite quickly as the data are readily available;
6. are useful as more than one risk factor can be identified at the same time in the same set of data;
7. are useful in studies of drug-induced illness if a medication is suspected as the side effects or adverse reactions can be seen immediately.

Disadvantages of Retrospective Studies   Retrospective studies and case control studies may not be as useful because

1. information required for the study may not be readily available;
2. information required for the study may not be accurately recorded;
3. when interviews are used, the person may not remember past information or facts;
4. when surveys/interviews are used the person may not remember past information or facts, or it may be entered into the form incorrectly;
5. when interviews are used the person may present slanted or biased answers;
6. patients and physicians may not remember past events or circumstances or may recall the circumstances differently;
7. individuals may fill in events in order to make the story complete or may give more importance to certain past events;
8. in serious diseases or in severe cases of some disease, affected individuals have a greater chance of strong biases;
9. bias can exist in the selection of controls;
10. built in bias in controls can occur due to controls being selected from medical records;
11. inadvertent underrepresentation or misrepresentation may occur due to the selection process for both cases and controls;
12. personal traits or behaviors may overrepresent the problems that contributed to the disease, condition, disability, or death.

CROSS-SECTIONAL STUDIES/SURVEY RESEARCH

Cross-sectional studies most often use a survey approach. Cross-sectional studies are also referred to as **observational studies**. Observational studies do not use clinical approaches or experimental designs. Relationships, differences in variables, and changes in characteristics within the study population with intervention or cause from the epidemiologist characterize observational studies. A change in one study characteristic is compared and studied in relationship to changes that occur in other characteristics.

A cross-sectional study is an interesting and valuable research approach. A **cross-sectional study** is a picture of diseases, health, medical, and psychosocial phenomena as they exist at a point in time. From a practical point of view, the point in time may be as short as a few minutes or as long as two or three months. The time frame of the "point in time," is based on the speed and efficiency in collecting the data. If a survey form is filled out in a college class of 600 people, the time frame is the time it takes for the class to fill out the survey form. If the survey is mailed, then the time frame is expanded to the time it takes to retrieve the questionnaires. Theoretically, for the individual filling out a survey questionnaire, the data represent the point in time covered by the time that it takes that individual to fill out the questionnaire. Thus, a cross-sectional study does represent a point in time from two different perspectives, the time frame of the individual and the time frame of the entire study.

A cross-sectional study is like using a camera to take a still picture of a health, mental, social, environmental, or other problem or event in a population, fixing the data at a certain period in time. The findings of longitudinal studies are often compared to cross-sectional studies as they often find the same results. The longitudinal study is difficult to conduct, since it has to follow groups in a population over time. The cross-sectional study can gather much the same information and can do so by establishing a population sample much like that of a longitudinal study. The researcher gathers data from the sample population all at once and does so at one point in time. Longitudinal studies do provide much better information and more accurate data in many ways, as they do follow the true progression of a phenomenon happening over time, taking into account the individual changes that can occur. Cross-sectional studies are limited to what data that has been gathered at one point in time.

A cross-sectional study can assess one or several variables at a time. Associations and correlation between variables can be easily evaluated in a cross-sectional study. Cross-sectional studies assess the relationships between (or among) health, disease, conditions, injuries, or other phenomena as they occur or presently exist in a population at a point in time or that particular time.

Case Example: High School Seniors' Health Knowledge: A Cross-Sectional Study

In the Lincoln County School District, personal health is taught for one semester in the seventh and tenth grades. The district director of health education was concerned about increases in smoking, drug use, lack of exercise, poor diet, and obesity in the county's high schools. The pressing question at hand was, Is health education, as it is being offered, doing any good for the high school student's health? How effective is the current approach to teaching personal health? How much health knowledge is being treated and translated into health behavior two years later?

Thus, a health risk questionnaire developed by the Centers for Disease Control and Prevention, was to be used to assess health risk behavior. The questionnaire was duplicated, Scantron sheets were included, and the packets were distributed to the health education department chairs in all ten high schools in the school district. Each health education chair was asked to give the questionnaire on exactly the same day to all seniors present in the high school. The department chairs were all successful in giving the questionnaire in the manner instructed, and 1,200 surveys were retrieved the same day.

Arrangements were made to have the Scantrons run at the CDC. Final results were returned, and the director of health education was able to create tables and graphs from the data. A final report was written and presented to the superintendent of schools.

The results showed that certain areas of health instruction were not working as expected, and some areas of instruction were badly needed. However, in some areas, such as drug and alcohol use and abuse, knowledge was quite high. A confounding variable was discovered when one of the students wrote a note that he had seen three different television programs on MTV about drug and alcohol use and abuse, that they were all rerun several times, and that he had watched them all.

Prevalence Studies and Cross-Sectional Studies

Because the concept of point in time is a part of a cross-sectional study, some epidemiological literature suggests that cross-sectional studies are prevalence studies. Prevalence

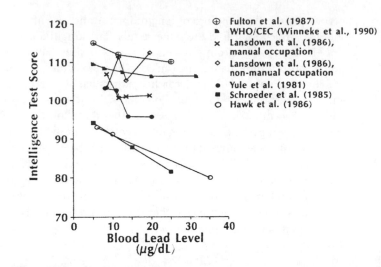

FIGURE 8.2   Comparison of blood levels and IQ scores of children from retrospective and cross-sectional studies. (Source: Centers for Disease Control and Prevention, *Preventing Lead Poisoning in Young Children*, Public Health Service, U.S. Department of Health and Human Services, October, 1991)

has been presented in detail in Chapter 5, including point prevalence and period prevalence. However, prevalence studies are but one form of a cross-sectional study (see Figure 8.2). Prevalence studies are used mostly with acute infectious communicable diseases. Cross-sectional studies include not only disease states, but conditions or states that could lead to disease, such as the amount of stress in a population. Need assessments are also done as cross-sectional studies. Incidence occurrences are not studied in cross-sectional studies.

Case Example: Pediculosis in Preschools: A Prevalence Survey

The head epidemiologist of Lincoln County's Department of Public Health, Division of Communicable Disease Control and Prevention, had received complaints of head lice from 15 of the county's 64 preschools. Thus, the epidemiologist decided that a random sample survey of all preschool children must be conducted in order to determine the extent of the problem and the prevalence of pediculosis among all preschool children within Lincoln County.

The epidemiological survey team decided that it must do an unannounced screening survey of all 64 licensed preschools. The sampling method would be a blanket survey/sample including all 64 preschools. A single public health nurse would be dispatched to each school. Ten public health nurses were identified as being able to work the survey, and it was determined that each nurse would be able to survey 3 to 4 schools in a day. The point prevalence time frame established would be no more than 3 days for completion of the prevalence survey. Children would be randomly examined in alphabetical order, with every fifth child being examined. To initiate immediate control of the spread of the head lice, the nurses would also examine all suspected cases and recommend the best treatment and control methods. The epidemiologist anticipated clustering cases of head lice and that dot maps would be produced. Followup and control measures would be done with all clusters, cases, and individual families. Family members and older siblings attending various schools would be investigated as well. Appropriate tables, graphs, charts, observed clustering, dot maps, and followup measures would be included in the report of the outbreak. The report would establish prevalence of pediculosis in preschools in the county.

Cross-Sectional Study Relationship Development

The absence or presence of a variable is assessed in a cross-sectional study. Each individual in a study group or a research sample that is representative of the study population is represented in the cross-sectional study for one point in time and the findings represent that particular time. The relationship between certain variables and the existence of a health factor, a disease, condition, or occurrence as well as the different levels of the condition can be studied and assessed. The same relationships, associations, and correlations can be assessed and analyzed in subgroups or various age groups. The epidemiological implication of cross-sectional studies is that the relationship of the absence or presence of a disease or cause of a disease can be studied. Another epidemiological implication is that the relationship of diseased to nondiseased persons or the variables implicated in the cause of the disease can be studied.

Advantages of Cross-Sectional Studies   Cross-sectional studies

1. are a one-stop, one-time collection of data (interview/examination/survey);
2. are less expensive and more expedient to conduct;
3. provide much information and data found useful for planning of health services and medical programs;
4. provide a one time glimpse at the study population, showing relative distribution of conditions, disease, injury and disability in groups and populations. (It is from this context cross-sectional studies are viewed as prevalence studies.)
5. provide the interrelatedness of attributes of disease and conditions in a group or population;
6. can be of some value in predicting future spread of certain disease through populations, such as cholera;
7. have one major advantage in that the studies are based on a sample of a major population and do not rely on individuals that present themselves for medical treatment.[3,4]

Disadvantages of Cross-Sectional Studies   Cross-sectional studies

1. fall short of showing strong cause-effect relationships if sample size is small;
2. only represent those individuals who filled out the questionnaire, took the survey, and participated in the study;
3. as used in disease studies, represent only those who are surveyed and/or have the disease;

4. when used as a prevalence of disease assessment, are not too effective if the level of disease rates is very small. Sampling techniques are used in cross-sectional studies and in the study of the prevalence of a disease in a population should be more accurate than some sampling approaches allow. Other approaches for disease prevalence are more effectively used, such as the reporting of every single case as in the notifiable diseases, especially with life threatening diseases such as rabies. Blanket surveys are also effective in studying the prevalence of a disease or condition in a population. The prevalence of some diseases in a population is unknown, as little effort is made to study them, such as cocksackie disease (a short-term viral infection causing sores in the mouth, most common in children under age 10).

5. recurrent conditions or disease or seasonal variations of them are not well represented in cross-sectional studies as when the study is conducted the condition may be dormant or inactive or at its peak. Incidence studies are more useful. Incidence and point and period prevalence concepts are presented in Chapter 5.

6. like most studies, have limited value in predicting future occurrences for some conditions or diseases;

7. are more effective in chronic diseases and behaviorally related conditions and less effective in communicable diseases with short incubation periods and short duration;

8. will show a high percentage of cases of a condition or disease of long duration while having the potential of not showing or having limited effect on diseases in a series of incident cases.[3,4]

SELECTION OF STUDY POPULATION

Some populations used for epidemiological studies may be based on ethnicity, race, potential to have a disease, higher prevalence of a disease in a group, probability to get the disease more than other groups, or other related reasons. For example, diabetes or alcoholism is often studied in the Navajo tribe as these conditions are more prevalent in this Native American population. One major study assessed alcohol and substance abuse in Native American adolescents. In 1979, Oetting and Goldstein surveyed 2,904 Native American adolescents in seven different locations in the United States and found that most had at least experimented with alcohol and drugs by age 17.[9] A self-report survey was given to 212 ninth- through twelfth-grade students who attend school on the Navajo reservation. The drug of choice was alcohol. Of the students who reported drinking beer, 47% of the seniors reported drinking at least monthly. The authors state that due to the cross-sectional nature of the study, one does not know whether or not the use of alcohol preceded or followed the onset of the use of marijuana or hard drugs. This statement shows at least one other limitation of a cross-sectional study. To overcome such limitations, questions can be included to address such issues. The questions would directly ask if they used beer first or marijuana first. Table 8.1 shows the findings from the study on alcohol and substance abuse in Native American high school students.[10]

For cross-sectional studies to be effective and valid, all subjects must have an equal chance to represent the population being studied. All members of the population study group should have an equal chance of being selected and filling out the survey form. By doing proper and objective sampling, all members of a population can be afforded an equal chance to participate in the study.

TABLE 8.1 Percentage of Native American high school students who experienced substance use/abuse at least once or twice a month by grade and gender

| | Percent Who Use Substances at Least Once or Twice a Month by Grade and Gender | | | | | | | |
| | Grade 9 (n = 48) | | Grade 10 (n = 66) | | Grade 11 (n = 54) | | Grade 12 (n = 37) | |
Substance	%M	%F	%M	%F	%M	%F	%M	%F
Cigarettes	57	43	38	26	52	26	33	19
Chew	48	17	41	9	44	15	33	38
Beer	48	43	34	26	56	48	47	43
Wine	14	13	7	11	16	11	13	10
Liquor	55	21	27	11	28	19	7	33
Pot	38	22	17	17	40	30	27	10
Inhalants	5	0	0	3	4	0	7	0
Depressants	5	0	0	0	0	0	0	0
Hallucinogens	0	0	0	0	0	0	0	0
Stimulants	0	0	0	0	4	0	0	0
Cocaine	0	0	0	0	0	0	0	0

(Source: Cole, G., Timmreck, T.C., Page, R. and Woods, S., "Patterns and Relevance of Substance Use Among Navajo Youth," *Health Values*, Vol. 16, No. 3, May/June 1992. Used with permission.)

SURVEYS IN CROSS-SECTIONAL STUDIES

One of the most common approaches to cross-sectional studies is through the use of survey methodologies. Many survey approaches are used to conduct epidemiological studies.

The survey approach is a widely used research approach in public health and government health studies. Survey research can be used in complex research designs or it can be as simple as a one-page questionnaire addressing a single variable or condition in the study population.

Several basic epidemiological survey research issues need to be considered. The first and most basic issue is to have a good research questionnaire. Previously developed questionnaires that are valid and reliable are available in published form. Researchers, consulting firms, and government agencies have spent much time and expertise in developing standardized questionnaires. Some questionnaires have been computerized. Special effort has been put into developing some survey forms so they can be computer scored and analyzed.[6,7]

If the questionnaire is developed by the epidemiologist or by an agency, then serious thought, time, and effort should be spent on question development. Questionnaires developed with much thought and effort better assure that a useful and effective study is the final product. Questions on the survey form should ask simple and straightforward questions. Questions should be asked in a manner that will get the information desired. Wording of the questions should be reviewed, tested, and edited to assure they are well prepared and ask what you want to know. Avoid writing double negatives into questions. (For example: "He has no immunizations, yes or no? There is no clinic near by, yes or no?") Good questions are presented in a direct and simplified manner and ask what one wants to know, what one wants to find out. Keep the questions and the questionnaires short and to the point.[5]

Retrieving the Questionnaires

A major problem in epidemiological research, or any research for that matter, is retrieving the questionnaires once completed by the participants. Thus, a system to retrieve survey questionnaires needs to be established by the epidemiologist in charge of the research.

Data gathering systems or methods (the way the survey is approached) should be coordinated with questionnaire retrieval. Some data gathering approaches lend themselves to questionnaire retrieval and solve the sample size and questionnaire retrieval matters; other approaches make retrieval more difficult. For examples, interviews and home visits solve data gathering problems and questionnaire retrieval problems. Mailed questionnaires are difficult to retrieve. Some seasoned researchers indicate that, in mailed questionnaires, a 50% return rate is considered quite good. If a survey is conducted in a large company, industry, or organization under the sanction of the organization's leaders, or under the control of the company's medical director, the return rates go up substantially. Returns increase if a company letterhead is used and the survey is sent through company mail.

FIVE DATA GATHERING APPROACHES

Several data gathering approaches are used in epidemiology, and five approaches are presented here. Any approach should keep imposition on the interviewee (subject) to a minimum. However, the epidemiological surveyor should be careful to not shortchange the interview nor the information gathering process either. The survey should be done in a manner that assures the information is obtained and that the questionnaires can easily be retrieved or sent in. Once the survey form is developed and tested, two of the major problems in survey research remain: (1) to obtain the participation of the subjects/respondents and (2) to retrieve the data (questionnaires).[5]

The five common approaches to survey research are

Person-to-Person Interviews   Using the survey form/questionnaire, an in-person interview is conducted. Interviews are often done in the subject's home, in a clinic, or in a center.

Drop Off Questionnaire   The survey form is left with the subject and the epidemiologist returns to retrieve it at a set time and date. This can be less of a burden on the person being interviewed as it allows the subjects to fill it out at their own pace and at their own convenience. A limitation is that this is a self-report process with no chance for clarification. The interviewee needs to be clearly informed of the time of retrieval and asked to have it ready and waiting. This approach works best in housing projects, senior high-rise apartments, or other housing arrangements with high density living and that are close by. The most difficult, due to transportation and distance, is a rural setting.

Mailed Questionnaires   The survey form is mailed to a list of predetermined individuals. Using sampling techniques, mailing lists are developed that represent all persons in the study population. For example, if the epidemiologist wished to study the immunization levels in the elderly in certain geographical areas, a proper sampling could be conducted from mailing lists obtained from senior high-rise apartments, government housing projects for the elderly, senior citizens centers, a county's Office On Aging, AARP chapters, churches, etc.

Telephone Interviews   Survey forms can be used in telephone interviews. In order to assure accuracy and consistency in the gathering of data, the survey form is followed precisely, providing standardized questioning processes. Names and phone numbers could be obtained from sources similar to those mentioned under mailed questionnaires.

Newsletter or Magazine Surveys   A short or abbreviated survey form can be included in a newsletter or regional magazine with a self-stamped mailing arrangement included. Include a folded survey form with the address and mailing stamp on the outside so the respondent can easily remove, fill out, fold, and mail.[5,6,7]

SAMPLING THE POPULATION FOR EPIDEMIOLOGICAL STUDIES

Good sampling is basic to and essential in all scientific research, and epidemiology is no exception. An epidemiological survey process has to have validity to it and should use recognized, standard, proved sampling approaches and methodologies. The number of individuals participating in the survey must be substantial enough in numbers to produce valid results, reliable findings, and outcomes that will give a true and accurate presentation of the epidemiological condition or concern. The epidemiologist should obtain as large a sample size as is feasible. The more participants in the survey, the more accurate the findings. In other words, the larger the sample size, the better. Small sample sizes can invalidate a study, resulting in a waste of time, money, and other resources.[5,6,7]

Sampling and Random Assignment

Types of concepts and activities that are basic to research are those of sampling and randomization or random assignment. Several random sampling concepts and approaches are used.

Random Assignment/Randomization

Random assignment and randomization are two terms that have been used interchangeably. **Randomization** is selecting and assigning individuals to groups with no intent to make assignments by any characteristic or category. Selection and assignment to research groups is done by chance only. Research groups and control groups, selected at the beginning of any research project, should be as much alike as possible and both groups should be representative of the general population. Equal representation can occur only if subjects are chosen by chance and assigned to the research study group by chance. Haphazard assignment is not a chance assignment and must be avoided. Logical and equal opportunity for assignment must occur for all, or at least be chosen only by chance in a logical fashion. A random sample is the result of a good sampling process combining randomization with sampling procedures.

Sampling methods and constructs are presented below. A random sample is selected by choosing sample units in such a fashion that each subject has a probable and fixed chance of selection. Random assignment is the assignment of subjects to treatment or study groups and control groups in a manner that allows each subject to have an equal opportunity to be included in the study group or control group.

Sampling and Sample Selection

Sampling and proper sample selection is fundamental to all research, and epidemiological survey research is no exception. Sampling should consider the kind of survey and approach to be used and the kinds of findings anticipated. Approaches to sampling as used in empirical research should be used. With regard to sampling, the size of the sample must be large enough to be representative of the study population. The reason for sampling is to get responses that show a true picture of conditions, disease, injuries, or disabilities and to have reliable data that can be analyzed without asking each and every person in the entire population. The main reason to use sampling is to cut cost and effort and yet predict need or determine problems (as opposed to surveying an entire population).[11]

Sample Size

A rule about sample size is to use the largest sample size that is possible or realistic, given the constraints of time and money. Statistical curves show that the smaller the sample size, the larger the error in predictability. The larger the sample the smaller the error in predictability. Budget and the predictability (level of confidence) also determine sample size. Ordinarily, several hundred questionnaires would be a good goal but should be based on population size.[4,5,6,7]

Sampling Approaches

Some of the sampling approaches that may be useful for need assessment type research include

Sample of Convenience   This sampling approach works well as long as the sample is large and includes a high percentage of the study population. This sampling approach usually includes recipients of a service, those involved in a clinic or available at a worksite. Generalizations are drawn from the findings and applied to the larger population. Even though this is one of the most commonly used approaches, it is one sampling approach that lends itself to much bias and is often criticized by behavioral science researchers.[4,5,6,7]

Random Sample   This approach will be valid as long as the sample is quite large and the selection process uses a true random approach, i.e., cutting up a list of names and selecting them out of a container and assuring that a set percentage are chosen. Another method is to select every fifth or seventh person from a computer printout of all persons in a study group.

Random has two dimensions. One is random selection and the other is random assignment. **Random assignment** is the assigning of people to groups so that each person has an equal chance of being selected to fill out the survey form. **Random selection** is the selection of individuals who will participate as subjects from the research population. Random selection is used in need assessment type studies more often than random assignment. Random assignment is used more in epidemiological surveys and is the more accepted form of research sampling.

Another sampling issue is that of generalizing to populations or generalizing *across* populations. The tendency in epidemiological studies is to generalize across populations. The epidemiologist needs to be aware that to generalize to a population is to do so at the risk of overlooking the conditions or diseases of subgroups within the study populations. This occurs even when using random samples, especially if the sample is small. To generalize across populations, the epidemiologist may (or may not) wish to take into account the sub-population's special customs, culture, traditions, health beliefs and practices, living circumstances, or lifestyles. An example would be in assessing food preparation practices of the elderly to determine how food preparation practices affect foodborne illness in the elderly. A random sample shows that certain food storage and food sanitation practices are ignored. If the population is further studied, it could be found that a major subgroup of Hispanics live within the study population. However, they were not well represented in the sampling process. In daily practice in the study group population, the Hispanics have more foodborne illnesses as they use more traditional and culturally motivated food preparation techniques that require handling the food more than usual and lack of sanitation practices contributing to foodborne illnesses. These important factors could be overlooked in the sampling process.[3,4,5,6,7]

Self-Selection/Volunteer Participation   In this sampling approach, a survey is given to patients at a public health clinic who are willing to fill out the form, making it somewhat of a sample of convenience. As a general rule, this sampling approach has more bias in it than other forms. Research has shown that certain types of persons will participate more than others in filling out research forms. Characteristics of the type of people who are willing to fill out a survey form are that they are usually more educated, have a higher occupational status, have a high need for approval, have high IQs, and are low in authoritarianism.[5,6,7]

Blanket Survey   This approach tries to interview all possible recipients of a service or program. A blanket survey is almost impossible to accomplish. Some need assessment programs sponsored by the Federal government in the past have completed need assessments of 75% to 80% of all elderly in a county in assessing health and social service needs.[5] This approach supports the notion that the larger the sample size, the smaller the error in predicting need. This is very costly, thus not used as often.

Stratified Sample   A stratified sample is done by dividing the study population into two or more segments, thus sampling a different proportion of each. This selection or stratification process is often based on economic, demographic characteristics, age or other variables that sensibly lend themselves to dividing the population into a strata or segments. Random sampling approaches are then used within each strata.[4,6]

Cluster Sample   This approach to sample selection is used if the study population is dispersed or in separated places or spread over a large geographic area. It lends itself better to mail surveys and is less practical for interview or telephone approaches. If travel time and costs are high for interviews, cluster sampling is more economical. Again basic random sampling is used. A large sample size needs to be maintained, if not, cluster sampling will not produce accurate results. Groups of people that cluster together are sampled, such as university students, church members, club members, public schools, a geographical area, housing tracts, etc. Sampling involves the initial sampling of groups of clusters and the sampling of each element of the clusters. Cluster approaches are used when it is impractical to compile a complete list of characteristics or influencing variables of a study population. In a city, a set of city blocks could be selected for sampling. From the selected city blocks, sampling is done for all of those living there. Sampling of subgroups within the city blocks based on race for example could also be done. This is also referred to as *multistage sampling*.[4,6]

Quota Sample   When a stratified sample is necessary or the desired approach, then a quota sample approach may be useful. If the interview approach is used, a quota sample may be a good approach. Random sampling should be used. Interviewers are assigned a quota of a given number of interviews from each segment or cluster. Problems arise in quota sampling if hourly wages are used. Assigned quotas and payment per number are more cost effective and productive, but efforts should be made to assure that honest and ethical filling out of the forms occurs, as they should be done by or with the subject.[4]

Density Sampling   Density sampling is often used in case control and longitudinal studies as a method of selecting controls. This approach conducts sampling from incident cases over a specific period of time. Sampling and assessment of controls is done through the entire study period. The aim of this sampling approach is to reduce bias by constant sampling of both subject and controls instead of using a cross-sectional approach of doing the assessment at a single point in time. As time passes, patterns of exposure to disease and health factors occur in both subjects and controls in longitudinal studies and the changes occur over long periods of time and sampling needs to account for such changes.

Whichever sampling approach is used, the epidemiologist must make every effort to assure the population is well represented. Subgroups or outliers should not over-influence the results nor be underrepresented. Sound, well-thought out scientifically founded sampling procedures should be used. If the epidemiologist desires in-depth information on complex sampling procedures, several books are available on the subject, as well as detailed coverage available in some texts on research methodology. If major epidemiology projects are to be conducted, a review of references on research and sampling references is recommended.

Sample Bias

Sample bias is important to consider and avoid. Many types of bias are encountered by the epidemiologist. One type is **visibility bias**; only those who are identifiable or are at hand are included and excluded are those not easily identifiable nor easy to access. A second type is **order bias**, which is when people are chosen by alphabetical order, numerical order, street address, or other sequential ordering. The tendency is to use people at the beginning too often and the end people (names) are rarely included. A third bias is **accessibility bias** which occurs most often when field workers are allowed to pick the sample. They tend to pick those persons who are most easily reached. Fourth is **cluster bias** which happens when the subject clusters are set too closely together, such as when those who live close to each other may interact and share information. Last mentioned is affinity bias, which is when people interview those to whom they tend to be drawn.[3,4,5,6]

Here is a summary and quick review of sampling and sampling concerns.

1. When conducting a sample for a study, be sure to sample equally the more visible and the more obscure portions of the study population.

2. Sampling should be conducted in an organized and systematic fashion in order to avoid an over sampling of some areas or groups and under sampling of others.

3. Sampling structure, approaches, and controls must be established to assure that all persons in the study group have an equal chance of being selected.

4. If the study population is clustered, there must be equal sampling within the clusters as well as between them.

5. If the survey workers are allowed to conduct their own sampling, a method of control must be established in order to assure sampling is properly done as well as control for the tendency for the surveyors to select people similar to themselves.

6. If the persons participating in the study are allowed to self-select as a sampling process, interaction with other participants in the survey should be restricted if possible.

7. Bias must be reduced and controlled. Are some survey participants more likely to respond than others or respond in a certain way and how can these factors be controlled?[3,4,6]

NATIONAL EPIDEMIOLOGICAL HEALTH SURVEY METHODOLOGY

In the United States, the National Center for Health Statistics and the Division of Health Interview Statistics have been collecting data continuously since 1957. The sample design of the survey has undergone changes following each census. Sample redesign allows the incorporation of the latest population information and statistical methodology into the survey design.

A multistage probability design is used, as it permits a continuous sampling of the civilian noninstitutionalized population in the United States. The survey is designed in such a way that each sample to be surveyed is representative for the study population with weekly samples added over time. High-frequency measures for large populations are more cross-sectional in approach and conducted in short time frames. For low frequency measures or smaller population groups, a longer time frame of data collection is used. In the National Health Interview Survey (NHIS), interviewing is done throughout the year, eliminating seasonal biases common in annual cross-sectional studies.

Sample Selection in the National Health Interview Survey

The study population is the civilian noninstitutionalized population of the United States. Primary Sampling Units have been established across the U.S. population, consisting of 1,900 geographically defined areas. Housing configurations are used from which to draw the samples from. Within each segment all occupied households are targeted for interview. If large numbers of houses are in one area, then subsampling is used in order to provide a manageable workload. Approximately 7,500 sampling segments are used that contain about 59,000 households, with 10,000 not usable. Of the 49,000 households interviewed about 127,000 persons will be sampled. In order to have better health status and disease related estimates for blacks, over sampling has been conducted starting in the late 1980s. Each person as a sample in the survey is weighted statistically to produce national estimates.[11]

Careful procedures are followed to assure the quality of data collected in the interview. Most households are contacted by mail before the interviewers arrive. Potential respondents are informed of the importance of the survey and assurance of confidence is extended. The home is visited until success is experienced, providing a response rate of between 95 and 98 percent. All members of the household 19 years and older are requested to be present during the interview.[11]

Focus Groups as a Sampling and Research Tool

Focus groups could be considered a cross-sectional research methodology and have some of the elements of survey research. Focus groups have been used mostly in marketing research. However, the use of focus groups has been used in selected settings and within limited areas of research. The common use of focus groups is to gather opinions or obtain information from persons affected by some experience. The nature of focus groups usually is more subjective in the process and then made objective in the analysis. Ten to 12 average persons who are consumers or potential consumers of a service are asked to participate in a session. Three to 15 different focus groups are held with new participants each time. Five or six well thought out and well-developed questions are used for every session. Each session is videotaped. When finished with all focus groups, the epidemiologist reviews the tapes and makes a grid of comments and develops an objective quantified database from them. Recurring comments, trends, problems, and concerns are noted and indicated in the grid which becomes the database.

A good facilitator is needed to conduct the focus groups. The facilitator is not to lead the group's comments or thinking. The participants should feel free to make any comment they wish. The facilitator needs to control the process by not letting one outspoken person control the time and comments, while drawing comments out of the more quiet persons. The responses must remain directed on the question under discussion and not allowed to drift into other areas. In summary, the use of focus groups may have some value in limited or certain circumstances, and may have limited value in tracking a disease. Focus groups would be of value in assessing consumer satisfaction with clinics or public health programs.

PROSPECTIVE STUDIES/LONGITUDINAL STUDIES

In epidemiology textbooks of recent times, the concepts of prospective studies seem to be blurred with and intermixed with cohort, incidence, and longitudinal research approaches. Some authors mix terms to create research designs such as *prospective cohort studies*. These terms need to be clarified, defined, and described. First, the general concept of prospective study needs to be explained. Lilienfeld and Lilienfeld refer to prospective and longitudinal studies as *concurrent studies* and call retrospective studies *noncurrent studies*, adding further confusion about research design concepts. Such renaming of terminology is often seen in fields ranging from law to medicine, and is seen as an effort to "epidemiologize" standard research designs by calling them new and different terms to fit in under the umbrella of epidemiology.[1]

The prefix *pro-* describes the concept of before, for, or in front of. *Prospective* is from the Latin *prospicere* which means *to look forward*. In English, prospective means to look forward in time, to look to the future or relating to the future. Thus, a **prospective study** is one that studies future happenings, events, and findings. Any study following a condition, concern, or disease into the future or over time is a prospective study. Any description of a forward looking research activity beyond this basic definition describes a special design or approach to the prospective study.

Some epidemiologists have modified and adopted the basic prospective study research design and intermixed the longitudinal study design for use within the field of epidemiology and labeled it a cohort study. Some epidemiology sources directly suggest and many others imply that the terms *cohort, prospective, concurrent, follow-up, incidence,* and *longitudinal* as used in epidemiological analytical studies are synonymous.

Longitudinal Studies

The **longitudinal study** approach used as a prospective study means the study occurs over time, often taking place over a long time period. In a longitudinal approach, time sequences pass for many of the subjects within the research period. Over a long time period, exposure to risk factors has time to run its course. Disease exposure and recovery, chronic disease development, changes occur due to the aging process, aging and exposure to environmental factors have to have time to run their course (see Figure 8.3).

Longitudinal studies usually have a pretest or initial assessment of health status or some determination of level or status of whatever condition or occurrence is being studied that

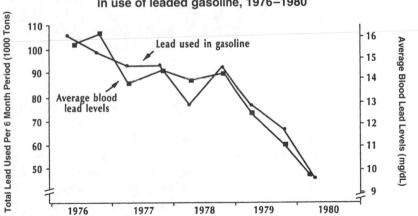

FIGURE 8.3 Example of the findings of a longitudinal study showing the changes in blood levels in relationship to a decline in use of leaded gasoline, from 1976 through 1980. (Source: Centers for Disease Control and Prevention, *Preventing Lead Poisoning in Young Children*, Public Health Service, U.S. Department of Health and Human Services, October, 1991)

can be repeated in a standardized fashion over time. It is essential that longitudinal studies use standardized tests that can be repeated in the same way over time so that validity and reliability of the study process exists. If any deviation from the study procedures occurs, the validity of the study will be in question.

A longitudinal study has built into it a gerontological study factor. As one follows people over time they age, thus by default the aging process is one factor of the study. One typical approach to a longitudinal study would be to select a large population, do proper sampling techniques in subject selection, and then place the study group participants into different age groupings. The study group then would be tested. Baseline data gathering as a starting point might include blood testing, medical exams and body function exams, pen and paper exams, interviews, filling out questionnaires, etc. The exact same tests are repeated at time intervals over set time periods. Usually followup exams and testing might be done every 6 months or yearly over several years. Another approach might be to do the testing over 20 years but only once a year. How often the repeated testing occurs depends on the type of condition being studied, how quickly changes in the condition occur, and funding. Chronic disease would be followed over many years, as would conditions dealing with the aging process. More acute diseases might be followed, tested, and retested over a few months or a few years. Testing would occur more often in shorter longitudinal studies.

Findings from longitudinal studies are similar to and in some cases almost identical to the findings of cross-sectional studies. Cross-sectional studies have the ability to produce like results to longitudinal studies but do so at one point in time.

An example of likeness of the two study approaches is shown in life span studies. As one goes through life and experiences the aging process, many psychosocial events are experienced. Life change experiences and transition periods have been studied both longitudinally and cross-sectionally. Levinson, et al., in a 10-year longitudinal study identified eight different periods of life change and transition periods across the life span.[12] A cross-sectional study of workers in the telephone industry in the mountainous west showed similar findings. A random sample taken from the 5,200 workers, who then were assessed with questionnaires for stress and life change events, showed almost identical findings as the 10-year longitudinal Levinson study. Using the work life span workers were placed in 9 age groups. From the nine age groups, the similar transition or life change periods emerged, showing some periods of life are more stressful than others. Ages 18–24, 40–44, and 60–65 were the most stressful and ages 30–34 and 55–59 are the least stressful time periods, according to the cross-sectional study.[13]

Case Example: Longitudinal Study/Prospective Research Design

An epidemiological researcher was challenged with the idea that workers with extremely high-stress jobs were more likely to gain weight, be prone to substance and alcohol abuse, smoke, have a limited education, and experience early heart disease. Metropolitan police officers were selected as high-stress employees, and garbage workers as low-stress employees, as test subjects for a longitudinal study to last ten years. Two or fewer years of employment was a limiting factor set on the study groups. Two years was chosen in order to include younger workers with limited years of stress, but because a large enough pool of subjects was needed, 75 new male employees were selected at random from all police employees and all male garbage workers. The subjects were placed in the two groups to establish a comparison/control group.

Attrition is one of the disadvantages of a longitudinal study and is of greatest concern to researchers conducting such studies. Because attrition was such a concern, 75 subjects were selected with the hope that 50 would finish the study. A loss of 25 subjects within the ten years was anticipated.

Paper-and-pencil measures of stress were used, body weight was taken, blood samples were drawn to test for drug and alcohol use, level of tobacco use was determined, education levels were noted, and complete medical histories, including EKGs and assessment of heart functioning and cholesterol levels, were determined. All measures were taken the first week of September in the first year of testing, to establish a baseline of data. The same measures were taken in both groups each September for the ten years of the study. The comparison group was compared to the study group in order to determine changes over time from the baseline of data. Final reports were written, with appropriate statistical analysis applied to the data, tables, and graphs, and summations were reported. Changes over time for each year were noted and presented. The study was to be continued for another ten years.

Advantages of Prospective and Longitudinal Studies   The advantage of a prospective/longitudinal study is

1. that the information gathered is more complete and accurate;

2. that the opportunity exists for the subjects to experience the risk factors, aging process, or condition or avoid the condition being studied;

3. there is a chance for control, and prevention measures can be tested and affirmed or rejected;

4. there is an opportunity for clinical intervention or immunization effectiveness can be proved;

5. the quality of the data is high due to the data not being a one-time exposure as in a cross-sectional study;

6. it takes into account seasonal variation or fluctuations or other changes affecting the data as they are not a problem over long term periods;

7. that the natural effects of the aging process can be tracked and assessed.[1,2,3,6,7]

Disadvantages of Prospective and Longitudinal Studies   The disadvantage of a prospective/longitudinal study is

1. that subjects are lost over time due to people dying, dropping out, moving out of the area, or moving and not informing the investigator/epidemiologist;

2. costs can be prohibitive. It is expensive to test and retest over time;

3. logistics of keeping track of subjects, developing a tracking system, and setting up the examination and testing processes over and over can be difficult to administer;

4. maintaining quality, validity and reliability within the testing and retesting process can be a problem;

5. deaths, relocating, changing jobs or loss of interest in the research are problems for the researcher.[1,2,3,6,7]

COHORTS AND COHORT STUDIES

Cohort as a general term means a group, a band, or body of people. As used in the context of epidemiology, it refers mostly to a group of persons being studied who were born in the same year or time period. As time passes, the group moves through different and successive time periods of life; as the group ages, changes can be seen in the health and vital statistics of the group. Health factors as well as deaths are tracked in cohorts (see Figure 8.4).

As one can see, cohort means to group persons by common characteristics, especially birth year. Thus, contrary to some epidemiology sources, cohort studies are not limited to nor are they necessarily prospective studies.[3,4] Cohorts of persons placed in a group can be studied as a group, backward in time (retrospectively), at a single point in time (cross-sectionally) as well as forward in time (prospectively). (See Figure 8.5.) Cohort studies are not limited to prospective studies; however, cohorts of individuals are often studied over time, especially grouped by age in longitudinal studies. Figure 8.4 is a pictorial presentation of how and where cohort concept fits into the different types of research designs.

A **cohort study** is an epidemiological method identifying a study population by age or by using other means or traits of grouping individuals for the purpose of research. Subgroups

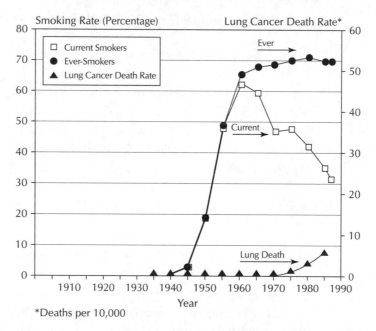

Changes in current smokers, ever-smokers, and lung cancer deaths, for white U.S. males born 1931 to 1940

*Deaths per 10,000

FIGURE 8.4 Smoking outcomes for two different birth cohorts. (Source: National Cancer Institute *Smoking and Tobacco Control Monographs—Strategies to Control Tobacco Use in the United States: A Blueprint for Public Health Action in the 1990's* Public Health Service, National Institutes of Health, U.S. Department of Health and Human Services, October, 1991)

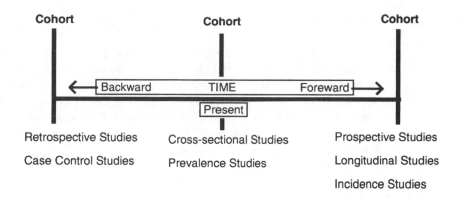

FIGURE 8.5 The relationship of *cohort* to various other types of studies.

of a study population can be established to assess if each group has or will be exposed to certain diseases or conditions. The unexposed are also studied. The extent of the exposure, probability of occurrence, types and levels of risk factors are all tracked in cohort subgroups across time and into the future. In summary, most cohort studies are longitudinal in approach, require large numbers of subjects, and are followed over time, usually for years.

Cohort Analysis

Another related term, *cohort analysis*, describes the way the cohort data is arranged and tabulated. **Cohort analysis** assesses morbidity and mortality and related risk factors data by ages of the subgroups or if a larger population, by cohorts of subjects. Time periods, retesting, reevaluation and followup activities are assessed as cohorts of individuals pass through time, age, and live life.

Once a cohort study is completed, (as in all studies) the data has to be analyzed, with rates, ratios and tables developed and presented. The morbidity and mortality data must be analyzed and tabulated by age groups and cohorts as they pass though time and the life span. The study population may be transient and will be subject to analysis only when they are present in the study population. Military personnel, college students, migrant workers, industries with high turnover rates may fall under such circumstances. (For an example, see Table 8.1.)

Cohort Effect

Cohort effect, also referred to as *generation effect*, is the changes and variation in the disease or health status of a study population as the study groups move through time. Any exposure or influence from environmental effects to societal changes which may affect the outcome of the study as these factors have, also affected the health status of the subjects as a cohort. As each group ages, passes through phases of the life span, and is exposed to the changes of life, such effects will be seen in each person within a cohort and will impact the results of the study.

Incidence in Cohort Studies

Cohort incidence is simply applying the concepts of incidence to the cohort groups and subgroups and the study population. As new cases of disease occur in the individuals of the cohort groups as they pass through time, the health status of the cohort is affected throughout the time period of the study. Incidence rates can affect the outcome of cohort studies and new cases must be tabulated and analyzed as they occur within the cohort. Incidence rates for the cohort subgroups and for the study population as whole can be developed. The end result would be in cohort incidence.

Odds Ratio in Cohort Studies

Odds ratio has been used as a means of analysis of cohort studies. From the findings of a cohort study the epidemiologist can estimate the chances of getting a disease if exposed, which then is compared to the chance of getting the disease, if not exposed. The 2×2, 4-celled epidemiology grid is useful in assessing exposed and nonexposed subjects compared to diseased and nondiseased, which provides the basic information necessary to do the odds ratio analysis. (Odds ratio and ratios are presented in detail in Chapter 5.)

Cohort Studies in Occupational Health Epidemiology

Mausner et al. suggest a historical prospective cohort study is a commonly used method in occupational health epidemiology. Also suggested is that occupational cohorts are often used in mortality studies as death records are more accessible and reliable than medical records that spell out the illness and related conditions. Work history of the subjects is also a unique element to be considered and studied.[2]

Confounding Variables in Cohort Studies

Kelsey suggests that confounding variables can have an effect on cohort studies and should not be ignored. In any study design, any factor that can cause change or influence an outcome must be considered. If confounding variables are not considered, a wrong conclusion can be made or misinformation provided in reports. Assessing risk factors or levels of exposure is done to determine their effect on health status or disease states.[3]

Selecting the Study Cohort

When selecting the study cohort the population of study should be reviewed to ascertain those people or groups that are susceptible and those not at risk. In clinical settings, the susceptibles can be screened for risk of exposure to infectious diseases by conducting serum antibody level assessments. Individuals with minimized risk of exposure must also be screened. For example women with hysterectomies would be excluded from a cohort of women being investigated for risks to cancer of the cervix. Persons with latent infections or recurring diseases such as the chronic fatigue immune deficiency syndrome caused by the herpes virus present a problem, as the disease may not be easily diagnosed. In the interest of saving time, money, avoiding unnecessary testing and effort, the preselection and screening of subjects for a cohort study must be given utmost attention and effort.

Cohorts representative of the general population such as the National Health Survey or the Framingham Heart Studies provide examples of good cohort sampling and study designs. If similar studies are to be conducted, such previous study examples could be reviewed for insights and ideas. Cohorts are often selected by disease states, the presence of certain conditions, regular exposure to risk factors, risk of having certain diseases or conditions by age and by age groupings that are then followed over time with many health and disease factors being studied within the population. Other risk commonalities of the cohort should be included in a study. Risk factors such as having a certain occupation or working in an industry in which subjects may be subjected to a certain type of exposure or condition, for example, lung disease in coke workers at steel mills, or brown lung in garment factory workers.

Another type of prospective longitudinal study is the **panel study**, also referred to as prospective cohort study. Data are retrieved from a cohort of subjects (panels) at different intervals in time and at multiple times. Panel studies do not require the subjects to be disease free as in standard cohort studies. Another way to view panel studies is to see them as a series of cross-sectional studies over time at various intervals. Changes in one variable can affect other variables as time passes or the life span is crossed. This type of research design has been found useful in large populations which are followed over time. The assessment of the health status and disease progression of exposed or at-risk persons with chronic diseases are tested as they progress. Diseases such as emphysema or scoliosis have been studied with panel studies. The effects over time of air pollution on lung and respiratory disease in university students is another example of the use of panel studies.[3]

Some techniques of panel studies include having the subjects keep diaries related to the issues being studied. Frequent interviews may be conducted in-person; frequent interviews over the telephone may be conducted. A combination of in-person and telephone interviews may also be used. Persons (subjects) may be requested to come to a center or clinic for tests or exams. Questionnaires and assessments most often cannot be done over the phone, so the epidemiology team has to either invite the subjects to a central location or visit them where they are, at home or at work.[3]

Most panel studies do not require recall of past events as the subjects are interviewed, examined, or tested at intervals. Thus, all that is required is to get the participants to cooperate. A limitation to this study approach is that cause-effect relationships are not always clear cut, as confounding variables may be present to influence the results.[3]

Another cohort related concept is that of **restricted cohorts** which are those groups or populations that have limited exposure, narrow behaviors or activities, or are from a limited work environment with restricted exposures or health problems. Workers placed in age groups and followed longitudinally would show progression of disease states or health status after exposures. Heart disease is a common condition studied longitudinally in cohorts of workers. Postmen, longshoremen, and other workers who have much physical activity are good examples of cohorts that have been studied for heart disease. Military personnel are also used as restricted cohorts.

Cohort studies need to come from populations where sampling can be effectively done. Large enough sample sizes have to be used, thus sampling has to come from a large population of cohorts. In some conditions or diseases, the low numbers of occurrences may not work well in the longitudinal cohort type study, thus the epidemiologist must predict the types and incidences of the disease possibilities within the study population to ascertain if it is a proper study design.

Cohort studies often place the individuals being studied into age groups. The epidemiologist must be sure to place the individual into logical group arrangements. The years must not be spread too far apart for each cohort group, nor should they be placed too close together. Additionally the epidemiologist must avoid placing subjects into two groups at the break point between groups of ages/cohorts. For example, the age grouping should be 20 through 24 and then start the next grouping with age 25 through 29. If the age grouping is done 20 though 25 and then 25 through 30 the person aged 25 is placed in both age groups and thus counted twice.

Advantages of Cohort Studies   The advantages of retrospective studies and prospective/longitudinal studies have been presented above. The uniqueness of cohort studies offers some advantages.

1. A captive study population located in an industry or work place provides easy access to the subjects and their records.
2. Large sample sizes are required, thus producing solid and credible findings.
3. Sampling is easier with a larger population and more representative samples can be obtained.
4. Certain disease states or risk factors can be targeted and closely studied.
5. Cohort studies prove cause-effect relationships because of the time span element.
6. Magnitude of risk can be shown in the cause-effect relationship of risk factors to the study group.
7. A baseline of rates can be established from which control, preventive, and health promotion programs can be developed and implemented.
8. A baseline of rates can be established from which future studies can be conducted.
9. Information on and a baseline for the prevalence of disease, condition or risk factors can be shown.
10. Data on new cases needing intervention, treatment, or control are discovered.
11. The number and proportion of cases which can be prevented or controlled when exposures to agents or risk factors are identified.
12. Inaccurate responses and inaccurate information are reduced due to not having to rely on memory or recall.
13. Different influencing or confounding variables can be estimated, studied and controlled.
14. Sample selection factors can be minimized as all persons are followed over time, both diseased and disease free; susceptibles and exposed.[1,2,3,4,13,14]

Disadvantages of Cohort Studies   The disadvantages of retrospective studies and prospective/longitudinal studies have been presented above. The uniqueness of cohort studies offers some disadvantages.

1. Large study populations are usually needed, which are not easy to find or access.
2. Because large groups are needed in the study populations, the expense of doing the research is quite high.
3. Individual dropouts in longitudinal studies are always a problem.

4. The introduction of unseen or unpredicted variables into the study population may cause the outcomes to be altered or influenced as time passes.

5. The study population often is not the general population and results cannot easily be extrapolated to the general population.

6. The study results are limited as the study is focused on a particular disease, condition, risk factor, or exposure.

7. Controls are not easily established in a cohort study.

8. Time to gather information, assess findings, and see results is long.

9. Time, effort, and coordination demands are high in cohort studies.

10. Acquiring and retaining study participants is most difficult due to the long-term commitment to the study and follow-ups.

11. Data analysis must be organized, and gathering systems and approaches must be adhered to in a dependable and consistent manner.[1,2,3,4,13,14]

SURVIVORSHIP STUDIES IN EPIDEMIOLOGY

Survivorship studies are used with chronic diseases and uses of life tables to study cohorts. Cohort life tables used in survivorship assessment show the chance that an event such as death from cancer will occur in successive intervals of time once a diagnosis has been made. The chances of surviving at each interval are also shown. The life tables are used to analyze the chance of survival for each time interval for those still alive at that time interval. The analysis yields a cumulative probability of surviving the projected time period, which is usually the period of the research study. Several criteria are used in assessing survivorship prognosis in chronic disease studies, such as death vs. survival, survival with recurrence, survival without recurrence, chance of living through certain intervals of the disease, etc.

For infectious diseases, case fatality rates are used for assessing survivability. (Case fatality rate is presented in Chapter 3.) For chronic diseases, cohort life tables are used to estimate the probability of surviving or dying within a specified time period after diagnosis. As in any study the researcher must assure all subjects are dealt with, diagnosed, tested, and followed up consistently over the study. For example, all subjects should be enrolled at the same time, such as at the time of diagnosis.

Life tables are useful epidemiology tools. **Life tables** are charts which summarize the patterns of survival and death in study groups of certain types of diseases such as chronic diseases. Survivorship is the number of persons out of a study population who would survive or remain disease free until a certain time interval is reached. Cohort life tables describe the actual survival rate of a study group. Mortality of cohorts is observed from the time of diagnosis until all die. In the case of a generation cohort, the time span is from birth until death. A *current life table* is another form of life table which presents the combined mortality experience by age of the study group for a set time period that is shorter than a life span.

In Figure 8.6 survival curves and risk of death curves, for males and females based on life tables, are presented for California for 1980. The dip at the beginning of life as shown in the chart is due to infant death rates (infant mortality) in the first year of life. As one reaches the later years of life the survival curve goes down and the risk of death curve goes up. The rate of change is dramatically seen as is the reduced survivability beyond a certain age.[17,18]

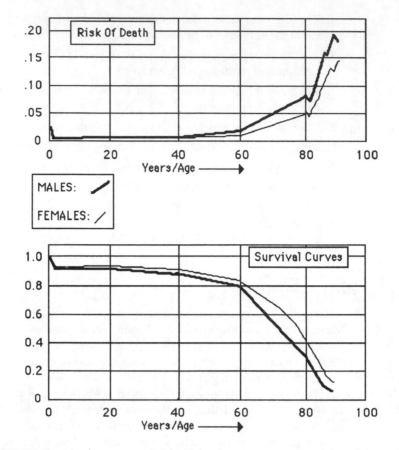

FIGURE 8.6   Survival curve and risk of death curve compared for white males and females in California, 1980.

PRETEST/INTERVENTION/POST-TEST DESIGN

This research design approach uses a basic experimental design plus additional features and methods. In its simplest design, the subjects are selected as a research group and a pretest situation is administered. Biomedical testing, psychological assessments, or paper/pencil test can be given to establish a baseline of pre-treatment data. The intervention or treatment is administered and a post-test is given at the correct time interval. The pretest baseline of data is then compared to the post-test data. The findings are analyzed with inferential (correlation) statistics and results are presented showing levels of significance of the findings. The results should show that the treatment caused any observed changes. In some research designs two or three post-tests may be given to assure that the changes endure over time and are not short-lived. Another design approach is to establish the procedure as presented above with modifications. For example, the study population would be broken into two groups, a treatment group and a control group. All procedures would be the same for both groups except that the control group would receive no treatment or intervention. Followup post-testing is conducted at various time intervals to check for

TABLE 8.2   A health education intervention quasi-experimental pretest/post-test research design

Gain scores* and standardized effect sizes† for selected self-reported behaviors among senior high school classes—Teenage Health Teaching Modules (THTM) evaluation, 1986–1989

	Classroom Type					
	Experimental			Naturalistic		
Behaviors	THTM (n = 39)	Control (n = 39)	Effect Size	THTM (n = 40)	Control (n = 40)	Effect Size
Mean cigarettes smoked	−1.49	3.18	0.47	0.87	1.57	0.14
Not smoking cigarettes	0.82%	−4.41%	0.32	−0.43%	−5.71%	0.50
Not chewing tobacco	−1.34%	−1.12%	0.04	−0.74%	−6.06%	0.65
Mean instances of illegal drug use	−0.23	0.30	0.58	0.05	0.26	0.32
Not using illegal drugs	−0.77%	−2.82%	0.14	0.57%	−4.05%	0.49
Mean number of alcoholic drinks consumed	0.08	0.62	0.19	0.16	1.14	0.50

*Gain score = post-test score minus pretest score.
† Standardized effect size = (THTM gain score minus control gain score) ÷ pooled standard deviation of gain scores.
(Source: Centers for Disease Control and Prevention, "Effectiveness of a Health Education Curriculum for Secondary School Students—U.S., 1986–1989," *Morbidity and Mortality Weekly Reports*, Public Health Service, U.S. Department of Health and Human Services)

lasting effects. A whole range of design possibilities exists for this research approach; an example is the quasi-experimental pretest/post-test control group design.

This research approach has had wide use in education, health education, health promotion, mental health, counseling and psychological interventions, to determine if educational or behavioral changes occur due to treatment or intervention.[6,7,8,13,14] Table 8.2 is an example of this type of study.

Effectiveness of a Health Education Curriculum for Secondary School Students—United States, 1986–1989

Risk behaviors affecting the health of young persons in the U.S. are drug abuse, alcohol use, tobacco use, poor dietary patterns, physical inactivity, unsafe sexual practices and injury-related behaviors. A curricula titled, Teenage Health Teaching Modules (THTM) was developed. THTM has 16 instruction modules that are used to develop five skills: self-assessment, communication, decision-making, advocacy, and self-management. A research study was developed to assess the effectiveness of the educational intervention. A quasi-experimental pretest/post-test control group design was conducted on 4,806 students in 149 schools in seven states. Pretest and post-test self-administered questionnaires assessing both knowledge and attitudinal changes due to the classes were analyzed for 2,530 students in the study group and 2,276 in the control group. Students in the treatment group were exposed to at least four to five health education modules, for 36 to 38 times in 45-minute class sessions for about 27 hours of instruction over a semester. Study results are shown in Table 8.2.

ETHICS IN RESEARCH

Researchers using experimental design must exercise much professional discretion and ethics in their work. People participating in experiments should not be unnecessarily exposed to harm or danger. Precautions should be taken to protect the health and safety of the subjects and to do no harm. Reporting research results must be done with the utmost honesty and clarity so as not to deceive the public or professionals in the field. Distorted or falsified results of some studies could cause harm or endanger not only the health of the subjects, but also large groups or populations, especially if such studies were on vaccines or drugs being developed to treat the masses. For experiments to be of value, believable, and used to help populations at risk, good scientific methodology and research control methods must be used (see Figure 8.7). Honesty in research and reporting the findings is basic expected professional behavior.

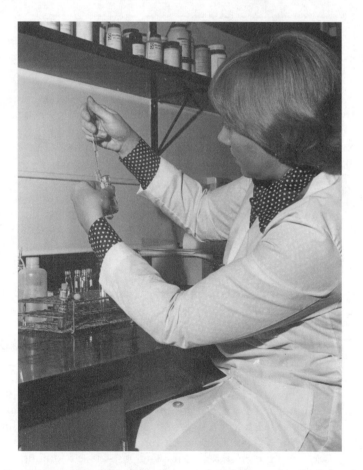

FIGURE 8.7 Epidemiologist/researcher at the Centers for Disease Control and Prevention (CDC). (Picture courtesy of Centers for Disease Control and Prevention, Atlanta, Georgia)

CONCLUSION

Several textbooks and other references are available that provide concepts and detailed instruction on the research designs presented above as well as other design approaches not presented in this book. The epidemiologist faced with a possible unusual research design should consult such references and textbooks or experts on research design.[6,7,8]

EXERCISES

Key Terms

Define and explain the following terms.

accessibility	independent variable
affinity bias	individual matching
analytical study	life table
antecedent	longitudinal study
antecedent variable	matching
category matching	observational epidemiology
clinical trial	observational study
cluster bias	order bias
cohort	panel study
cohort analysis	prospective study
cohort effect	quasi
cohort incidence	random assignment
cohort study	random selection
community trial	restricted cohorts
confounding variable	retrospective study
cross-sectional study	stratification
dependent variable	subject
descriptive study	survivorship study
experimental study	variable
ex post facto	visibility bias
frequency matching	

Study Questions

8.1   Certain advantages and disadvantages exist for each of the various research designs. Contrast and compare the *advantages* and *disadvantages* of a longitudinal study with a cross-sectional study design on the following factors:

a.   time factors
b.   sample size needed
c.   cost of conducting the research
d.   usefulness as a research design to epidemiology
e.   design structure
f.   bias related problems
g.   data analysis and tabulation
h.   the presentation of the results

8.2   As an epidemiologist you have the responsibility of studying people who died of pneumonia after surgery in the last 7 years in Mt. View Hospital. You are to use the medical records of the hospital. Design a study that will allow you to successfully complete the project and meet the responsibility given you. Explain the study type or design and provide a detailed structure of the research study as well as its organization and actual research design characteristics.

8.3   As the hospital epidemiologist you have been requested by the hospital administration to study the effects of administering antibiotics to patients at different time frames in hours (2-hour intervals up to 24 hours) just prior to having surgery that requires opening the chest cavity. The study is aimed at reducing infections caused by surgery as well as reducing deaths by investigating mortality prevention from this type of surgery through the preventive use of antibiotics. The study is to take place over the next 15 years. Design a study that will meet the responsibility given to you. Explain what type of design you will use and provide in-depth details of the research study structure, organization, and design.

8.4   You have been asked to study the effects of stress across the life span of family members with a close family member with HIV/AIDS. The study is to be from the time of diagnosis until the death of the family member. Explain what type of design you will use and provide in-depth details of the research study structure, organization, and design.

8.5   Certain advantages and disadvantages exist for each of the various research designs. Contrast and compare the *advantages* and *disadvantages* of a pretest-intervention—post-test design with a cross-sectional study design on the following factors:

   a.   time factors
   b.   sample size needed
   c.   cost of conducting the research
   d.   usefulness as a research design to epidemiology
   e.   design structure
   f.   bias related problems
   g.   data analysis and tabulation
   h.   the presentation of the results

8.6   Contrast and compare the *advantages* and *disadvantages* of a retrospective study with a longitudinal study design on the following factors:

   a.   time factors
   b.   sample size needed
   c.   cost of conducting the research
   d.   usefulness as a research design to epidemiology
   e.   design structure
   f.   bias related problems
   g.   data analysis and tabulation
   h.   the presentation of the results

8.7   a.   From the information found in Figure 8.6 identify, explain, and discuss the research design used in this study, and explain how it was used, how sampling was done, how controls were used, and how the study was conducted.
       b.   Identify, explain, and discuss the dependent and independent variables of this study.

REFERENCES

1. Lilienfeld, A.M., and Lilienfeld, D.E. 1980. *Foundations of Epidemiology*. New York: Oxford University Press.
2. Mausner, J.S., and Kramer, S. 1985. *Epidemiology: An Introductory Text*. Philadelphia: Saunders.
3. Kelsey, J.L., Thompson, W.D., and Evans, A.S. 1986. *Methods in Observational Epidemiology*. New York: Oxford University Press.
4. Slome, C., Brogan, D., Eyres, S., and Lednar, W. 1982. *Basic Epidemiological Methods and Biostatistics: A Workbook*. Monterey, CA: Wadsworth.
5. Timmreck, T.C. 1991. *Handbook of Planning and Program Development for Health and Social Services*. San Bernardino, CA: Health Care Management Development Associates.
6. Alreck, R.L., and Settle, R.B. 1985. *The Survey Research Handbook*. Homewood, IL: Irwin.
7. Kerlinger, F.N. 1986. *Foundations of Behavioral Research*, 3rd edition. New York: Holt, Rinehart and Winston.
8. Neale, J.M., and Liebert, R.M. 1986. *Science and Behavior*, 3rd edition. Englewood Cliffs, NJ: Prentice Hall.
9. Getting, E.R., and Goldstein, G.S. 1979. "Drug Use Among Native American Adolescents." In *Youth Drug Abuse: Problems, Issues and Treatment*. Toronto, Ontario: Lexington Books.
10. Cole, G., Timmreck, T.C., Page, R., and Woods, S. 1992. "Patterns and Prevalence of Substance Use Among Navajo Youth," *Health Values*, Vol. 16, No. 3.
11. National Center for Health Statistics. 1990. *Vital and Health Statistics: Current Estimates from the National Health Interview Survey, 1989*. Hyattsville, MD: Centers for Disease Control and Prevention, Public Health Service, U.S. Department of Health and Human Services.
12. Levinson, D.J., Darrow, C.N., Klein, E.B., Levinson, M.H., and McKee, B. 1979. *The Seasons of a Man's Life*. New York: Ballantine Books.
13. Timmreck, T.C., Braza, G., and Mitchell, J. 1984. "Growing Older: A Study of Stress and Transition Periods," *Occupational Health and Safety*, Vol. 53, No. 9, pp. 39–48.
14. Rothman, K.J. 1986. *Modern Epidemiology*. Boston: Little, Brown and Company.
15. Monson, R.R. 1990. *Occupational Epidemiology*, 2nd edition. Boca Raton, FL: CRC Press.
16. Friedman, G.D. 1978. *Primer of Epidemiology*. New York: McGraw-Hill.
17. Selvin, S. 1991. *Statistical Analysis of Epidemiologic Data*. New York: Oxford University Press.
18. Wray, J.A., and Todd, J.J. 1983. *Vital Statistics of California 1981*. Department of Health Services, State of California.

9

Time, Place, and Person

CHAPTER OBJECTIVES

This chapter on the epidemiological elements of time, place, and person

- addresses the effect of time, place, and person on the study and control of disease in populations;

- reviews the role of time, place, and person on the causation, effect, and spread of diseases in groups and populations;

- presents the importance of the various facets and aspects of the element of *time* on epidemiological study and analysis;

- presents the importance of the various facets and aspects of the element of *place* on epidemiological study and analysis;

- presents the importance of the various facets and aspects of the element of *person* on epidemiological study and analysis;

- presents the relation of *time* to *place* in epidemics and their investigation, while addressing the *where* and *when* questions;

- develops a comprehensive review of the elements and aspects of *person* with regard to age, race, sex, occupation, religion, education, and related variables that address the *who* question;

- presents terms and exercises that assist in reviewing chapter concepts and materials.

INTRODUCTION

In the study of epidemiology, two basic and distinct activities must take place. The first is the study of the amount and distribution of disease, conditions, injury, disability, and death within a population. To conduct these studies the epidemiologist explores all facets of time, place, and person. Detailed assessment of each of these three elements is completed and analyzed in epidemiology studies. Some epidemiologists refer to this as descriptive epidemiology. The second activity of epidemiology is often referred to as analytical epidemiology. (See Chapters 7 and 8 for a review of analytical epidemiology concepts.) The epidemiologist must also answer the when, where, and who questions in all investigations.

The *when* question is answered by investigating and studying all aspects of time elements associated with the cause, outbreak, spread, distribution, and course of diseases and conditions. Also studied is the effect upon and interaction between time and *where* of disease cause, outbreak, spread, and distribution. The study of the *place* of occurrence is as essential as any other phase or aspect of an epidemiological investigation. The *who* aspect is affected by the spread, distribution, and course of diseases and conditions and is always investigated extensively due to the toll that diseases have on human lives and suffering. Various aspects of the *person* have to be considered, analyzed, and investigated. Persons can do an array of behaviors, have a variety of beliefs, and can be influenced by tradition, culture, and societal expectations to such an extent as to cause unnecessary deaths, cause the spread of disease, and promote unhealthy conditions and actions in families, groups, and populations. The range of experiences and environmental exposures one can have across the life span are broad and different, thus producing a different health status in each person or population group.[1,2,3]

TIME

Basic to any epidemiological study is the assessment and analysis of time and its effect on the occurrence of disease, disorders, and conditions. The time aspects of epidemiology investigations range from hours to weeks to months to years to decades. Short-term disease incubation periods of a few hours can be as important to the epidemiologist as longitudinal studies spanning two or three decades. Another term used occasionally to describe time factors in epidemiology is **temporal**, which means **time** or refers to time-related elements or issues.

Any or all time sets, configurations, or segments that relate to diseases or risk factors can be of value to epidemiological studies. The type of disease or condition with its surrounding characteristics will dictate what time elements need to be considered and used. Certain infectious diseases such as cholera have short time elements (incubation periods) and certain chronic diseases such as emphysema have long duration time elements. (Incubation periods, point prevalence, period prevalence, incidence, time factors in the course of a disease, and other important time-related factors of communicable and chronic diseases are presented in detail in Chapter 2.)

Quick analysis of epidemiological data or phenomena are easily understood if they can be seen in pictorial form, as in a graph, chart, or map. *Time* is best understood if presented in graphic form. The standard way to present time in a graph is to show the frequency (numbers) of cases or occurrences on the vertical, or *y-axis* (for example, rate per 1,000; number of cases; number of exposures). Time is laid out along the horizontal, or *x-axis*, and can be presented in a variety of increments. Hours to days or weeks to years are all commonly used, and the time frame chosen depends solely on the time increment that is appropriate. (Figure 9.1 shows time presented along the *x*-axis in days, Figure 9.2(A,B) shows years, and Figure 9.6 shows groupings of dates.) Time can be presented as days by actual date or as straight days, weeks, months, or years. It can be placed in groupings by day, week, month, or year. When an appropriate time frame for the disease or condition being shown is used, it should be labeled as such, as days, weeks, months, and so on. The epidemiologist making a time-related graph should provide the reader with all the important labels and information needed to study and analyze the graph. Studying a graph of time plus *place* or *person* can provide epidemiologist and layperson alike with many insights and observations about cause-effect relationships, sources of cause, and various types of trends that have occurred and are occurring.

In both retrospective and prospective studies, it is common to track disease occurrences in ten-year blocks of time. The time period often used indicates the beginning and end of ten-year time periods. The years are referred to as **decennial years** (1970, 1980, 1990, 2000). Charts, exhibits and other figures used to present data may use decennial years. Weeks, months, years, and five-year increments are also used.[1,2,3]

Time as a basic element in epidemiological measures and as a basic investigation consideration is used in looking at causation of disease, disorders, and conditions. An episode of a disease can be localized by where it occurs (**place**) and by the *time* in which it occurs and is of equal importance. When time and place elements quickly merge in a disease outbreak, together they become useful in demonstrating etiological connections. The merger of these two elements is of special concern when the time intervals between exposure and onset of the disease are closely related, as seen in cholera epidemics. In the historical cholera epidemic in the Broad Street-Golden Square area of London as set forth in the Snow case in Appendix I, the elements of time and place were most helpful in the investigation. The time factors of the incubation period of cholera and the duration of the epidemic together allowed Dr. John Snow to determine onset, peak of the outbreak and the downturn of the epidemic. Figure 9.1 shows the duration of the disease outbreak as a time factor in the cholera epidemic in the Board Street area of London in 1854. The time factor in producing an epidemic curve is also observed in Figure 9.1.[4]

Four Time Trends Used in Epidemiology

Four factors of time are used in the assessment of epidemiological events. Time in the context of disease outbreaks is looked upon in the long-term, as well as the short-term. To help in study and to understand disease related variations four time configurations or elements are used. The four are *secular trends, short-term trends, cyclic trends*, and *seasonal trends*.

Secular (Long-Term) Trends   Changes in disease, conditions, disability, and mortality which occur slowly over long time periods are referred to as **secular changes** or **secular trends**. A term that has recently emerged in some epidemiology literature that is used interchangeably with secular trends is *temporal variation* or *trends*, also *temporal distribution*. Changes seen over extended time periods, even several decades in certain or selected diseases, are of concern in epidemiology, especially for control and prevention programs in public health. Secular trends are usually considered to last longer than one year. An example of a major secular trend related to smoking is the tracking of lung cancer deaths in both males and females over the years. In 1988–89, for the first time in history, female smoking rates had surpassed that of males, which means that lung cancer rates of females will eventually surpass males.

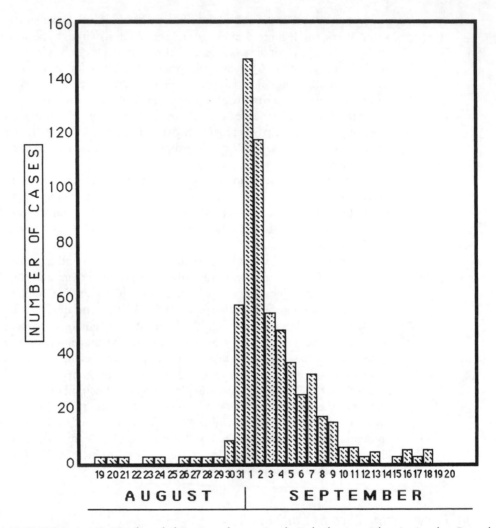

FIGURE 9.1   Example of the *time* factor in the cholera epidemic in the Broad Street–Golden Square area of London in the 1800s, showing the epidemic curve of the outbreak. (Source: Snow, John, *Snow on Cholera*, The Commonwealth Fund: New York; Harvard University Press: Cambridge, MA, 1936)

Another secular trend related concept is that of **secular cycles** of diseases, also referred to as secular cyclicity. Cycles of disease on a secular trends basis involve observing the cycle of the incidence of a disease over a long time period. Hepatitis A has been observed to have a 7-year cycle and measles to have a 2-year cycle. The level of immunizations in a population as well as the number of susceptibles help determine such cyclic trends. Chronic disease may be observed in secular cycle trends. For example, oral cancer cycles have been observed in birth cohorts based on the social popularity of using or not using chewing tobacco.

Cancer rates for most types of cancer are tracked over time, with secular trends being identified over years and decades. Lung cancer trends provide the most dramatic cancer rate changes and are made distinctly visible on line graphs. Figure 9.2(A,B) shows the

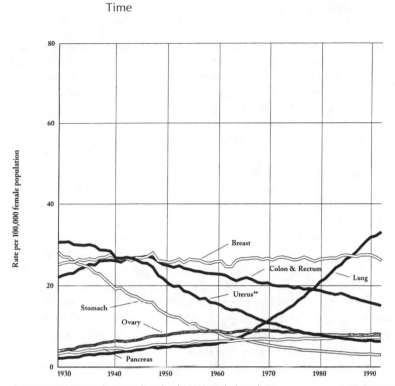

FIGURE 9.2A
Age-adjusted cancer
death rates,* females
by site, United States,
1930–1992. (Source:
Vital Statistics of the
United States, 1995)

*Rates are per 100,000 and are age-adjusted to the 1970 standard population.   **Uterine cancer death rates are for cervix and corpus combined.

Note: Due to changes in ICD coding, numerator information has changed over time. Denominator information for the years 1930–1967 and 1991–1992 is based on intercensal population estimates, while denominator information for the years 1968–1990 is based on postcensal recalculation of estimates.

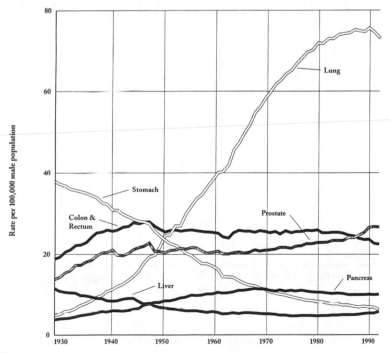

FIGURE 9.2B
Age-adjusted cancer
death rates,* males
by site, United States,
1930–1992. (Source:
Vital Statistics of the
United States, 1995)

*Rates are per 100,000 and are age-adjusted to the 1970 standard population.

Note: Due to changes in ICD coding, numerator information has changed over time. Rates for cancer of the liver are particularly affected by these coding changes. Denominator information for the years 1930–1967 and 1991–1992 is based on intercensal population estimates, while denominator information for the years 1968–1990 is based on postcensal recalculation of estimates.

secular trends of cancer occurrence at seven different sites in the body. In 1930, lung cancer was the second least common site of all cancers in males. By 1960 lung cancer had surpassed the other sites and continues to climb rapidly. Smoking is the most common contributing factor to lung cancer. Leukemia has risen only slightly and breast cancer has shown little change. The various cohorts of smokers have changed over the years as most have increased their tobacco consumption, contributing to the increases in lung cancer. Little behavior has been seen that affects the cause of breast cancer, thus, little change in breast cancer is seen.[5]

On June 5, 1981, the first cases of acquired immune deficiency syndrome (AIDS) were reported by health care providers in California and the Centers for Disease Control and Prevention. Since then AIDS has been a disease of concern not only to medical and public health officials, but to almost every member of society. As of May 31, 1991, CDC had reported 179,136 cases of AIDS in the United States. AIDS has been transmitted mostly by homosexual sex acts, intravenous-drug use with contaminated needles, and heterosexual activities by persons with multiple partners. AIDS has also been transmitted from mother to child in the process of giving birth (perinatal acquired pediatric AIDS cases) and from blood transfusions. Epidemiologists have been concerned about the secular trends of persons infected with AIDS and public health agencies at local, state, and national levels have been following the trends over the years. In Figures 9.3 and 9.4 are two examples of secular trends of AIDS, over one decade. Figure 9.3 shows perinatally acquired pediatric AIDS cases, and Figure 9.4 shows the AIDS cases among recipients of blood transfusions or blood products.[6]

The key factor in the leading causes of death, especially cardiovascular disease, and cancer in the United States is smoking. In 1930 few people smoked, but by 1965 cigarette consumption had reached its peak of over 4300 cigarettes per year per person on the average

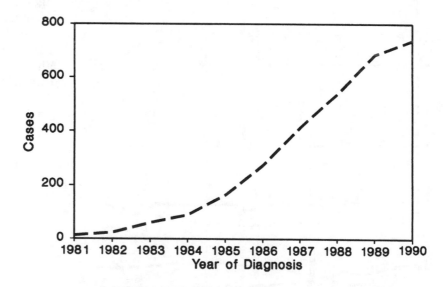

FIGURE 9.3   An example of secular trends in perinatally transmitted AIDS in pediatric cases. (Source: Centers for Disease Control and Prevention, "The HIV/AIDS Epidemic: The First 10 Years," *Morbidity and Mortality Weekly Report,* Vol. 40, No. 22, June 7, 1991, p. 361)

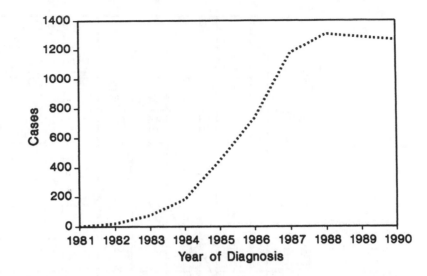

FIGURE 9.4 An example of secular trends of AIDS transmitted by blood transfusion or blood products. (Source: Centers for Disease Control and Prevention, "The HIV/AIDS Epidemic: The First 10 Years," *Morbidity and Mortality Weekly Report*, Vol. 40, No. 22, June 7, 1991, p. 361)

for adults over 18 years of age. The use of cigarettes, in contrast to other tobacco products, has been a widespread 20th-century phenomenon. The changes in cigarette consumption have had a direct association with mass production techniques using machines and high technology, changes in social values, extensive advertising, and with lung cancer (see Figure 9.2). Figure 9.5 shows the 90-year secular trends of cigarette consumption for adults, aged 18 and over from 1900 to 1990. When the secular trend of cigarette consumption is compared to lung cancer secular trends, the upward trends of both are obvious and directly associated.[7]

Short-Term Trends One short-term time factor of first consideration to epidemiology is that of incubation periods in communicable diseases, and where applicable the equivalent risk factors in chronic diseases. Examples of short-term risk factors of chronic disease concern would be attacks of asthma from allergies or a chronic obstructive pulmonary disease (COPD) event from excessive smoking of cigarettes. (Incubation periods and related time factors are presented in Chapter 2.)

Short-term trends obviously are of short-time intervals or limited time frames. Even though seasonal and cyclic trends occur within short-time frames, due to their unique features they are used as separate categories. Most short-term trends are limited to hours, days, weeks, and months. Thus, events of limited duration are included in the short-term trends category. An example of a short-term time frame would be the cholera epidemic studied by Dr. John Snow in the early 1800s (Figure 9.1).

A chemical spill in the Sacramento River in Northern California that caused dermatitis among workers is a good example of a noncommunicable disease environmental exposure event depicted in short-term trend charts used in an epidemiology study. On July 14, 1991, a train tanker car derailed spilling 19,000 gallons of the solid fumigant metam sodium

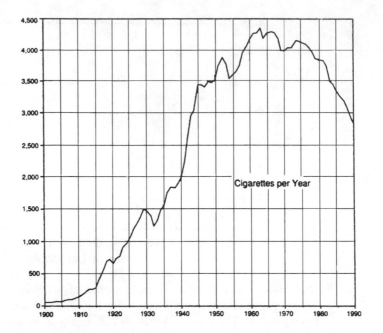

FIGURE 9.5   Example of secular trend of per capita cigarette consumption for adults, 18 years and older in the United States from 1900 to 1990. (Source: National Cancer Institute, *Strategies to Control Tobacco Use in the United States: A Blueprint for Public Health Action in the 1990s*, Smoking and Tobacco Control Monographs, National Institutes of Health, Public Health Services, U.S. Department of Health and Human Services, October, 1991)

into the Sacramento River north of Redding in north central California. The chemical is known to be a skin irritant. As the chemical drifted down the river killing fish, a cleanup effort was undertaken. During the cleanup an outbreak of dermatitis occurred among Shasta County jail inmates and crew leaders who assisted in the cleanup by removing dead fish from the river. A retrospective cohort study was conducted of 42 inmates and 27 crew leaders who presented themselves for medical treatment for dermatitis. Rashes occurred in 25 out of 33 workers or 76%. Rash onset was 0–18 days after exposure in the river, peaking at 3 to 4 days. The rash affected the exposed parts of the body. The prevalence of water contact and the duration of time in the river was similar for inmates and crew leaders as compared to other workers. Figure 9.6 is an example of a short-term trend of dermatitis cases among workers participating in the cleanup in the Sacramento River, by data of onset over the time period of part of July and August.[8] Figure 9.6 shows the epidemic curve and time trends in a dermatitis outbreak.

In August 1991, 16 persons had been confirmed with St. Louis encephalitis out of 24 possible exposures. Onset of symptoms for the 24 patients occurred from July 14 through August 17. All persons lived in Jefferson County in central Arkansas. The crude attack rate for the persons in Pine Bluff was 39 per 100,000 population. Cases were clustered in low socioeconomic status census tracts. The public was recommended to curtail evening outdoor activities and apply insect repellent when outdoors, as St. Louis encephalitis is vectorborne and transmitted by the mosquito. In Figure 9.7 the short-term time trends of

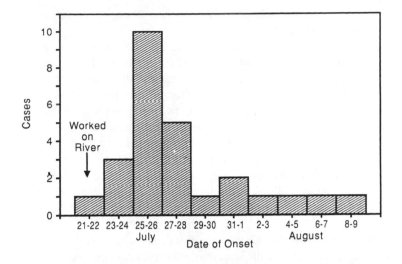

FIGURE 9.6   Example of short-term time trends showing numbers of dermatitis cases among workers participating in chemical spill cleanup in the Sacramento River in Northern California by date of onset for part of July and August, 1991. (Source: Centers for Disease Control and Prevention, "Dermatitis Among Workers Cleaning the Sacramento River After a Chemical Spill—California, 1991," *Morbidity and Mortality Weekly Report*, Vol. 40, No. 48, December 6, 1991, pp. 821–827)

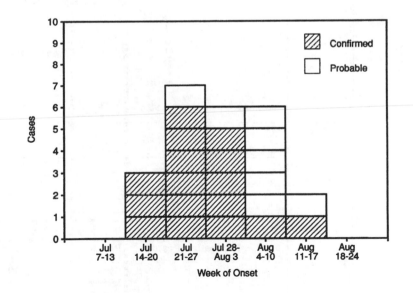

FIGURE 9.7   Example of short-term time trends of cases of St. Louis encephalitis in Pine Bluff, Arkansas, shown by week of onset in July and August, 1991. (Source: Centers for Disease Control and Prevention, "St. Louis Encephalitis Outbreak—Arkansas, 1991," *Morbidity and Mortality Weekly Report*, Vol. 40, No. 36, September 6, 1991, pp. 606–607)

cases of St. Louis encephalitis in Pine Bluff, Arkansas, are shown by week of onset in July and August, 1991.[9]

Polio has been one of the most devastating and disabling diseases to beset mankind. Thousands of people have died from this highly infectious disease. Polio crippled thousands more, until the development and distribution of vaccines in the early 1950s, which finally halted the devastating effects of this disease. Polio has a whole range of effects on the human body from minor muscular involvement to full paralysis of major vital muscle groups. Iron lungs were invented to help those persons breathe who were disabled with paralysis of respiratory muscles. The course of the disease and the time factors of the disease had to be understood in order to intervene through control and prevention measures.

Figure 9.8 shows the course of polio which demonstrates the short-term time factors implicated in this disease. The disease process can cease at any stage, depending upon the response of the immune system and the host's ability to resist the disease.

Cyclic Trends   Short-term as well as secular trends of some diseases have been known to be **cyclic**. Some disease cycles are seasonal, while cycles of other diseases may be controlled

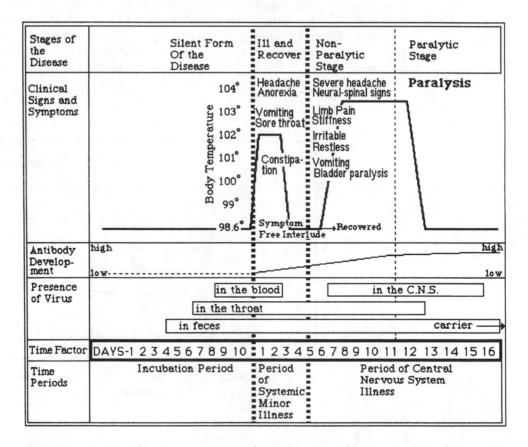

FIGURE 9.8   Graphic representation of time factors in the course of the disease poliomyelitis. (Adapted from: Reagan H. *"Schematic Representation of Major Findings in the Typical Course of Clinically Biphasic Poliomyelitis,"* unpublished handout)

by other cyclic factors such as the school year calendars, immigration patterns, migration patterns, duration and course of diseases, placement of military troops, and wars. Other phrases used to describe trends of disease cycles are *secular* and *seasonal cyclicity*. Cyclic changes refer to recurrent alterations in the occurrence, interval, or frequency of diseases. Seasonal trends are presented below. Secular cyclicity is a combination of following diseases over the long term combined with observing the cyclic nature of the disease. Some disease outbreaks occur only at certain times but in predictable time frames or intervals, over long terms, thus epidemiologists track cyclic changes over time. The study approach is quite straightforward. Cases of the disease under study are followed and tabulated by time of onset according to a diagnosis or proof of occurrence. Short-term fluctuations should use shorter time elements. The appropriate rates, charting approaches, and calculations are calculated by the epidemiologist as seen fit.

One disease that is very cyclic on a short term basis is chickenpox (varicella). As outbreaks of chickenpox are viewed over time, major cyclic variations are evidenced on a yearly basis. A similarly and dramatically portrayed annual cycle is seen in outbreaks of salmonella food poisoning. The cycle of chickenpox is also seasonal in its cycle. Chickenpox is one of the notifiable diseases and is more easily and accurately tracked than some diseases. Figure 9.9 presents the cyclic nature of chickenpox.[10]

Seasonal Trends and Variations   A consistent pattern of diseases can be seen for some diseases or conditions falling within a calendar year. An increase in incidence of a disease or condition during certain months, with cyclic variations by time of year and season indicates a **seasonal trend** in a disease.

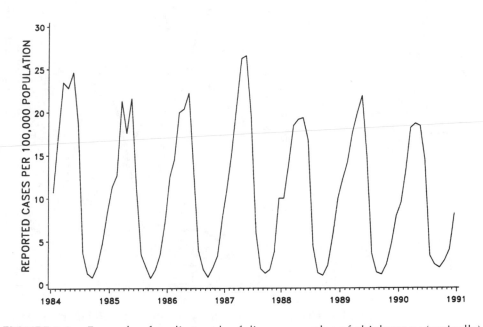

FIGURE 9.9   Example of cyclic trends of disease—cycles of chickenpox (varicella) outbreaks over an 8-year period by month. (Source: Centers for Disease Control and Prevention, "Summary of Notifiable Diseases, United States—1990," *Morbidity and Mortality Weekly Report*, Vol. 39, No. 53, October 4, 1990)

Seasonal trends and variations are interesting to study and provide dramatic visual epidemiological presentation when epidemiological activities are plotted on a chart or graph. Extremes in difference are readily seen. For example, influenza peaks in January and February and is lowest in the middle of the summer. In contrast, aseptic meningitis peaks in the summer, which may be related more to behaviors of the populations than to the weather. More people go swimming in the summer, exposing themselves to contaminated water in swimming pools, ponds, and lakes, all of which may have high bacteria levels or other abundant pathogens such as amoebas.

Seasons show many factors of health interest, such as children born in the summer achieve higher mean scores on IQ tests than winter-born children. High cholesterol readings in accountants are related to the tax calendar. Suicide rates are tied to seasonal variation and times of year. Mental retardation varies some with season. The high peak of births of children with mental retardation is in February with lowest rates in the summer. Admission rates to hospitals are cyclic and seasonal. Figure 9.10 is a chart comparing seasonal fluctuations between two different communicable diseases, meningococcal infections and encephalitis. Figure 9.10 is an example of the observed dramatic seasonal fluctuations of diseases (as is Figure 9.9).[3]

Seasonal change or variation has a profound effect on diseases. The plotting of such diseases affords the epidemiologist much opportunity to search for cause-effect relationships.

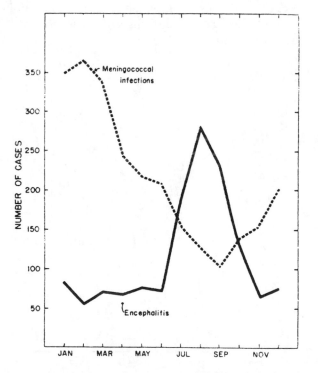

FIGURE 9.10   Example of seasonal variation of different diseases. Meningococcal disease occurs most in the winter months and encephalitis, transmitted by the mosquito, is highest in summer months. (Source: Centers for Disease Control and Prevention, "Reported Cases of Meningococcal Infections and of Primary Encephalitis by Month: United States—1968," *Morbidity and Mortality Weekly Report*, Vol. 17, 1971)

If a disease occurs only in the summer, then that is when the epidemiologist searches for the causative factors that would be available in that time period. Is the increase due to the exposure of new water sources, for example, drinking from a stream in the mountains, and if so at what time of year? Is it from summertime swimming in a contaminated public swimming pool or a lake? Is it a vectorborne disease from an insect that is active only in the summer? What vectors are available for disease transmission in the given time period and are missing at other times of the year or seasons? Are vehicles of transmission present during the time period that are not present during other time periods? Are the cases/subjects exposing themselves to environments, situations, places, or circumstances during this time period that are not available at other times of the year or in other seasons? Are the cases hiking or camping in the woods in the summer when insects are present that are implicated in vectorborne diseases? Are foodborne diseases from summertime camping, hiking, fishing, hunting trips, or picnics considered? Are certain fomites used during certain time periods that might not be used during other seasons, such as shared drinking glasses or containers?

Overall, the epidemiologist must consider seasonal fluctuations in recreational and occupational activities that may implicate or account for exposures or variations in outbreaks. The epidemiologist also must recognize the limits of seasonal variation implications. For example, chickenpox attack rates are predictable in their seasonal trends and cyclic nature. However, once a household has been exposed to chickenpox, the attack rate cycles no longer hold true.

TIME CLUSTERING

For the epidemiologist to gain insights into the cause and spread of certain diseases, the clustering of related events of the disease along an axis of time must be studied and plotted with little regard for the population at risk and comparisons to the unaffected population group. *Clustering* is a term with broad application and many names as used in epidemiology. Clustering of time-related events is when a group of cases of a disease occur close together and have a closely patterned and well aligned distribution pattern (see Figure 9.11). Clustering of a disease does not occur only in a time-oriented pattern or distribution, but also occurs in a certain or limited geographical area or place. Thus, both time and place variables, relations, and concerns have to be analyzed and plotted. Terms that have been used interchangeably with time clustering in epidemiology are **time-place cluster** and **disease cluster**.

An aggregate of rare or special disease events often is analyzed using time and/or place clustering. Multiple sclerosis and leukemia are two diseases that have unusual time and place clustering, as well as being the subject of much speculation about being zoonotic diseases, transmitted from small dogs and from cats. Multiple sclerosis has been hypothesized as being associated with ownership of small dogs which have been kept indoors, and it occurs more often in northern climates. House cats have been implicated in leukemia clustering in certain geographical areas.

Cluster analysis is an epidemiological method of plotting and analyzing, through appropriate statistical approaches of the grouping of variables or epidemiological observations into highly related subgroups of the study population. One approach of measurement of clustering is by assessing the time interval between the suspected cause of the disease and the onset of a series of cases of the disease. Mean and variance of the time interval are analyzed. The variance of the time interval may be shorter if the measurement is derived from the data of occurrence of the event that brought on the disease.

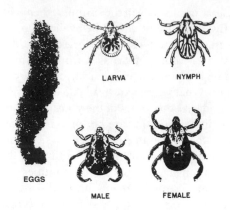

FIGURE 9.11   The life cycle of the tick; eggs, larva, nymph, adult male and female. The tick is a vector of disease and seasonal variation determines its life cycle, which is an important element of *time* in the transmission of diseases such as Lyme disease and Rocky Mountain spotted fever. (Picture courtesy of Centers for Disease Control and Prevention, Atlanta, Georgia)

According to MacMahon, clustering of causal events along the time axis, when studying cases of a disease, will be less apparent when the time interval between cause and effect is variable, and will be less apparent if there is a consistent change in the time interval during the observation period. If the interval between exposure and disease onset decreases as an outbreak progresses, it is possible that the dates of the onset of the cases may be more closely grouped about the mean than the time intervals between exposure and onset of the disease. Time clustering does indicate that a certain preceding event and the disease onset are associated in time. However, as in any epidemiological study the cause-effect relationship must be carefully and scientifically established.[1,3] Place clustering is also a part of spot/dot map activity. (See spot/dot maps as presented later in this chapter.)

Time/Place Clustering Analysis Using the Poisson Model

The Poisson probability distribution is an inferential statistics probability measure. The Poisson distribution is also referred to in some sources as the *Poisson spatial distribution* and the *Poisson spatial/nearest neighbor distribution*. The **Poisson distribution** is used to describe objects or events as they are distributed geographically (spatially) at random, with possibility of showing how the events cluster.[11] Poisson distributions do have limited use in epidemiology, but the concept is presented here to encourage creative and unique application of the concept, if not the method. Time and space clustering of cases can indicate that some disease causative agents or other etiological factors were introduced into the area at the time of the outbreak of an epidemic.

The Poisson distribution is applied to epidemiological studies to show the distribution and geographical clustering of patterns of disease outbreaks, exposures, and the occurrence of individual cases. To provide for a clearer analysis, the geographical area is divided into a series of square areas, with all having an equal amount of space in each square. For example, a city or county could be divided into one mile squares, showing where each case occurred on the map, as in cases of pediculosis (Figure 9.12). The equality of the square sizes

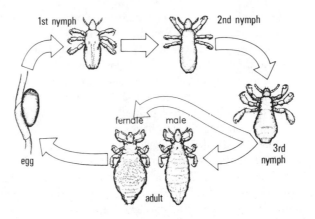

1st nymph 2nd nymph

female male

egg

adult

3rd
nymph

FIGURE 9.12   The life cycle of the head louse (Pediculus). The head louse is a microscopic pest that infests the hair, resulting in irritation, itching, and skin disease (secondary bacterial infection) and is transmitted from person to person. Head louse outbreaks are still common in all levels of elementary and secondary schools. (Picture courtesy of Centers for Disease Control and Prevention, Atlanta, Georgia)

and placement allows for randomization of the cases as they occur. Randomization is used in Poisson distributions to make them accurate and scientific. *Random*, in reference to the Poisson distribution, indicates that each case has a probability of falling into each square with an equal proportion of all the squares. The size of the square rather than the location influences the probability associated with each case or point. From a scientific perspective, for the Poisson distribution to be accurate, the probability that each case falls in a specific square must be small and the chance to do so must be constant.[11]

When geographical (spatial) clustering exists, then the probability for each square differs. Where cases cluster close together the probability of cause-effect relations goes up. When the clustering is low then the probability goes down. If it is not obvious whether or not a high enough level of assurity about a clustering is occurring, then a statistical test of significance could be used. Many biostatistics texts contain formulas for Poisson distribution analysis.[11]

There are many limitations to using the Poisson distribution to assess clustering. As time passes and a disease progresses in a cluster in a certain area, straight counts of the events may not be enough to deal with the constant changes that are occurring. Since distance is a continuous measure, the actual distance between points may be assessed by the **nearest-neighbor analysis**. The nearest neighbor is the closest next case. The distance from a target case, the index case, or any one case to the nearest other case(s) is calculated. The nearest neighbor is the closest case, distance-wise and geographically. Mean distances can be calculated and the variance of the distribution for a set of nearest-neighbor values can be derived as long as the distribution occurred at random.[11]

The limitation of the Poisson distribution and the nearest neighbor approaches is that the pattern of the disease as well as the time frame in which it occurs may not occur at random in the community. The occurrence of diseases is controlled by the susceptibility and risk levels of the population. That is, how many of the population have been immunized? How many susceptibles exist in the population? How many subjects have been exposed? How many behaviors or job exposures contain risk factors? Populations do not live in nice random positions in squares on a map. However, in population areas with high-density living, Poisson and nearest neighbor approaches do have some value, as the clustering of cases can be easily seen. Map transformation is a technique used in such cases.[11]

Geographic distribution around a point is another use of the Poisson type clustering of time and place analysis. If an index case is identified, then clustering may be seen around the index case point and may be seen spreading out from it. Nearest neighbor distances can be calculated, time frames of the disease transmission assessed, and predictions of the continuation of the outbreak plotted.

Poisson distributions have limited use in many communicable disease epidemiological studies. Most epidemiology sources do not even cover Poisson distributions and the concept is found most often in inferential statistics and biostatistics books. If Poisson distributions are not readily useful, traditional epidemiological spot maps (dot maps), though a simplified approach, can be of value in assessing communicable disease outbreaks in geographical areas, plotting both time and place clustering.

Case Example: Time and Space Clustering in Guillain-Barre Syndrome and Its Relationship to Swine Influenza Vaccination

In 1976, it was observed that the use of the killed swine flu vaccine was associated with an increased incidence of Guillain-Barre syndrome. The Centers for Disease Control and Prevention established a surveillance of persons in Michigan with the syndrome who had the disease with an onset between October 1, 1976 and January 31, 1977. Neurologists, medical record departments at hospitals, and physical therapists throughout Michigan were contacted to see if new cases were being seen. Hospitals had the highest rate of response. Hospitals saw 36%, physical therapists saw 36%, and physical therapists 5%. The 24 percent remaining were reported by primary care physicians, patients, and families. A total of 132 cases were confirmed. Approximately 2,300,000 persons were vaccinated during the time period of October 5 to December 16, 1976. Figure 9.13 presents the time factors and the time clustering of the disease outbreak as well as the course of Guillain-Barre syndrome by cases in Michigan in 1976–1977. Figure 9.14 presents the time-place clustering of Guillain-Barre syndrome in the State of Michigan.[1,2,3,12]

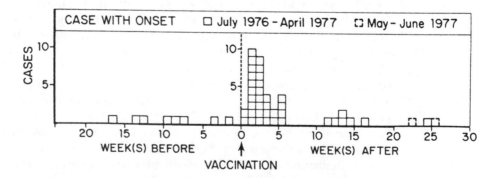

FIGURE 9.13   An example of the time factors and the time clustering of the outbreak in Michigan of Guillain-Barre Syndrome by cases—July, 1976–June, 1977. (Source: Breman, J.G., and Hayner, H.S., "Guillain-Barre Syndrome and Its Relationship to Swine Influenza Vaccination in Michigan, 1976–1977," *American Journal of Epidemiology*, Vol. 119, No. 6, 1984, pp. 880–889)

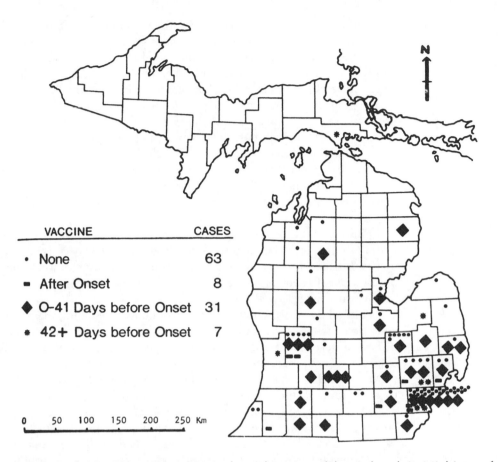

FIGURE 9.14 An example of time-place clustering of the outbreak in Michigan of Guillain-Barre Syndrome by cases in July, 1976–June, 1977. (Source: Breman, J.G., and Hayner, H.S., "Guillain-Barre Syndrome and Its Relationship to Swine Influenza Vaccination in Michigan, 1976–1977," *American Journal of Epidemiology*, Vol. 119, No. 6, 1984, pp. 880–889)

PLACE

Useful to the epidemiologist is the plotting of diseases, conditions, and maladies and their clustering on maps and the use of other related tools for locating various cases of diseases. Maps and clustering assessment tools are valuable, especially during an outbreak, especially if the disease is of general consequence to the public, affects a large population, and is widespread geographically. When considering **place**, the geographic location of the source of the disease as well as the reservoir of the organism should be considered in the analysis. The location of the case at the time the infection occurred, the clustering of the cases, as well as time factors related to the disease onset should be considered. The establishment of effective prevention and control measures is dependent upon identifying place-related issues and concerns. When control measures are implemented at the site where the infection occurred, the control of additional cases may or may not be prevented. Following the hosts to further locations and implementing controls where they are found would further prevent outbreaks.

Stopping the infection at the source is important but may not stop an outbreak of a disease if the infected hosts are then widely distributed geographically. Each case and source would have to be located. The initial source would also have to be identified and controlled. For example, if food was contaminated in a food processing plant, and then distributed to grocery stores and restaurants, the closing of the stores would only partially prevent the continuation of the outbreak. The food processing plant would also have to be closed and the sale of food products dealt with as well.

The occurrence of certain diseases and conditions can be identified relative to place in terms of location or geographical area established by natural topography of the land or natural barriers on the earth's surface. For example elevation, large rivers, seas, oceans, or mountain ranges may serve as natural demarcations of where a disease might begin or end. Elevation can also be a natural barrier as some pathogens or vectors may not survive as well at high elevations.

The idea of the location of people and their relationship to getting some disease is not new. In the mid 1850s Dr. John Snow observed that cholera occurred more at seaports than inland. In 1883 Dr. A. Hirsch published a three volume set of works on epidemiological observations. The volumes were titled, *Handbook of Geographical and Historical Pathology*, which associated place with disease.

Political boundaries, mostly borders of countries, establish the place at which certain conditions, diseases, and disorders occur or do not occur. An underdeveloped country can be next to an advanced industrialized nation and just a few miles away different sets of diseases can exist. Immunization programs, protected water supplies, removal of liquid waste (sewage) and solid waste (garbage), all rely on regulations, government organization, and financial support through taxation. Mostly these public health and governmentally supported measures are seen in the industrialized nations, while the conditions just across the border of an underdeveloped country can be just the opposite, as are the types and amounts of diseases seen. The contrast between Mexico and the United States is but one example.

Within the United States' boundaries, diseases fail to recognize the borders of cities, counties, and states, as social, transportation, and political conditions are basically the same across the political lines. Unfortunately not all cities, counties, and states are funded equally in public health, disease prevention, and control and thus some differences are seen. However, generally the differences across the various borders within the United States are not as readily discernible as they are in places like Africa. In the United States, the natural barriers play a much larger role in limiting disease outbreaks and place of occurrence than political borders.

It is well established that some diseases occur more in some places than others. Japan has lower levels of coronary artery disease, mostly due to diet. In West Texas lower levels of coronary artery disease are seen, mostly due to the hardness of the water and the minerals found in it. Nevada has high levels of lung cancer. Across the state line, Utah has lower levels of lung cancer than most other states due to the health behaviors and religious beliefs against smoking and using alcohol of many of the residents. A major portion of the state of Utah is inhabited by members of the Church of Jesus Christ of Latter Day Saints (Mormons) whose doctrine, called the "Word of Wisdom," forbids the use of tobacco and alcohol. Rabies occurs at a much higher rate in the United States along the U.S.-Mexico border than elsewhere, due to infected dogs and other animals crossing the border from Mexico. Multiple sclerosis occurs mostly in the northern United States. Some studies suggest MS is mostly likely caused by small dog ownership and sick dogs being kept indoors in the cold months. The multiple sclerosis virus and the distemper virus are similar to each other. Further study and more profound cause-effect relationship verification is needed to substantiate these hypotheses. Leukemia occurs mostly in northern states and least in the southeastern United States.

Five Criteria or Characteristics Peculiar to Place

Immigration and migration activities affect the disease rates and levels both in the place from which the people leave and the new place to which they go. As sick people leave a place, the health status goes up. If sick people move into a place, then the disease rates not only go up but can be widely spread, as well as new diseases being introduced into places where the disease never previously existed.

Below are five characteristics that are peculiar to place which epidemiologists study and are geographical criteria that should be considered when associating place and diseases.

1. High frequency rates of the disease are observable in all ethnic groups that inhabit the area.
2. High frequency rates of the disease are not observed in persons of similar groups inhabiting other areas.
3. Healthy persons entering the area become ill with a frequency similar to the indigenous population.
4. Inhabitants who have left the area do not show the same high rates of the diseases as those persons who remained in the area.
5. Species other than man inhabiting the same area show similar levels of infestation to that of man (of the applicable zoonotic diseases).

It is recognized that these criteria have limitations; however, they are useful to consider. The more of the above criteria that a disease satisfies, the more probability that the frequency of a disease is related to place (see Figure 9.15).[3]

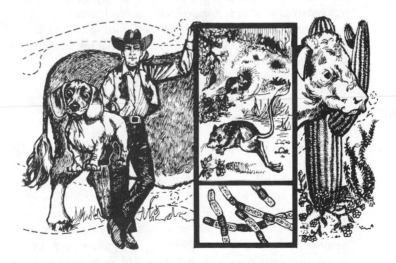

FIGURE 9.15   The life cycle of valley fever (coccidioidomycosis). Also called San Joaquin fever or desert fever, this infection is caused by inhaling spores of the bacterium *Coccidioides immitis*, which are suspended in the air during dust storms. This disease is a good example of the *place* aspect of disease, as it occurs in the United States only in the Southwest and is endemic in hot, dry areas. The unique *person* aspect of this disease is that it is most common in females ages 15 to 25. (Picture courtesy of Centers for Disease Control and Prevention, Atlanta, Georgia)

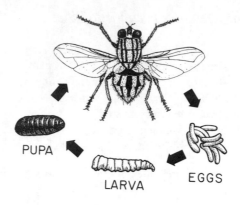

PUPA   LARVA   EGGS

The life cycle of the housefly. The housefly is a notorious vector of disease, spreading pathogens to humans from feces, garbage, and decaying food and animals. (Picture courtesy of Centers for Disease Control and Prevention, Atlanta, Georgia)

Ecological Environment and Place

Topography, climate, and ecological character have much influence on place aspects of the existence and spread of diseases. Temperature, rainfall, winds, water, humidity, cold, heat, hours of sunshine, and other conditions affect the ability of pathogens, especially bacteria, molds, fungi, and parasites, to survive in the environment. The ecological aspects of the environment affect the ability of pathogens to thrive and be transmitted. Various aspects of the ecosystem consist of vectors, vehicles, reservoirs, and hosts for a range of communicable diseases (see Chapter 2). Foliage, animals (both small and large, domestic and wild) and the insects (mosquitoes, flies, lice, fleas, ticks) that transmit the diseases are all part of the ecological environment of place and disease.

Physical Environment and Place

Water and air are two important components of the physical environment essential for the survival of man and other forms of life on earth. Drinking water and air quality can vary from place to place and can affect one's health status. The chemical and mineral makeup of water (hardness) has affected the health of people who live in areas where hard water is prevalent. In West Texas, the water contains many minerals and is very hard. Fluoride is one of the minerals common in the ground water. In places where fluoride is abundant as in parts of West Texas, mottling of teeth is seen, as are fewer trips to the dentist. Low levels of heart disease in West Texas are attributed to the hard water as well. Endemic occurrences of goiter have long been associated with low levels of iodine in the soil, food, and water of certain areas. High levels of lung cancer occur in certain places where air pollution (often combined with smoking) is a problem. Examples are the inland valleys of Southern California, Southern Nevada, the Hudson River area of New York, and the Mississippi River delta area of Louisiana. Figure 9.16 shows the places where lung cancer has high occurrence and the clustering of diseases is also observed.

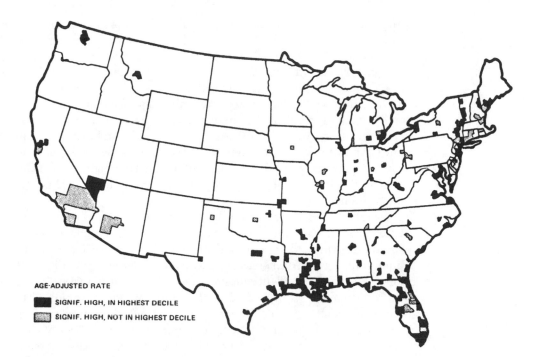

FIGURE 9.16 A spot map of the highest occurrences of lung and bronchial cancer in the United States (the 48 continental states). The disease clustering effect is also observed. (Source: National Center for Health Statistics, Centers for Disease Control and Prevention, Public Health Service, U.S. Department of Health, Education and Welfare, 1982)

Social and Cultural Environment and Place

How people in a society or population group use food, water, chemicals, and how they practice sanitation, hygiene, personal health has a great effect on the health status of that population. Other forces affecting health status such as health beliefs, traditions, social and cultural interactions all have an effect on the development and spread of diseases. The Fore tribe in Papua New Guinea, is but one example of cultural beliefs and behaviors contributing to an epidemic and unnecessary deaths. The Fore people suffered for years from Kuru, a disease affecting the brain and nervous system. Kuru causes shaking, paralysis, crippling of the limbs, and mental impairment, and occurred mostly in women and children. It was eventually discovered after an extensive epidemiological investigation that the cause of Kuru is a slow virus transmitted to the Fore women and children by the cultural tradition of eating the brains of the dead family members.

Social interactions and cultural practices have long been studied in both modern and primitive societies of which many have been linked to disease, disability, and death. The traditional church or school potluck picnic has long been known to be associated with epidemics of food poisoning from staphylococcal food poisoning, salmonellosis, or typhoid fever. Sexual activity with many partners is often implicated in the spread of sexually transmitted diseases, including AIDS. The gathering of large bodies of people in a confined environment is a hotbed for the transmission of communicable diseases as in Legionnaire's disease. Childhood diseases such as chickenpox can spread like wildfire through a school district when most children are susceptible. Head lice (pediculosis) do not require susceptible status as all children are susceptible. Head lice continue to be an epidemic in school children across the United States and are a social interaction driven condition among children. Children study, play, and interact under close conditions and like to try on and wear each other's clothing, which can be infested with head lice. The same is true for measles if immunization levels are low (see herd immunity in Chapter 2). Conjunctivitis has spread through institutionalized populations with an equal amount of vigor. Many case examples exist where this disease has infected almost every patient in a nursing home.

People of the same race, ethnicity, and culture, especially of minority groups, tend to desire to live close to each other. The concentration of races and ethnic groups also has an effect on the types and amounts of diseases found in a place. Unfortunately some concentrations of races in certain areas bring with them poor living conditions due to low socioeconomic status, low levels of education, and lack of occupational skills. Thus, some diseases identified by place are influenced by these other person conditions. This phenomenon, though commonly observed in central city areas and migrant camps, is not limited to the United States. Refugee camps due to migrations and wars, barrios of cities, and tent cities where populations of poor and deprived people gather are places of disease infestations and are often sites of severe epidemics. One such example was a slum barrio of Lima, Peru. The small city of Acapulco, a suburb of Lima, is mostly a slum of makeshift huts, with no fresh water supply, sewage running in the streets, ditches and streams and into the ocean without treatment, garbage not collected nor controlled. The end result was that in 1991, the first epidemic of cholera in 100 years occurred hospitalizing tens of thousands and killing thousands. Public health activities, or the lack of them, as well as social and cultural environments have a major impact on the epidemiology of the place.

MAPS AND SPOT/DOT MAPS IN EPIDEMIOLOGY

Epidemiologists use maps for locating cases of a disease during an outbreak or an epidemic. The dot map approach is especially useful if the disease is widespread, of general consequence to a large population, and if it has a clustering effect.

With some diseases, the plotting of the location of individual cases on a map may be of limited value. At that point, the locating of centers of exposure and occurrence maybe more useful. For example, limited information may be gained when trying to plot every case of measles occurring in elementary age children if the places of exposure are public schools and not the home or neighborhood. The assessment of clustering may be of more importance in such situations. Thus, the identification of elementary school locations as the place of exposure may be of more value, or in some cases, the plotting of both cases and schools. Plotting on a map the preschool children who became cases and were exposed by older siblings may be important as well.

Following are several examples of the epidemiological use of maps to show the distribution and occurrence of various diseases, both communicable and chronic. Also presented are dot maps or spot maps which are used to show how they are used in the context of epidemiology in the identification and location of cases of a disease with regard to place, and where appropriate, the effects of clustering of the disease can be seen.

Use of Maps in Epidemiology

Several maps are presented on the following pages as used in epidemiological studies and investigations. General maps of disease on the national level are presented. Spot/dot maps are also presented including building mapping for use in epidemiological investigations.

One disease of interest to most every member of society is AIDS, a sexually transmitted disease that has devastated the African continent, and by 1990 had infected or killed 161,073 persons in the United States, with 41,595 cases occurring in 1990 alone in the United States. One place question often used is Where do most of the cases of AIDS occur in the United States? The place concern related to AIDS has been of concern to lay persons and epidemiologists alike. Figure 9.17 shows the occurrence of AIDS in the United States.

Another sexually transmitted disease, but one thought to be under control by some segments of the general public, is syphilis. Syphilis is still occurring in epidemic proportions in certain places in the United States. To identify where the concentrations of syphilis occur, an epidemiological map is useful. Figure 9.18 shows the geographical concentration and distribution of syphilis in the continental United States in 1990.

Measles has been of great concern to public health in modern times, a period when most people should be free from the risk of getting the disease. Immunizations are readily available yet are not being acquired by certain segments of the population. In 1988 the largest age-specific increase in rubella incidence occurred among persons aged 15 years and older and under age one year. In 1989, a greater proportion of cases occurred among the 1- to 14-age group. Religious communities with unvaccinated children contributed in part to this increase in this group. Figure 9.19, an epidemiological map, shows the changes of incidence rates of reported rubella in the United States for the years 1988, 1989, and 1990.[13]

Heart disease is the number one cause of the death in the United States for all races. A study of ischemic heart disease that used epidemiology maps to present the findings showed a marked difference in the geographical distribution of this disease in California. When black males are compared to white males, place of occurrence is markedly different as well. Figures 9.20 and 9.21 show the difference in place for ischemic heart disease for the two races. Place of occurrence is highly influenced by where the different races live and are concentrated. People of same ethnic backgrounds prefer to live with each other, regardless of efforts to integrate populations. Thus when looking at place and race together, maps may reflect where races concentrate and thus where diseases occur unique to the merging of the above factors.[14]

Although estimates of alcohol-related mortality have been determined for the United States, they have not been well defined for smaller geographic areas. Efforts have been made at the national level to determine the percentile ranking of each county in order to assist in ranking metropolitan areas that overlap state boundaries, such as the tri-state metropolitan area including New York City and parts of Connecticut and New Jersey. Figure 9.22 is an epidemiological map showing the comparison of U.S. percentile rankings for alcohol-related deaths for the Connecticut, New Jersey, and New York metropolitan area from 1979 to 1985.

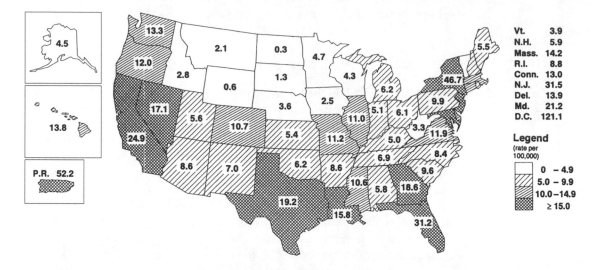

FIGURE 9.17   Epidemiological map showing the occurrences and distribution of AIDS in the United States—1990. (Source: Centers for Disease Control and Prevention, "Summary of Notifiable Diseases, United States—1990," *Morbidity and Mortality Weekly Report*, Vol. 39, No. 53, October 4, 1990)

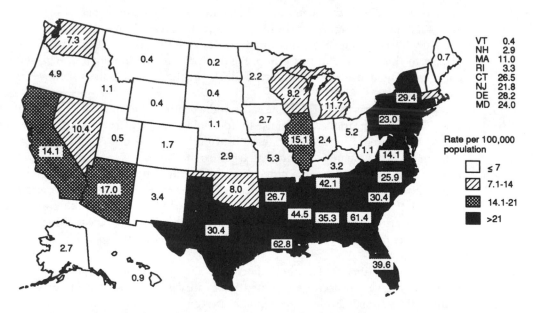

FIGURE 9.18   Epidemiological map showing the occurrence and distribution of syphilis in the United States—1990. (Source: Centers for Disease Control and Prevention, "Summary of Notifiable Diseases, United States—1990," *Morbidity and Mortality Weekly Report*, Vol. 9, No. 53, October 4, 1990)

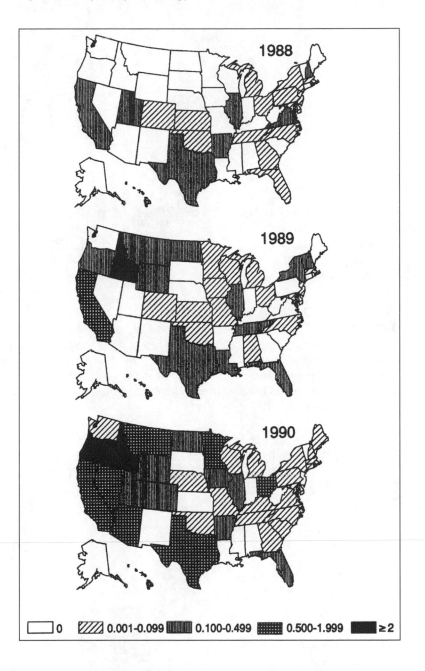

FIGURE 9.19 Epidemiological map showing the dramatic changes in incidence rates of reported rubella per 100,000 population in the United States for 1988, 1989 and 1990. Mississippi requires reporting of congenital rubella syndrome but not rubella cases. (Source: Centers for Disease Control and Prevention, "Increase in Rubella and Congenital Rubella Syndrome—United States, 1988–1990," *Morbidity and Mortality Weekly Report*, Vol. 40, No. 6, February 15, 1991)

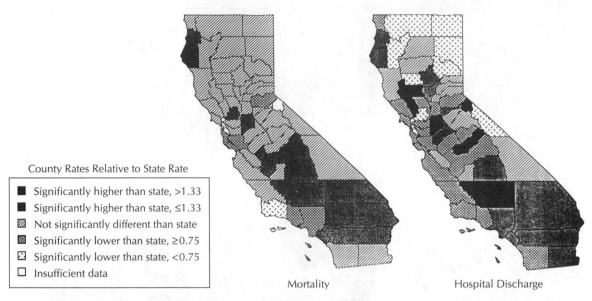

County Rates Relative to State Rate

- ■ Significantly higher than state, >1.33
- ■ Significantly higher than state, ≤1.33
- ▨ Not significantly different than state
- ▩ Significantly lower than state, ≥0.75
- ▧ Significantly lower than state, <0.75
- ☐ Insufficient data

Mortality   Hospital Discharge

FIGURE 9.20   Epidemiological map showing *place* of mortality and hospital discharges related to ischemic heart disease among white males in California 1983–1987. (Source: Technical Report No. 2, *Ischemic Heart Disease, Hypertension and Cerebrovascular Disease Deaths and Hospitalizations—California, 1983–1987*, California Chronic and Sentinel Disease Surveillance Program, California Department of Health Services, October 1990)

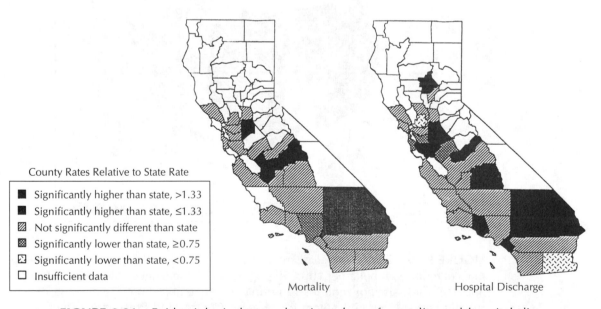

County Rates Relative to State Rate

- ■ Significantly higher than state, >1.33
- ■ Significantly higher than state, ≤1.33
- ▨ Not significantly different than state
- ▩ Significantly lower than state, ≥0.75
- ▧ Significantly lower than state, <0.75
- ☐ Insufficient data

Mortality   Hospital Discharge

FIGURE 9.21   Epidemiological map showing *place* of mortality and hospital discharges related to ischemic heart disease among black males in California 1983–1987. (Source: Technical Report No. 2, *Ischemic Heart Disease, Hypertension and Cerebrovascular Disease Death and Hospitalizations—California, 1983–1987*, California Chronic and Sentinel Disease Surveillance Program, California Department of Health Services, October, 1990)

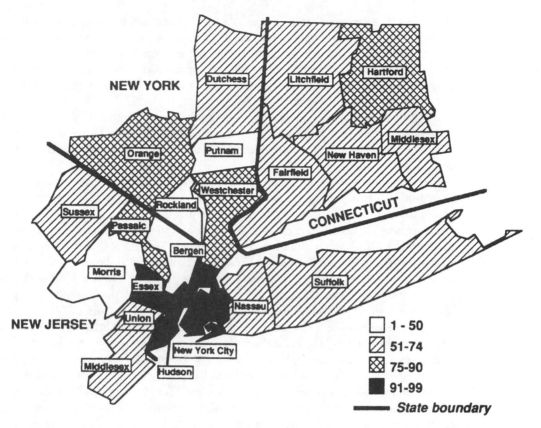

FIGURE 9.22   Epidemiological map showing the U.S. percentile ranking of alcohol-related deaths for Connecticut, New Jersey and New York metropolitan areas from 1979 to 1985. (Source: Centers for Disease Control and Prevention, "County Data on Alcohol-Related Mortality—United States," *Morbidity and Mortality Weekly Report*, Vol. 40, No. 32, August 16, 1991)

Application of Spot/Dot Maps in Epidemiology

What is a **spot (dot) map**? How is it used in epidemiology? What value are spot maps to the epidemiologist? The word *spot*, as in spot map, suggests the location or spot where the disease or exposure actually occurred with a dot placed on the map signifying the place of each occurrence. *Dot* refers to plotting of the disease or exposure on a map with a dot being drawn on a map for each case. A dot is more appropriate for single cases and the clustering of dots indicates the spots where the epidemic is occurring. Thus, either the term, *spot map* or *dot map*, seems appropriate.

An important facet of epidemiology map use is that the epidemiologist must feel free to be creative in map construction and plotting. The epidemiologist should use whatever method or approach that makes common sense in its development—whatever approach aids in the assessment and analysis of the outbreak so that it leads to some conclusion as to the source of the outbreak.

A dot map is a graphic presentation of where certain diseases, disabilities, conditions, or deaths occur or where the exposure took place. To develop a dot map, the epidemiologist places dots on an appropriate sized map, identifying the location of each individual case of a disease, the place of exposure or the place of residence of individuals with a specific condition or attribute. The dot map has a whole range of uses, from identifying the location of cases of Lyme disease in rural areas to the location of unusual patterns of cancer occurrence in industrial areas and the place of the homes of elderly with disabilities in a city, to the location of population centers in a state or county.

Dot map development in epidemiology has been used effectively with infectious diseases of short duration with localized outbreaks and with chronic diseases on a national basis. Dot maps more recently have been used to identify sources of industrial pollution and chronic disease occurrences.

The plotting of a dot map is one of the most basic epidemiological processes, and has been used historically to investigate the occurrence of epidemics of communicable diseases and is still used today. The value of the dot map is that it enables the epidemiologist to visually assess the actual physical location of individual cases of disease, the clustering of cases, and identification of the sources of infection or risk factors. The observation of the clustering of cases is one of the most valuable aspects of dot maps. The inferences made from a dot map depend on the potential that exists for a population to develop the disease, the number of susceptibles in the community, and on the cases of chronic or industrially related disorders or conditions, and the potential for exposure to risk factors.

In some diseases and conditions, dot maps prove to be of little value. For example, when investigating smoking in adults, it would be meaningless to try to plot on a map the cases or exposures or sources from which the risk factors (the cigarettes) were obtained as smoking is evenly distributed and is widespread. Cigarettes are sold everywhere in the community and smoking is done at random in society, thus to plot cases of cigarette smoking or where the cigarettes were obtained or smoked by using a dot map would, in general, be of little value epidemiologically. If a study were to focus on school children in certain areas, the use of a dot map might be of value. When studying smoking the person issues are of more value to the epidemiologist than the geographical location. However, the concept of place should not be ignored as some place-related issues may prove to be worthwhile, especially if combined with other respiratory disease exposures. For example, if subjects who smoke are living in an area with high levels of air pollution, then place issues are of great importance in such an investigation.

Dr. John Snow's Use of a Dot Map in the Cholera Epidemic in London

Historically, the first printed and consequently the most widely published use of a dot map in an epidemiological study was the one plotted by Dr. John Snow of the cholera epidemic in the Soho District and Golden Square areas of London in the early 1800s. Dr. Snow plotted both numbers of cases and location of cases by place of residence on a map. He also identified the location of the potential sources of cholera, which he believed to be water. The water pumps in the district were also located on the dot map, as were the distances one would have to travel to the pumps to get water. The place where persons were not getting the illness were also plotted (i.e., the brewery). The dot map of the cholera epidemic in London plotted by Dr. Snow is shown in Case Study I.

Dot Map Showing Populated Areas of Idaho   One of the general uses of a dot map is for locating population centers within a state. Figure 9.23 is an example of a dot map for the state of Idaho and is presented as an example of a dot map used to show population centers.

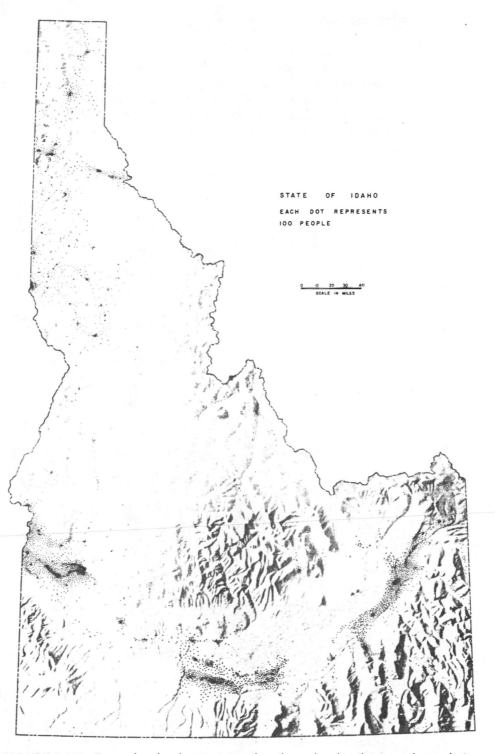

STATE   OF   IDAHO

EACH   DOT   REPRESENTS

100   PEOPLE

0   10   20   30   40
SCALE IN MILES

FIGURE 9.23   Example of a dot map, used to show the distribution of population centers across the state of Idaho. Each dot represents 100 people. (Source: Vital Statistics for the State of Idaho, 1978)

Dot Maps in Disease Investigation

Maps and dot map activities are often used in current epidemiology practice. The most common use for dot maps has been in infectious disease investigation to identify both sources of infection and cases. Many waterborne disease outbreaks lend themselves to being plotted on dot maps. Case examples serve well to illustrate the point and afford the opportunity to examine some actual case usage of dot maps as used in some epidemiological investigations. Figures 9.24 and 9.25 are but two examples.

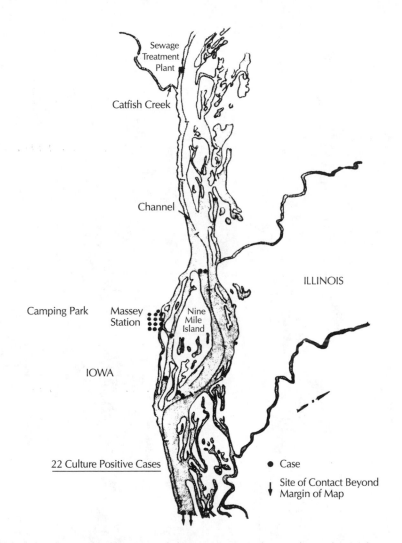

FIGURE 9.24   Example of map and dot map use in the epidemiological investigation of a shigellosis outbreak caused by swimming in the Mississippi River showing locations of where persons swam within three days of the onset of illness. (Source: Rosenberg, M.L., Haziet, K.I., Schaefer, J., Wells, J.G., Pruneda, R.C., "Shigellosis from Swimming," *Journal of the American Medical Association*, Vol. 236, No. 16, October 18, 1976, pp. 1849–1852—used with permission)

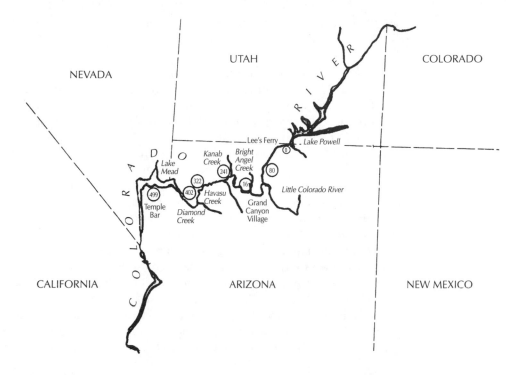

FIGURE 9.25   Example of map and dot map use in the epidemiological investigation of a shigellosis outbreak on river raft trips down the Grand Canyon on the Colorado River. (Source: Merson, M.H., et al. "An Outbreak of *Shigella sonnei* gastroenteritis on Colorado River Raft Trips," *American Journal of Epidemiology*, Vol. 100, No. 3, 1974, pp. 186–195 — used with permission)

Shigellosis Outbreak from Swimming in the Mississippi River   Epidemics of shigellosis (*Shigella sonnei*) have occurred from swimming in contaminated river water. *Shigella* is a gastroenteritis that is rapidly spread among humans by the fecal-oral route. Only a small number of pathogens from contaminated water or food need to be ingested. In Dubuque, Iowa, 45 members of 29 families were exposed to shigellosis and tested positive with disease onset between July 9 and August 9, 1974. Symptoms of shigella include diarrhea, fever, chills, abdominal pain, nausea, vomiting, and headache. Of the 43 persons consulting a physician, 18 cases were hospitalized. The patients were not clustered by place of residence nor by sex or age. When most cases had reported swimming in the river, suspicion of swimming in Mississippi River water motivated an epidemiological study. Figure 9.24 shows the map of the river and the place where the cases were exposed, and is presented here as an example of a dot map used in epidemiological studies. It was found that those persons who held river water in their mouths were the ones who were the most at risk of getting the disease. Person-to-person transmission of the disease was seen among family members in some families but not found to be transmitted between different families. The map assisted in locating the source of contamination. A small creek that emptied into the river upstream was implicated. The shigella pathogens could also have come from the sewage treatment plant that is located upriver from the swimming areas. Without the assessment of such maps, important sources of infection might be overlooked. Dot maps are of great assistance in such epidemiological investigations.[15]

Shigellosis from River Raft Trips down the Grand Canyon on the Colorado River   In the summer of 1972, a major outbreak of *Shigella sonnei* gastroenteritis occurred on the Colorado River among people participating in river raft trips. In 1972, 14,000 persons made the trip down the Colorado river with 21 different companies conducting trips. The boatmen were men, 20 to 30 years of age and were responsible for food and water handling, yet had no food sanitation and handling training. The symptoms shown in the cases were characteristic of shigella. The epidemiological investigation indicated that the illness originated among boatmen and spread to passengers primarily by person-to-person transmission. The investigation found no common water or food source for the outbreak. The river water as well as the tributaries showed that the water was not suitable for drinking unless purified. Retrospective as well as prospective studies were conducted. No common exposure point could be identified for the 109 ill persons. Human fecal contamination was evident at only one creek (Kanab Creek) and it was rarely used for drinking water. The kilometer points were used to pinpoint the location of exposure. Forty percent of the ill persons became ill after kilometers 43 and 64. The time factor as well as the location of place should also be considered in such a study. One item that the study did not address was incubation period in relationship to the kilometer/place of onset of the illness. Figure 9.25 is the map showing kilometers downriver from Lee's Ferry, used to assess place of exposure.[16]

USE OF BUILDING MAPS IN EPIDEMIOLOGY

Two approaches to use of building maps have been used in epidemiology. The first approach is mapping the inside of a building, which can include the location at the time of exposure of cases who acquired the disease while inside the building, and the sequence of air flow through the building via air conditioning and heating systems, personnel flow, or traffic. The locations of related disease reservoirs on site are also identified and plotted on the building map. The second approach is mapping the location of buildings and the structures implicated in the place of the occurrence of disease outbreaks. Building maintenance workers, engineers, and architects can assist the epidemiologist in investigating building-related epidemics. In the case of an outbreak in a large public building or a complex of buildings, not only should guests of a hotel, students in a school, or patients within a hospital be assessed for exposures, but building workers and visitors should not be overlooked as potential cases.

Legionnaire's Disease Using Dot Maps and Hotel Maps   In 1976 the first major common-source outbreak of Legionnaire's disease that received national attention, occurred in a Philadelphia hotel at a convention for the American Legion. In the summer of 1979, another major outbreak of Legionnaire's disease occurred at a hotel in Eau Claire, Wisconsin. As in the Philadelphia epidemic, the air-conditioning cooling tower was implicated in transmission of the disease. In Eau Claire, 8 persons in a city of 50,000 were admitted to hospitals with atypical pneumonia. Clinical and laboratory tests showed the *Legionella pneumophila* pathogen to be present and a four-fold rise of the antibody titer was shown in the patients. Several hotels and their guests located close by were investigated. Hotel ventilation systems were examined, with environmental samples collected from the cooling towers, source water, fan filters, and rainwater puddles from hotels

A and B. Thirteen cases were found and ten patients had been exposed in hotel A. A 3- to 8.5-day incubation period was discovered. No cause-effect relationships could be found between food or water consumption. A map of hotel A was used in the epidemiological investigation of the Legionnaires' disease.[17]

In 1980–1981 two major outbreaks of Legionnaires' disease were experienced in a regional medical center in Burlington, Vermont. In the two outbreaks, 85 cases of Legionnaircs' disease were diagnosed. All cases had been within the city of Burlington at least 10 days prior to the onset of symptoms. Exposures were both hospital and community based. No common in-hospital exposure was associated with the onset of the disease. Water systems in the community were evaluated as a possible source for the *Legionella* pathogen. A cooling tower located 150 meters upwind from the hospital was implicated as the source of the pathogen's reservoir. Maintenance workers who did work on the tower had higher titers for *Legionella* than other tower workers who worked at a similar cooling tower 1.6 kilometers away. The epidemiological use of a spot map included wind direction assessments for the months of May and July. Figure 9.26 shows location of Tower A in relationship to wind direction influence and other structures as well as where the cases occurred.

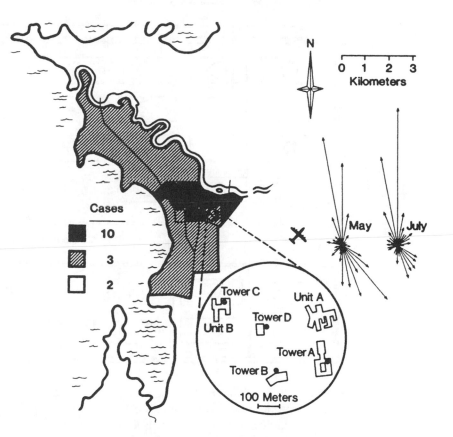

FIGURE 9.26   An example of a spot map showing cases, building and wind direction as used in an epidemiological study of Legionnaires' disease in Burlington, Vermont. (Source: Klauke, D.N., et al. "Legionnaires' Disease: The Epidemiology of Two Outbreaks in Burlington, Vermont, 1980," *American Journal of Epidemiology*, Vol. 119, No. 3, 1984, pp. 382–390— uscd with permission)

Use of Building Map in Tuberculosis Outbreak Investigation Exposure to tuberculosis in buildings and their closed environments has been reported. TB has been shown to circulate throughout a building via the central air circulation system. A clerk in an insurance company visited her physician concerning a cough of one month's duration. Her chest x-ray showed a shadow in the right lower lobe of her lung consistent with pulmonary TB. Sputum tests confirmed the diagnosis. Ten months earlier during a screening test for TB, the clerk had a tine test which showed negative for TB. It was concluded that she was a new case with primary TB and the case was referred to the local public health department. The epidemiologist at the public health department began an investigation. All contacts were investigated, including roommates, an elderly couple, her social group, and fellow workers, for a total of 31 persons being contacted. All 31 were given clinical tests. The group with the largest numbers of exposures were her fellow employees, thus the investigation was focused on the insurance company worksite. An office map of the claims department she worked in was drawn up and desk locations noted. The infected clerk occupied desk number 10 on the map (see Figure 9.27). The flow of the air throughout the entire floor of the building needed

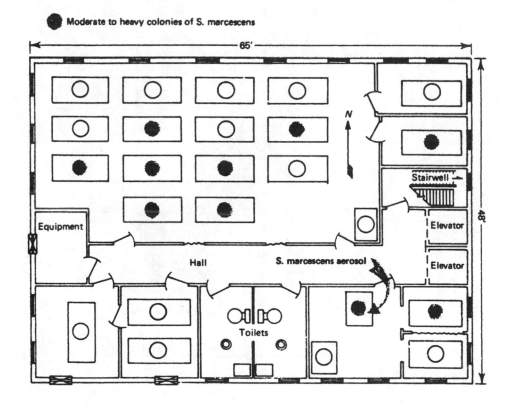

FIGURE 9.27 Building map of the floor plan of the claims department being investigated for an outbreak of tuberculosis. Also shown are the locations of culture plates showing colonies of the organism used in a test to show the role of the ventilation system in disease transmission and to confirm that the receptionist was the source of infection/tuberculosis. (Source: Adapted from Shindell, S., Salloway, J.C., and Oberembt, C.M., *A Coursebook in Health Care Delivery*, Appleton Century Crofts: New York, 1976—used with permission)

investigation. Thus, a map of the ventilation system and air flow throughout not only the claims department but the entire floor was also developed, all done in order to aid in the epidemiological investigation[19] (see Figure 9.28).

Upon investigating the receptionist, it was discovered that she had been treated for tuberculosis in a sanitarium five years earlier. Tests showed that the receptionist had advanced stages of TB. Two vice-presidents also tested positive for TB. The receptionist was considered to be the source of the outbreak. To confirm the suspicion, during a weekend when the building was vacant, culture plates were placed on all desks. A nonpathogenic bacteria aerosol was released at the point where the receptionist sat. Nine of the culture plates became infected including the one placed on desk number 10, the clerk (the index case) who presented herself to the physician, starting the investigation. Figure 9.27 is a building map showing the location of the petri dishes and cultures, verifying that the ventilation system was the source of transmitting the TB pathogens to other persons within the building.[19]

Use of Spot/Dot Maps in Investigating Typhus   A classic use of a dot map in the investigation of a major disease outbreak was that of an epidemic of typhus in Montgomery, Alabama, in 1922–1925. The use of a dot map showed that the place of residence and the

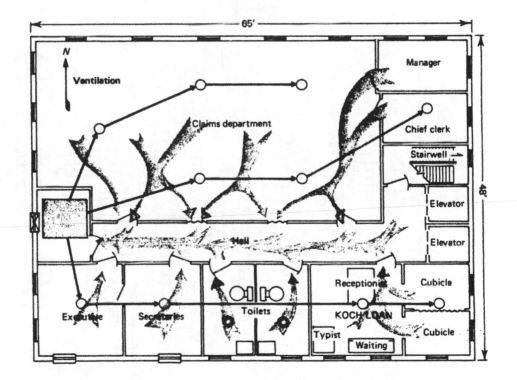

FIGURE 9.28   Example of use of a building map to plot the ventilation and air flow of the claims department and entire floor being investigated for an outbreak of tuberculosis. (Source: Adapted from Shindell, S., Salloway, J.C., and Oberembt, C.M., *A Coursebook in Health Care Delivery*, Appleton Century Crofts: New York, 1976—used with permission)

place of work are different sources of infection and that the worksite could be implicated as the source of a disease outbreak. The worksite exposures showed that the cases were clustered in one area of the business district. The clustering was around food-handling establishments and feed stores in a rat infested area near the river. The rat and rat flea were implicated in the transmission of murine typhus. A dot map was plotted to aid in the epidemiological investigation. Figure 9.29 is an example of a dot map of Montgomery, Alabama, showing the place of employment (unemployed are plotted on the map according

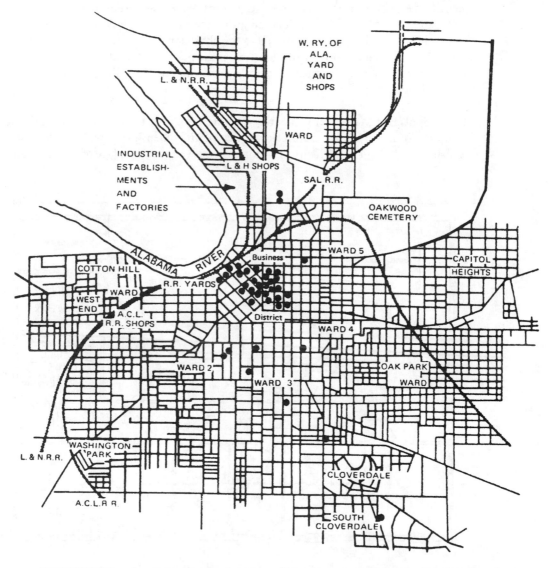

FIGURE 9.29   An example of a dot map of Montgomery, Alabama showing the place of employment of cases in a typhus epidemic in 1922–1925. (Source: Adapted from Maxcy, K.F., "An Epidemiological Study of Endemic Typhus (Brill's Disease) in the Southeastern United States," *Public Health Reports*, Vol. 41, pp. 2967–2995, 1926)

Mapping in Epidemiology

New Computer Mapping Software Technology Useful in Epidemiology

Several new software-driven mapping programs have been developed recently, some especially for epidemiology and others adapted for use in public health and epidemiology. Epi Info is a statistical and questionnaire development software program, developed by the Centers for Disease Control and Prevention. It has a companion software program called Epi Map, which is used to create various kinds of epidemiological maps.

Other mapping software programs have been adapted for epidemiological use. Several business software companies make mapping programs for market research that can be adapted to epidemiology. Disease dot maps, spot maps, case clustering, and zip code marking can be done easily on the marketing versions. Other business programs are used to identify locations of target populations or service providers. Geo/Navigator, developed by Visuals Solutions in Reno, Nevada, allows you to scan in a topographic map, onto which important information and place markings can then be added or drawn over. Geo/Navigator runs on a Macintosh and handles various forms of pictures and graphics, such as EPS and PICT files. Geo/Navigator has been used in analyzing movement of physicians' offices from lower-income parts of town to wealthier areas in Birmingham, Alabama (*Business Geographics* March/April 1994, pp. 38–37). Environmental Systems Research Institute in Redlands, California, using digital mapping software in combination with the Global Positioning System (GPS), has been mapping various environmentally related projects, including tracking plumes of contaminated water in local aquifers. The National Center for Health Statistics has produced a 1997 government map book, *Atlas of United States Mortality*, which details geographical views of death in the United States, and looks at 18 different causes of death in 805 clusters of counties for the entire country. The report details *place* of death rates from 1988 to 1992. Samples of the maps can be seen on the Internet at http://www.cdc.gov/nchswww/nchshome.htm The book is available through the U.S. Superintendent of Documents.

to place of residence). Figure 9.30 is a dot map showing the place of residence of all cases of typhus in Montgomery, Alabama.[20]

Clustering in Time and Place

When faced with a possible epidemic the epidemiologist looks at the pattern of cases and how they fall within a given geographical area and they are then plotted on a map. The time pattern of occurrence is also plotted but on a graph. Time and place patterns are thoroughly

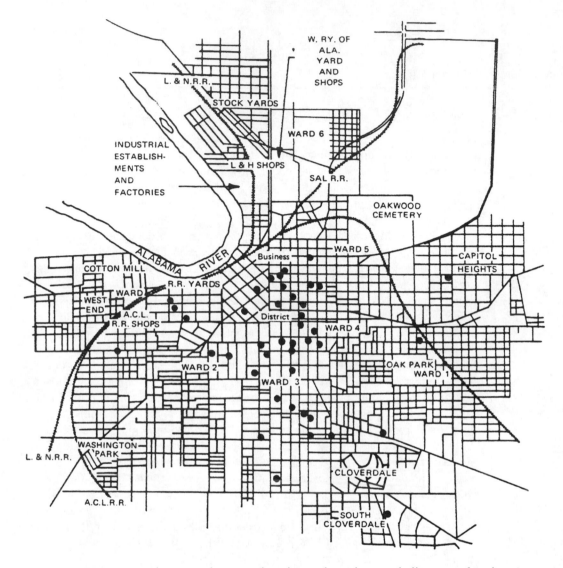

FIGURE 9.30   A dot map showing the place of residence of all cases of typhus in Montgomery, Alabama. (Source: Adapted from Maxcy, K.F., "An Epidemiological Study of Endemic Typhus (Brill's Disease) in the Southeastern United States," *Public Health Reports*, Vol. 41, pp. 2967–2995, 1926)

examined for evidence that the distribution of cases is piling up in one place and that they are not occurring randomly.

When the clustering of disease is investigated, it often involves smaller numbers of cases and limited geographical areas. The analysis of disease clustering may not fit well into sophisticated statistical approaches due to the limited number of subjects. Several new computer software programs have been developed to assist the epidemiologist in the analysis of disease clustering. One program is called *Cluster Analysis and Computer Software* or *CLUSTER*. This program examines if the cases are placed at random or not; it also is used to determine other important factors such as if the disease clusters are grouped closely in space; if the cases are grouped close in time; if the cases are an aggregate, closer in time and space than would be normally expected; if some geographical areas such as zip codes have more cases than others; if some subgroups or ethnic groups have more cases than others.[22]

PERSON

Much of the focus of epidemiology is aimed at the *person* aspects of disease (see Figures 9.31 and 9.32), disability, injury and death. **Person**-related issues have previously been presented in Chapters 4 and 5. The discussions of cohorts and research designs also should be reviewed as they have many person-related implications. Populations of people have been characterized according to a number of standard variables and traits. From a practical point of view, the traits used to describe the *person* aspects of epidemiology have been limited according to the purpose and resources of concern to a particular study or investigation. The information already available from common sources such as public health departments and government agencies, plus the information gathered from studies, has its limitations.

Epidemiological studies usually concentrate on several major demographic characteristics of the person: age, sex, race/ethnicity, marital status, education, occupation, and others; as appropriate or if any other trait has any value or implication for the study at hand.

The characteristics of the person are presented below separately, however, in practical use it is difficult to separate the various traits. It is common use in epidemiology to compare age and sex, or age and race, or race and sex, or sex and occupation, or sex and race/ethnicity, or other combinations of the various characteristics of the person.

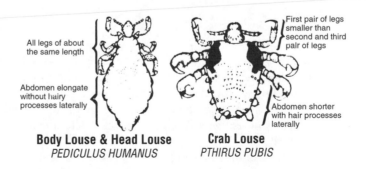

FIGURE 9.31   The two types of lice found on humans. Both types are transmitted directly from *person* to *person*. Infestation by *Pthirus pubis* is considered a sexually transmitted disease, as it is found in the pubic area. (Picture courtesy of Centers for Disease Control and Prevention, Atlanta, Georgia)

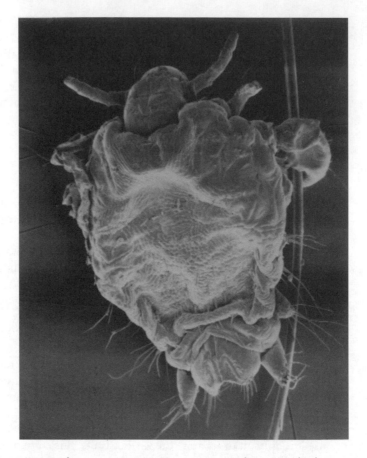

FIGURE 9.32   An electron microscope micrograph (magnified 200 times) of the crab louse (*Pthirus pubis*). (Picture courtesy of Centers for Disease Control and Prevention, Atlanta, Georgia)

Age

Of the many traits of *person* that can vary the outcomes of a study or that better determine cause-effect relationships with regard to relationships of disease, conditions, injury, chronic disease, and other maladies that beset man, *age* has the greatest influence. *Age* alone has more of a confounding effect than any other single trait. Age has to be considered in all studies; age is the most significant determinant of differences in traits among all person variables.

Because of the strong influence that age has as a variable on the outcomes and findings of studies, it has to be considered and if necessary controlled for. A basic control measure to account for the differences in age is that of standardization of rates, and the use of age-specific rates and age-adjusted rates.[1,2,3]

Scientists in a variety of fields from the biomedical/public health to the social-behavioral sciences have long recognized the differences age has on the person. Diseases and conditions of old age are different from diseases of youth. Middle-aged persons have different accident patterns than persons in their early twenties. Jean Piaget, a Swiss zoologist, began studying and observing behavior and intellectual development in children. He studied the different levels and ages at which children and people adapt to and cope with their environment. Piaget determined that there were four major stages of intellectual development. All stages reflect how well the child can master certain stages of abstract thinking and perception of size, weight, and volume of objects, liquids in containers, etc. The four stages include the sensory motor period, which is observed in the 18- to 24-month-old period of a child's life. The second stage is the pre-operational stage, which ranges from 4 to 5 years. The third stage of intellectual development is termed the stage of concrete operations and occurs around ages 6 or 7. The final state of Piaget's four periods is called the stage of formal operations, showing the mastery of abstract thinking.

Erik Erikson took the development steps further by suggesting eight stages of development. Erikson looked beyond abstract thinking and intellectual development to consider all facets of development, which may be initiated by a crisis or conflict.[24] In a longitudinal study Levinson identified transition periods across the life span.[25] Timmreck, Braza, and Mitchell in a study of the worklife span identified periods of high levels of stress and a period of little stress, all at different ages in the worklife of individuals. In their study, three age periods were found to be highly stressful and one period had negative stress.[26]

How long a person lives is one of the most basic aspects of the person with which epidemiologists are concerned. Longevity or life expectancy continues to be a measure of the health status of various populations, differing in various races and different countries.

The average life expectancy for Americans is 75 years. White women live the longest in the United States, 78 years on average. White men and black women both live the same average length of time, 72 years. Black men live to age 65, on the average. Figure 9.33

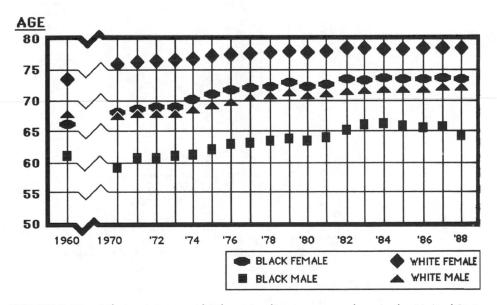

FIGURE 9.33 Life expectancy at birth, according to race and sex in the United States for 1960 and the years 1970 through 1988. (Source: Centers for Disease Control and Prevention, *Health—United States—1990*, Public Health Service, National Center for Health Statistics, U.S. Department of Health and Human Services)

shows the changes and trends in life expectancy since 1960. Life expectancy has increased for all races in the United States. The causes of death which have contributed most to the disparity in life expectancy between white and black males and females are cardiovascular diseases, homicide, cancer, and infant mortality. These causes of death accounted for about 60% of the differences in life expectancy at birth between blacks and whites, males and females.

Age is the one strongest variable to predict differences in diseases, conditions, and health events, and as these are compared, the power of the age variable is easily seen. Two communicable diseases that can cause death and are on the list of notifiable diseases are pertussis (whooping cough) and tetanus (lockjaw). A common immunization many have received includes vaccines for both pertussis and tetanus. Figure 9.34 presents the effect of age on the numbers of cases of pertussis per 100,000. For comparison and contrast Figure 9.35 presents a graph on the numbers of reported cases of tetanus by age group. Pertussis is most common under age 4 with the under 1 year age group having the preponderance of cases.[10] This is probably due to the lack of immunizations in the early years of life, with the majority of immunizations lacking under age 1 and secondly under age 4. With tetanus the opposite is true. Most have tetanus vaccinations early in life, yet fail to continue with booster shots or the revaccinations required for this disease throughout life. Before immunizations for infectious diseases, if persons acquired a disease, they either recovered or

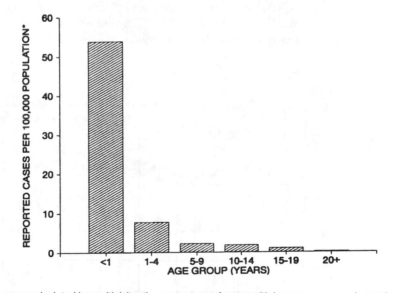

Rates were calculated by multiplying the percentage of cases with known age group by total reported cases and dividing by the population in that age group.
Census population figures modified by age were used for the age groups.

FIGURE 9.34   Age factor in the incidence of pertussis (whooping cough) in the United States—1990 by age group. (Source: Centers for Disease Control and Prevention, "Summary of Notifiable Diseases, United States—1990," *Morbidity and Mortality Weekly Report*, Vol. 39, No. 53, October 4, Public Health Service, National Center for Health Statistics, U.S. Department of Health and Human Services, 1990)

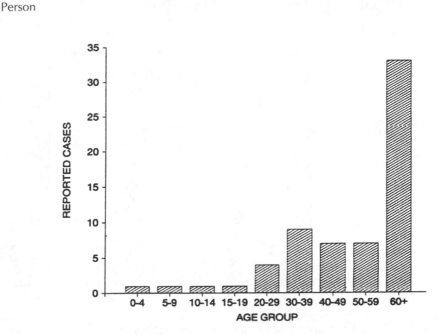

FIGURE 9.35   Age factor in the incidence of tetanus (lockjaw) in the United States for 1990. (Source: Centers for Disease Control and Prevention, "Summary of Notifiable Diseases, United States—1990," *Morbidity and Mortality Weekly Report*, Vol. 39, No. 53, October 4, Public Health Service, National Center for Health Statistics, U.S. Department of Health and Human Services, 1990)

died. Those who recovered had a lifelong immunity to the disease. Now childhood diseases are controlled, but at later ages in life some diseases are reoccurring and booster shots are required. At one time polio was thought to be gone. Now, post-polio syndrome has occurred in polio victims. Cases of tuberculosis thought to be in remission at an early age are recurring in the later years of life. The severity of a disease can also be age-related. Influenza, pneumococcus, and salmonella can be more severe to the very young and the elderly. Generally it is common knowledge that certain bacterial infections such as *staphylococcus aureus* and diseases caused by coliform pathogens are more common and more severe in the older and more frail, as well as in the very young.[1,27]

Almost all diseases can occur at all ages, however, certain diseases occur more at certain stages in life than at others. This fact is especially true for chronic diseases, and since chronic disease usually takes time to develop, many occur in later years of life. As age increases so does the percentage of persons experiencing chronic diseases. By age 65, 45% of the population has some limitation of activity due to a chronic condition. Arthritis is ten times more likely to occur among persons aged 45 to 64 than under age 45. The rate for arthritis doubles for those over 65 years of age.[1] Age plays a major role in heart attacks, with 55% of all heart attacks occurring in persons over age 65. Of the persons who die from heart attacks, four out of five who die are over age 65. In the older age groups, women who have heart attacks are two times more likely than men to die from them within a few weeks. Figure 9.36 shows by age, based on a 26-year follow-up study in the Framingham Heart Study, the number of Americans who experience heart attacks each year.[28]

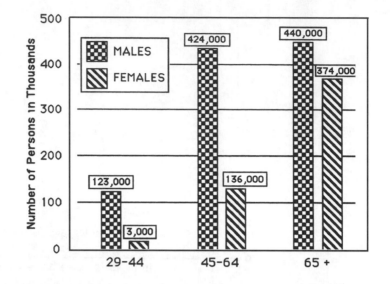

FIGURE 9.36   The number of heart attacks that occur each year, by age and sex. (Source: Adapted from *1991 Heart and Stroke Facts*, American Heart Association National Center: Dallas, Texas, 1991)

Age and Population Pyramids

Population or age **pyramids** have been used for many years by demographers and epidemiologists to track the changes in population age groups over time. The numbers of persons in various age groups in a selected population such as a state or country are affected by birth rates, fertility levels, wars, death rates, and migration. Thus, the population is dynamic and changes over time. Large or small cohorts of people born in the same year can be seen to move up the life span and the population pyramid over time. Male age groups are presented in a bar graph on one side and female age groups are presented on the opposite side in a similar bar graph arrangement, but going in the opposite direction. Thus, males in one age grouping will somewhat mirror females within the same age group. A population pyramid uses two person characteristics and is an age/sex comparison. The age and sex traits are collected at a specific point in time, usually through the ten-year census.

The value of the population pyramid is in the comparison over time among different populations, the changes in the shape of the pyramid. The shape is caused by the numbers of persons born in the years of the age groups. Some years, as in the baby boom years, large numbers of births are seen and in other years such as the zero population growth years of the 1970s, the birth cohorts are smaller.

Social and health related changes in populations can be seen in birth cohorts when plotted on a population pyramid. Some examples are the effect of wars, famines, droughts, use of birth control measures, fertility levels (number of females between ages 15–45 available to have children), the reduction of marriages and falling apart of the family structure in a country. The higher the birth rate in a country, the younger the population. Poor development of public health systems and little control of infectious disease such as sanitation of water supplies and food, control of sewage and garbage, low levels of immunizations and poor medical care can lead to increased deaths and fewer people growing into older age groups. All of these factors affect not only the shape of a population pyramid, but the events of society can also be reflected in the pyramid as time passes. As the events affect a population the events move up through the different age groups in the pyramid.[1,30,31]

Population pyramids are graphic representations dramatizing events that affect the health status and mortality of age groups in large populations. Changes can be seen over time as they affect the gender and size of a population in the different age cohorts. The pyramid is constructed using 1-year or 5-year groupings, with males traditionally plotted on the left and females plotted on the right against a vertical central axis. Since the pyramid is used to compare cohorts of age and sex over time for a select population, the proportions of males and females are used. In plotting a pyramid on a graph, usually 18 different age groups are used in 5-year increments, with the top (oldest) being 85+ (which now should possibly be expanded to include age groups for the older ages as the life expectancy in these age groups continues to rise and grow) and the bottom (youngest) being 0 to 4 years. Thus, the bottom of the chart used in the development of the pyramid would present 0–4 years, 5 to 9, 10 to 14, 15 to 20, and so forth, on through to the top of the chart where the last two groupings are 80 to 84 years and 85+ years. A horizontal bar graph representing the numbers of males in each age group is drawn to the left of the center vertical line and a bar graph representing the numbers of females in each age group is drawn to the right of the center line. Changes in the pyramid shape represent any major changes in births, deaths, and migration in the various age cohorts (see Figure 9.37).[1,30,31]

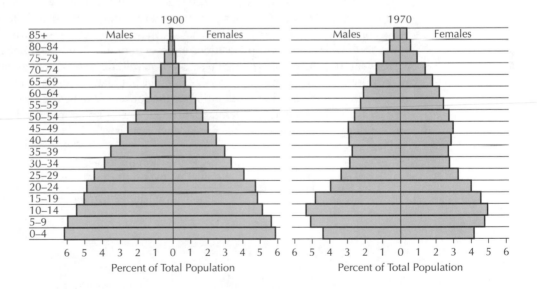

FIGURE 9.37 Population pyramids for the United States comparing age cohort groupings and sex for 1900 and 1970. (Source: From, Mausner, S., and Kramer, S., *Epidemiology: An Introductory Text*, W.B. Saunders: Philadelphia, 1985—used with permission)

A tall, pointed pyramid shape represents a population with a high birth rate, a high death rate, and public health, socioeconomic and medical care conditions that do not allow cohorts to live into old age. The pointed top and a very broad based bottom shows that many babies are born and that infant mortality is high. This pointed top shape also shows that many persons are dying in each birth cohort each year so that very few persons are in the older age cohorts at the top of the pyramid. The cohorts have rapidly diminished over time, leaving smaller numbers of people in the older age groups. A beehive shaped pyramid indicates that the population is having low birth rates as well low death rates. If an hourglass shape is seen, it indicates a transitional type population moving through the population due to low levels of births in the cohort of that time period. If a large protrusion area is seen this is also a transitional population, but one of a large birth cohort moving through the population pyramid. If the pyramid is fairly block shaped with only a small point (somewhat close to the beehive shape) this represents a more industrialized society, with high levels of effective public health measures in effect, good socioeconomic conditions, and good medical care; life expectancy is high with large numbers of age cohorts living into the older age groups. This block-shaped pyramid would be representative of the United States in modern times.[1,30,31]

The ability of a population to support itself economically is of concern to public health and political officials. How dependent certain segments of a population are on others predicts how well these groups or subgroups can contribute to society. The ability to contribute or the dependency a group has on others is measured by a dependency ratio. The dependency ratio reflects the worklife span. **Dependency ratio**, though actually a rate, describes the relationship between the potential to be self-supporting by age and the dependent segments of the population by age, in other words, those segments of the population not in the work force. The beginning period of economic self-sufficiency ranges from age 15 to 20, depending on who is defining the age. Mostly age 18 should be used. Many leading industries require a person to be 18 years of age in order to seek full employment. The upper age for being considered in the work force has changed in recent times and will probably be reevaluated as the older cohorts of populations increase in number and the numbers of younger persons entering the work force decline, as workers will still be needed. Retirement at 65 had already been eliminated in certain work areas of the population. Age 70 is now viewed as the age of retirement by many and will influence the concept of dependency in society.[1,30]

To assess the amount of potential dependency in a population, the dependency ratio was developed. The formula for the dependency ratio is[1,30]

$$\text{Dependency ratio} = \frac{\begin{array}{c}\text{Population under age 18}\\\text{Population over retirement age (65)}\end{array}}{\text{Population ages 18 through 64}} \times 100$$

SEX

Next to age, sex (or, gender) makes the second most significant difference in health events or risk factors of disease. The first and most outstanding observations about sex or gender differences are those of mortality and morbidity differences. A few facts point to the differences between males and females. More males are born each year yet more males die within the first year of life (have higher infant mortality) and throughout life than females. Females outlive males by 5 to 7 years. Females have higher levels of mental health problems than males. Males have more accidents and acquire AIDS more than females. However, levels of morbidity and use of health care services are higher for females than for males.[10,29]

The association of disease to sex is shown by the difference in disease rates, males compared to females in incidence and prevalence of diseases. Males do not have 50% of the cases of a disease and females the other 50% of the cases. Even though this may be the case in certain epidemics of communicable disease, it does not hold true for chronic diseases nor all infectious diseases.

Sex (Gender) and AIDS

AIDS is a good example of the differences in the rates of cases for males and females. Figure 9.38 shows the annual rates for AIDS per 100,000 in the adult population. It can be observed that males have a much higher rate for AIDS than females. Age groups can also be seen in this chart. Combining age and sex person characteristic differences in epidemiological charts is a common and useful way of presenting and comparing the differences.

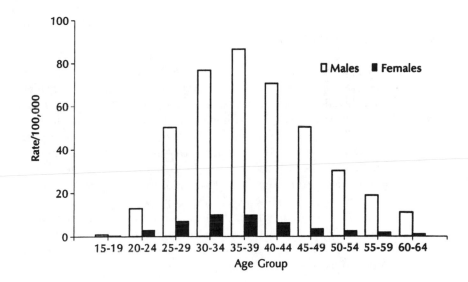

FIGURE 9.38 Example of male and female comparison of annual rates of AIDS per 100,000 in the adult population in the United States in 1990. Sex and age comparison are shown for reported cases. (Source: Centers for Disease Control and Prevention, "Summary of Notifiable Diseases, United States—1990," *Morbidity and Mortality Weekly Report*, Vol. 39, No. 53, October 4, 1990, Public Health Service, National Center for Health Statistics, U.S. Department of Health and Human Services)

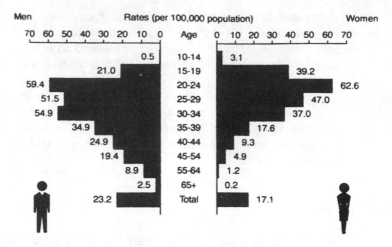

FIGURE 9.39   Example of male and female comparison of annual rates of primary and secondary syphilis per 100,000 in the adult population in the United States in 1990. Sex and age comparison are shown for reported cases. (Source: Centers for Disease Control and Prevention, *Sexually Transmitted Disease Surveillance 1990*, Public Health Service, National Center for Prevention Services, Division of STD/HIV Prevention, U.S. Department of Health and Human Services, 1990)

Sex (Gender) and Sexually Transmitted Diseases

The difference in disease rates for sexually transmitted diseases (STDs) shows marked differences in male and female comparisons. Males have a slightly higher rate of incidence for syphilis and gonorrhea than females. Gonorrhea rates for men and for women have declined over the last decade. Rates for women fell below the 1990 objective by the year 1987.

The rates of congenital syphilis and rates of syphilis in women have increased since 1984. (See Figure 9.39.) Overall primary and secondary syphilis rates have steadily declined to 2.4 cases per 100,000 in whites in 1990. In contrast, rates among blacks have increased dramatically from 51 per 100,000 in 1983 to 135 per 100,000 in 1990. Large increases have occurred both for black men (157 cases per 100,000) in 1990 and for black women (116 per 100,000), suggesting that heterosexual transmission is primarily responsible for the epidemic. Figure 9.39 presents a male/female comparison of rates of primary and secondary syphilis. Again, more than one person trait is shown, with age and gender both presented for comparison.

Sex (Gender) and Effect of Heart Disease Risk Factors

Figure 9.40 shows how risk factors affect both males' and females' danger of a heart attack at age 55. As risk factors like smoking, high cholesterol, and high blood pressure are added, the risk increases proportionally. Males not only have a greater risk of a heart attack than females, but also have a greater risk at a younger age. After menopause, females risk of death from heart disease increases, but still not as much as males for the same age.

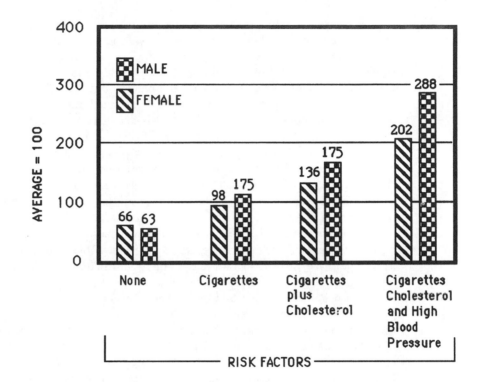

FIGURE 9.40   Example of the effect of sex (gender) and age and risk factors on the chance of heart attack in 55 year old people. (Source: Adapted from *1991 Heart and Stroke Facts*, American Heart Association National Center: Dallas, Texas, 1991)

RACE AND ETHNICITY

In recent years, some effort has been made at the national and state levels to be more sensitive to the presentation of data on race and ethnicity. It is clear even to the average person that many major differences exist between culture, behavior, health events, and related activities. Even though some good efforts are recognized, still, in the United States, the diversity of races and ethnicity goes unrecognized in the statistics and reports published by state and national health agencies and organizations. The traditional approach of presenting charts on "white, black, and other" leaves much information out and provides an incomplete picture. The differences and diversity among Asians, Native Americans, Latinos/Hispanics, blacks, and other minorities need to be recognized. About 52 different tribes of Native Americans are registered in the United States today, representing 52 different cultures, backgrounds, and possibly genetic makeup. The same is also true for African Americans. All blacks have been lumped into one category. Genetic and genealogical investigations are beginning to show a great deal of diversity among blacks. Like Native Americans, blacks historically come from different tribes and locations and all are not the same. Are all whites the same genetically and culturally? Is an Irishman the same as an Italian? Are Swedes the same as Spaniards?

On the other hand, some epidemiologists, in trying to show ethnic diversity among Hispanics, have confused the issue even more by using such vague and unfamiliar terms as "non-Hispanic black," and "non-Hispanic white," or "Hispanic non-white," or "Hispanic-white." It is recognized that the diversity of the whites' and blacks' backgrounds are too complex to be easily separated in data and reports, but the differences in backgrounds should be taken into account when possible. Even though more effort is required, a call is made for epidemiologists, public health officials, and demographers to make a major effort to separate race, ethnicity, and culture in reports and data assessments. Research studies need to be designed so that diversity in races (and religions, presented below) can be captured in the data collection process and then more correct information will be available and can be reported in a more complete manner. Planned effort on the epidemiologist's part in recognizing race and ethnicity differences will cost little and require little effort. The recognition of such a need is a first step in the right direction.

In epidemiology, race is often reported in association with age, sex, education, and occupation, as well as selected diseases and risk factors. (See the section on STDs on page 315.) The place variable of race and ethnicity has taken on important public health meaning in recent years. The merging of the person variables of race and place are important for epidemiologists and public health officials to consider. Races and ethnic groups cluster together in certain locations. Many reports from government sources list the location of races by four general areas, which fall short of recognizing the clustering of races. The four general areas used are Northeast, Midwest, South, and West. For example, the broad expanses of low populated areas of Nevada, Wyoming, Arizona, and Oregon make the statistics for the West low in numbers of blacks and high in whites. However, if the Southern California region is assessed for clustering of races, it is discovered that in certain regions, blacks, Hispanics, and Asians are in the majority. For example, in San Bernardino County, California, the San Bernardino School District reports that whites are 33% of the population attending school. Thus, if race is reported only for the West, the report fails to present an accurate picture of race distribution, i.e., Idaho compared to California.

TABLE 9.1 Distribution of race in the United States population and the increase (change) in each racial group for the decade of 1980 to 1990

Race	Percent of Population		Change
	1980	*1990*	
Total	100.00	100.00	9.8
White	83.1	80.3	6.0
Black	11.7	12.1	13.2
Native American, Eskimo, Aleut	0.6	0.8	37.9
Asian or Pacific Islanders	01.5	02.9	107.8
Hispanic	06.4	09.0	53.0
All other races	03.0	03.9	45.1

(Source: U.S. Bureau of the Census, *1990 Census Profile*, No. 2)

Race and Demographic Changes

The location of concentrations of blacks, Hispanics, and Asians has been changing over the last decade and will continue to do so. Meanwhile the minority populations have increased while the number of whites has declined. Blacks, Hispanics, Asians, and Native Americans continue to increase in numbers. Table 9.1 presents recent changes in race and ethnicity in the United States and the percent of change for each racial grouping.

Race and High Cholesterol Levels

Coronary heart disease and related causes of death increase as blood cholesterol levels increase. Hispanics have lower serum cholesterol than whites and blacks, with Cubans having the lowest for both males and females. Figure 9.41 shows the gender comparisons by race for serum cholesterol levels for ages 20–74 in the United States for the years 1976 through 1980.

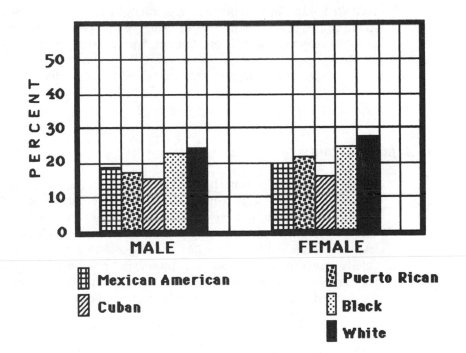

SOURCE: National Center for Health Statistics, National Health and Nutrition Examination Survey II, 1976–80 and Hispanic Health and Nutrition Examination Survey, 1982–84

FIGURE 9.41   Example of race implications of percentage with serum cholesterol among persons ages 20–70 years in the United States from 1976–1980 and 1982–84. (Adapted from Centers for Disease Control and Prevention, *Health—United States—1990*, Public Health Service, National Center for Health Statistics, U.S. Department of Health and Human Services)

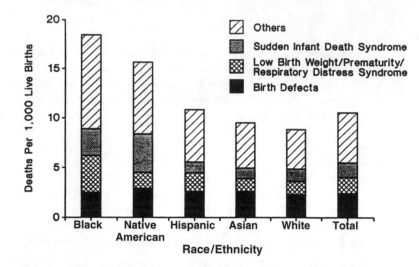

FIGURE 9.42 An example of race/ethnicity by underlying causes of infant mortality in the United States 1983. (Source: Centers for Disease Control and Prevention, "Reports on Selected Racial/Ethnic Groups. Special Focus: Maternal and Child Health," *Morbidity and Mortality Weekly Report,* Vol. 39, No. SS-3, Public Health Service, National Center for Health Statistics, U.S. Department of Health and Human Services, July 1990)

Race and Infant Mortality

Infant mortality varies greatly by racial and ethnic group and is a good example of the person characteristic of race and the impact it makes on health status. Birth defects contribute to infant mortality and also vary among racial and ethnic groups. Infant mortality rates due to birth defects were highest among Native Americans (2.9 deaths per 1,000 live births), followed by Asians and Hispanics (2.6), and blacks (2.5). Infant mortality rates due to birth defects were high among minority infants of low birth weight. Birth defects are an important contributor to infant mortality among all racial and ethnic groups. Figure 9.42 presents the underlying causes of infant mortality by race and ethnicity in the United States.[32]

MARITAL AND FAMILY STATUS

For the past decade or so the field of public health and epidemiology has slowly and continually excluded and diminished the role of marital status and family status in overall implications on health status of individuals and society. A review of several years of epidemiological and public health reports produced by federal and state agencies showed little focus or mention of the effect of marital status and the effect of intact families as preventive influences of disease, conditions, or risk factors. Gangs, drug abuse, unwed mothers, teenage pregnancy, sexually transmitted diseases, AIDS, nutrition problems, suicide, and a variety of other factors are plaguing society. In the 1990s many studies have drawn much attention to the poverty level and the health of children. Reports of concern for adolescents and their health status have been published by private research foundations as well as governmental agencies. The reports on the poverty stricken child ignore the fact that the child originally came from some sort of a family structure and would be best raised in a healthy family environment. Meanwhile public health agencies and official reports continually focus more on solving most of these concerns with after-the-fact treatments, with little or no focus on prevention within the family structure or even encouraging the maintenance of and strengthening of the family. Functional, intact families have been shown in Asian cultures and in the past in the United States to reduce and prevent many of the above-mentioned problems. Yet, little has been done in the last two decades by public health and government agencies to encourage strengthening the family structure in the United States.

Other family-related factors useful to epidemiologists include family size and placement of members within the family structure. Maternal age is of much concern to the medical and public health community. Higher levels of Down's syndrome babies are born to mothers after age 40. Teenage births have the highest risk to both the baby and the mother. More health care dollars are spent on premature births, which are often to unwed mothers.

The absence of one parent in the family has been a major concern in the last 10 to 15 years. Divorce and cohabitation have risen to the highest levels known in the history of the United States. Disrupted families are common, and children of these families suffer the most in terms of social, emotional values, and health development. More effort is needed in the study of the effects of the disrupted family on health status and how to prevent the destruction of the family in America. Table 9.2 presents statistics on various aspects of marital status and marital arrangements.

TABLE 9.2   Marital status and related statistics

Marital Status of the United States by Sex—1990							
Never Married		*Married and Together*		*Divorced*		*Widowed*	
Male	*Female*	*Male*	*Female*	*Male*	*Female*	*Male*	*Female*
25.8%	18.9%	61.3%	56.0%	7.2%	9.3%	2.7%	12.1%

Married Couples—Black/White Race		
	1980	*1990*
Total Couples Married	49,714,000	52,924,000
Total Black/White	167,000	219,000
Husband Black Wife White	41,000	155,000
Husband White Wife Black	45,000	64,000

(continued)

TABLE 9.2   *(Continued)*

Population Never Married by Age and Sex

Age	Male 1980	Male 1990	Female 1980	Female 1990
65+	4.9	4.2	5.9	4.9
55–64	5.3	5.8	4.5	3.9
45–54	6.1	6.3	4.7	5.0
40–44	7.1	10.5	4.8	8.0
35–39	7.8	14.7	6.2	10.4
30–34	15.9	27.0	9.5	16.4
25–29	33.1	45.2	20.9	31.1
20–24	68.8	79.3	50.2	62.8

Marriages and Divorces per 1,000 in the United States

Marriages 1980 = 10.6   Divorces 1980 = 5.2
Marriages 1985 = 10.1   Divorces 1985 = 5.0
Marriages 1990 = 9.8   Divorces 1990 = 4.7

(Source: U.S. Bureau of the Census, *Marital Status and Living Arrangements*, March, 1990)

FAMILY STRUCTURE AND GENEALOGICAL RESEARCH

In epidemiology the family is viewed from the family of procreation, the reproductive years when a head of the household ought to be present; the family of origin, the close and immediate family in which a person is born, is nurtured, taught, given values, goes through childhood and the formative years; the extended family, which includes not only the influence of grandparents, aunts, uncles, cousins, and in-laws, but the physiological and genetic results and family influences.

A person inherits many traits, both good and bad from parents, grandparents, and past family members. Genetically, intelligence levels may be passed down from generation to generation as well as some diseases. For example, some forms of muscular dystrophy are genetically transmitted. Family trees have been used to study the genealogy of both genetically transmitted and communicable diseases. Family trees were used to investigate Kuru, a disease caused by a slow virus. Genealogical family trees have been used to trace alcoholism in a family's past. Facial/scapular/humoral dystrophy has been studied using the genealogy of large extended families with a polygamy history in the 1880s in Utah. The Church of Jesus Christ of Latter Day Saints maintains one of the largest genealogy libraries in the world in Salt Lake City, Utah, aiding genealogists and epidemiologists in family history studies.

OCCUPATION

The person characteristic of occupation can be reflective of income, social status, education, socioeconomic status, risk of injury, or health problems within a population group.

Selected diseases, conditions, or disorders occur in certain occupations. Brown lung has been identified in workers in the garment industry, black lung in coal miners, and certain accidents and injury to limbs in farm workers.

Occupation is requested on many research questionnaires and is used to measure socioeconomic status. It is also a determiner of risk and exposure peculiar to certain occupations and is a predictor of the health status of and conditions in which certain populations work. Occupations have been divided by five broad classifications. The five classifications are

1. Professional
2. Intermediate
3. Skilled
4. Partly skilled
5. Unskilled

Subclassifications of the five main classifications have been used in various epidemiological reports.

Standard mortality ratios (SMR) for specific occupations have been developed, based on risks that might be associated with the physical and chemical exposures common to certain occupations. For example, coronary artery disease has been found to be lower in several active occupations than in sedentary occupations. Persons who work for larger organizations have medical insurance and access to health care providers and medical institutions, and thus benefit from better health status.[3,23]

It has also been observed that health status and mortality of a population can be affected by the levels of employment within the population. The term **healthy worker effect** has been used to describe this observation. That is, employed populations tend to have a lower mortality rate than the general population. Workers tend to be a healthier lot to begin with and persons who are unhealthy or who may have a life-shortening condition are more likely to be unemployed. As workers go through the life span, the chance of death increases and the healthy worker effect decreases. Unhealthy workers tend to leave the work environment or retire earlier than healthy employees. Leaving work early in life also reduces exposure to occupational hazards. Instead of exposure to risk factors causing disease, disease causes those at risk to leave work. Absence due to disease produces lower work-related risk exposure levels than would have occurred if workers remained at work.[23]

EDUCATION AS A CHARACTERISTIC OF THE PERSON

Education, like occupation, can be valuable as a measure of socioeconomic status. Persons with training, skills and education made substantially more money per year than persons with no training or skills. Persons with higher education levels are more prevention oriented, know more about health matters and have a better health status. In females, the higher the level of education, the lower infant mortality and maternal mortality rates.

In recent years epidemiologists and demographers have not readily reported education as a characteristic of the person as much as in the past.

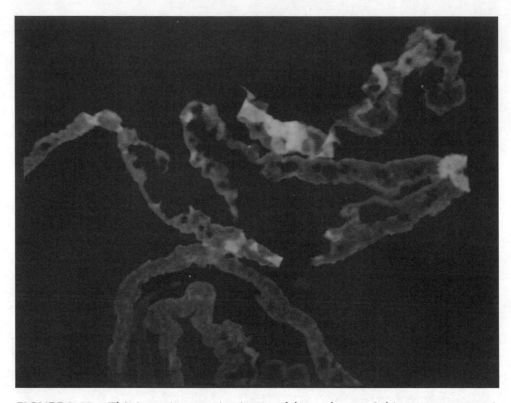

FIGURE 9.43   This is a microscopic picture of the pathogen *Schistosoma mansoni*, that causes the parasitic disease schistosomiasis. Schistosomiasis is a disease that well exemplifies the concepts of *time, place,* and *person*. It is a parasitic infection caused by a blood flukeworm, transmitted to humans via an intermediate host, the freshwater snail. In freshwater tropical climates (*place*), the worm enters the body through skin exposed when swimming, wading, bathing, working, or washing in infested waters (*person*). The disease occurs most in the warm summer months (*time*). Drugs are not very effective in treating the disease, and prevention is the best approach. (Picture courtesy of Centers for Disease Control and Prevention, Atlanta, Georgia)

Some disease variables may not show much of a cause-effect association when correlated with education. Yet, education as a trait of the person does have an effect on the health status of the population and this variable should not be overlooked in epidemiological research and reports.

When combined with other traits of the person such as age, much information can be learned about populations. For example, when educational attainment and age are compared, different age groups show different levels of education. Table 9.3 presents educational attainment and age groups.

TABLE 9.3   Educational attainment in the United States—1989

	Male	*Female*
Four or more years of high school	77%	76%
One or more years of college	41%	35.3%
Four or more years of college	24.5%	18.1%

	White	*Black*	*Hispanic*	*Other*
Four or more years of high school	78.4%	64.6%	50.9%	76.1%
One or more years of college	39.3%	28.1%	23.0%	48.6%
Four or more years of college	21.8%	11.8%	9.9%	34.2%

Age	*4 Years of High School*	*4 Years or More of College*
75+	46.2%	10.1%
65–74	60.4%	11.7%
55–64	69.1%	16.2%
45–54	78.4%	22.0%
35–44	86.6%	27.9%
25–34	86.6%	24.2%

(Source: U.S. Bureau of the Census, *Current Populations Survey*, March, 1989)

EXERCISES

Key Terms

Define and explain the following terms.

cyclic trends	person	secular trend
decennial year	place	short-term trend
dependency ratio	Poisson distribution	spot map
disease cluster	population pyramid	temporal
dot map	seasonal trend	time
healthy worker effect	secular change	time-place cluster
nearest neighbor analysis	secular cycle	

Study Questions

9.1   Using the data presented in Table 9.4, using a computer spreadsheet, develop two population pyramids, one for an industrialized nation (Sweden) and one for a developing country (Mexico). Use the information presented under population pyramids and Figure 9.37 to

TABLE 9.4 Data for Sweden and Mexico showing sex (gender) for each country plus age groups in the middle

| Age-Sex Structure for Sweden and Mexico, 1974 (percentages) | | | | |
| Sweden | | Age Group | Mexico | |
Male	Female		Male	Female
.4	.6	85+		
.7	1.0	80–84		
1.2	1.6	75–79	.5	.6
1.8	2.3	70–74	.5	.5
2.4	2.7	65–69	.6	.7
2.9	3.0	60–64	.7	.8
2.9	3.0	55–59	.9	1.0
3.3	3.3	50–54	1.3	1.3
2.9	2.9	45–49	1.6	1.7
2.7	2.7	40–44	2.0	2.0
2.9	2.8	35–39	2.4	2.4
3.6	3.3	30–34	2.9	2.9
4.2	4.0	25–29	3.6	3.5
3.6	3.4	20–24	4.4	4.3
3.3	3.2	15–19	5.5	5.5
3.4	3.2	10–14	6.6	6.4
3.7	3.5	5–9	7.7	7.5
3.4	3.3	0–4	9.3	9.0

(Source: Adapted from United Nations, *Demographic Yearbook,* United Nations Publications: New York, 1975)

understand how to construct a population pyramid. The use of computer spreadsheets in this exercise is encouraged. (Hint—Use negative numbers on males and positive numbers on females to get a nice graphic/bar chart/pyramid.)

9.2   Using the information from Figure 9.44 and Figure 9.38, explain and discuss the known risk factors and the potential they present to AIDS and explain the role of gender and age as risk factors in acquiring AIDS. Compare and contrast the risk of getting AIDS for 6th graders, seniors in high school, and 35-year-old persons, and include potential sources of exposure and mode of transmission.

9.3   After reviewing and studying the map in Figure 9.16, explain and discuss the following:

a. Compare and contrast the high rates of these two respiratory tract cancers in Louisiana, Southern California, New York, and Southern Nevada.
b. What are the risk factors of lung and bronchial cancer in each of these places? How do they differ and how are they alike in these four different locations?
c. Explain the limitations of and the value of a spot map such as Figure 9.16 in locating and identifying the place of chronic diseases.

ACQUIRED IMMUNODEFICIENCY SYNDROME (AIDS)—Reported adult/adolescent cases, by exposure category, United States, 1990

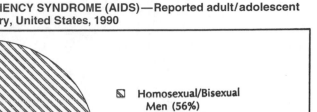

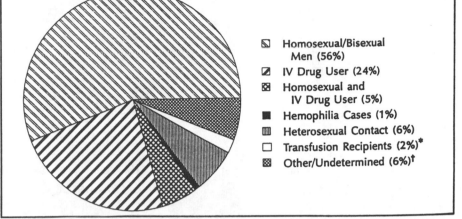

*Includes 14 transfusion recipients who received blood screened for HIV antibody, and 1 tissue recipient.

†"Other" refers to 4 persons who developed AIDS after exposure to HIV-infected blood within the health care setting, as documented by evidence of seroconversion or other laboratory studies. "Undetermined" refers to patients whose mode of exposure to HIV is unknown. This includes patients under investigation; patients who died, were lost to follow-up, or refused interview; and patients whose mode of exposure to HIV remains undetermined after investigation.

FIGURE 9.44 Person risk factors in acquiring AIDS. (Source: Centers for Disease Control and Prevention, "Summary of Notifiable Diseases, United States—1990," *Morbidity and Mortality Weekly Report*, Vol. 39, No. 53, October 4, 1990)

9.4 Compare and contrast Figure 9.34 on the disease pertussis with Figure 9.35 on the disease tetanus with regard to all of the *time*-related elements of these two communicable diseases. First list all of the time-related elements to be considered, then compare and contrast the two diseases.

9.5 From the information in Figure 9.45, list all related time and person factors related to this figure. Discuss and explain the role that time and person factors play in suicide in youth and adolescents as presented in the figure.

9.6 Explain and discuss the concept of *time clustering*. Using Figure 9.10, explain the significance of time clustering in meningococcal disease and encephalitis.

9.7 Contact your local vital statistics office, use maps or other sources, and obtain the population for a city in your community. Acquire or draw a map of your county. Develop a population spot map for your county, based on the population statistics, using one dot for every 100 people.

9.8 From the data in Table 4.1, using "Rate per 100,000 Population: Male–Female," use a computer spreadsheet and graphics package to create a population pyramid for the United States.

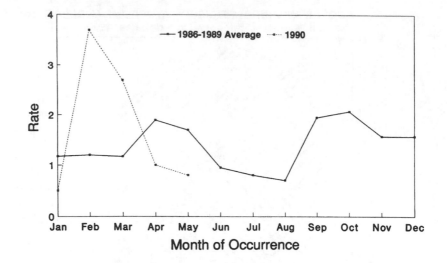

FIGURE 9.45   Rate of suicide attempts among 10- to 19-year-olds by month in Santa Fe County, New Mexico, from January 1986 through May 1990. In 1989 there was a population of 13,625, of 10- to 19-year-olds. There were 165 suicide ideation/attempts and twelve suicides occurred from 1985 through 1990. (Source: Adolescent Suicide and Suicide Attempts—Santa Fe County, New Mexico, January 1985–May 1990," *Morbidity and Mortality Weekly Report*, Vol. 40, No. 20, pp. 330–331, May 24, 1991)

REFERENCES

1. Mausner, J.S., and Kramer, S. 1985. *Epidemiology: An Introductory Text*. Philadelphia: Saunders.
2. Lilienfeld, A.M., and Lilienfeld, D.E. 1980. *Foundations of Epidemiology*. New York: Oxford University Press.
3. MacMahon, B., and Pugh, T.F. 1970. *Epidemiology: Principles and Methods*. Boston: Little, Brown and Company.
4. Snow, John. 1936. *Snow on Cholera*. Cambridge, MA: The Commonwealth Fund of New York; Harvard University Press.
5. American Cancer Society. 1991. *Cancer Facts & Figures—1991*. Atlanta, GA: American Cancer Society.
6. Centers for Disease Control and Prevention. 1991. "The HIV/AIDS Epidemic: The First 10 Years," *Morbidity and Mortality Weekly Report*, Vol. 40, No. 22, June 7, 1991, p. 361.
7. National Cancer Institute. October 1991. *Strategies to Control Tobacco Use in the United States: A Blueprint for Public Health Action in the 1990s*. Smoking and Tobacco Control Monographs, National Institutes of Health, Public Health Services, U.S. Department of Health and Human Services.
8. Centers for Disease Control and Prevention. 1991. "Dermatitis Among Workers Cleaning the Sacramento River After a Chemical Spill—California, 1991," *Morbidity and Mortality Weekly Report*, Vol. 40, No. 48, December 6, 1991, pp. 821–827.
9. Centers for Disease Control and Prevention. 1991. "St. Louis Encephalitis Outbreak—Arkansas, 1991," *Morbidity and Mortality Weekly Report*, Vol. 40, No. 36, September 6, 1991, pp. 606–607.
10. Centers for Disease Control and Prevention. 1990. "Summary of Notifiable Diseases, United States—1990," *Morbidity and Mortality Weekly Report*, Vol. 39, No. 53, October 4, 1990.

11. Selvin, S. 1991. *Statistical Analysis of Epidemiologic Data*. New York: Oxford University Press.

12. Breman, J.G., and Hayner, H.S. 1984. "Guillain-Barre Syndrome and Its Relationship to Swine Influenza Vaccination in Michigan, 1976–1977," *American Journal of Epidemiology*, Vol. 119, No. 6, pp. 880–889.

13. Centers for Disease Control and Prevention. 1991. "Increase in Rubella and Congenital Rubella Syndrome—United States, 1988–1990," *Morbidity and Mortality Weekly Report*, Vol. 40, No. 6, February 15, 1991.

14. Technical Report No. 2. 1990. *Ischemic Heart Disease, Hypertension and Cerebrovascular Disease Deaths and Hospitalizations—California, 1983–1987*. California Chronic and Sentinel Disease Surveillance Program, California Department of Health Services, October 1990.

15. Rosenberg, M.L., Haziet, K.I., Schaefer, J., Wells, J.G., and Pruneda, R.C. 1976. "Shigellosis from Swimming," *Journal of the American Medical Association*, Vol. 236, No. 16, October 18, 1976, pp. 1849–1852.

16. Merson, M.H., et al. 1974. "An Outbreak of *Shigella sonnei* gastroenteritis on Colorado River Raft Trips," *American Journal of Epidemiology*, Vol. 100, No. 3, 1974, pp. 186–195.

17. Band, J.D., et al. 1981. "Epidemic Legionnaires' Disease," *Journal of the American Medical Association*, Vol. 245, No. 23, June 19, 1981, pp. 2404–2408.

18. Klauke, D.N., et al. 1984. "Legionnaires' Disease: The Epidemiology of Two Outbreaks in Burlington, Vermont, 1980," *American Journal of Epidemiology*, Vol. 119, No. 3, 1984, pp. 382–390.

19. Shindell, S., Salloway, J.C., and Oberembt, C.M. 1976. *A Coursebook in Health Care Delivery*. New York: Appleton Century Crofts.

20. Maxcy, K.F. 1926. "An Epidemiological Study of Endemic Typhus (Brill's Disease) in the Southeastern United States," *Public Health Reports*, Vol. 41, pp. 2967–2995.

21. Centers for Disease Control and Prevention. 1989. *Homicide Surveillance*. Division of Injury Epidemiology and Control, Center for Environmental Health, U.S. Department of Health and Human Services.

22. Aldrich, T., and Griffith, J. 1993. *Environmental Epidemiology and Risk Assessment*. New York: Van Nostrand Reinhold.

23. Monson, R.R. 1990. *Occupational Epidemiology*, 2nd edition. Boca Raton, Florida: CRC Press.

24. McConnel, J.V. 1974. *Understanding Human Behavior*, 2nd edition. New York: Holt, Rinehart and Winston.

25. Levinson, D.J., Darrow, C.N., Klein, E.B., Levinson, M.H., and McKee, B. 1979. *The Seasons of a Man's Life*. New York: Ballantine Books.

26. Timmreck, T.C., Braza, G., and Mitchell, J. 1984. "Growing Older: A Study of Stress and Transition Periods," *Occupational Health and Safety*, Vol. 53, No. 9, pp. 39–48.

27. Beneson, A.S. 1985. *Control of Communicable Diseases in Man*, 14th edition. Washington, D.C.: American Public Health Association.

28. American Heart Association. 1991. *1991 Heart and Stroke Facts*. Dallas: American Heart Association National Center.

29. Centers for Disease Control and Prevention. 1991. *Health-United States-1990*. Public Health Service, National Center for Health Statistics, U.S. Department of Health and Human Services.

30. Weeks, J.R. 1981. *Population*, 2nd edition. Belmont, CA: Wadsworth.

31. Hartley, S.F. 1982. *Community Populations*. Belmont, CA: Wadsworth.

32. Centers for Disease Control and Prevention. 1990. "Reports on Selected Racial/Ethnic Groups. Special Focus: Maternal and Child Health," *Morbidity and Mortality Weekly Report*, Vol. 39, No. SS-3, Public Health Service, National Center for Health Statistics, U.S. Department of Health and Human Services, July 1990.

10

Observational Methodology, Association, and Causality Development

CHAPTER OBJECTIVES

This chapter on the elements of observation methodologies, association, and causation development

- addresses the methods used in observational and epidemiological analysis in populations at risk of outbreaks of disease and conditions;
- reviews the role of and the understanding of causation;
- reviews cause-effect relationships in the spread of diseases in groups and populations, and related terminology;
- presents the importance of the various facets of association and their development in epidemiological study and analysis;
- presents the various webs of causation as tools of analysis in epidemiology;
- presents the importance of the various facets and aspects of hypothesis development in epidemiological studies and analysis;
- reviews the basic concepts of surveillance in epidemiology;
- presents the various aspects of screening, screening tests (including the sensitivity, specificity of tests), and the analysis of such tests;
- presents the various aspects of risk measurement and assessment analysis in epidemiology;
- presents the relationship of causation and risk to association in understanding, controlling and preventing epidemics in populations.

INTRODUCTION

Observational methods used in epidemiology include the study of the natural course of events that have occurred in the past (retrospective studies) and the study of events when and as they occur (cross-sectional studies) and events as they happen in the future (prospective studies). When nature is allowed to take its course, and differences that occur or changes that take place in one or more of the variables or subjects are observed and noted, scientific observations are made and are considered observational methods of study or **observational study**. Observational method of study is based on the concept that changes which are observed in one trait or variable can cause changes in other related characteristics or variables, and those changes occur without the events being altered by the epidemiologist or without intervention by a researcher. Observational study searches for *causation*, **causation of disease** or *causality*; cause-effect relationships. In observational study, **association** is also sought. Association usually refers to events that occur more frequently together than they would by chance and gives reason to determine the strength of the association. Distant and disassociated events affecting one common factor need to be considered in association and causality and how they eventually affect the outcome in the subject. A set of disassociated events can be studied to see how the events fall together and is called a *web of causation*. Hypotheses need to be considered and developed using logical and scientific approaches in order to study association and causality. Risk assessment and screening are also tools to study epidemiological events but other tools may include intervention tactics which can take the study methodology from an observational study design to experimental design approaches.

CAUSALITY IN EPIDEMIOLOGY

The process of studying a series of events leading to a disease outbreak in a community involves developing a relationship of causes to effects which produce results. **Causality** or causal association deals with cause-effect relationships, which is used to ascertain how different events or circumstances are related to each other and/or how the events are related. For example, how does a certain type of exposure lead to a certain disease, moreover, how do certain exposures lead to disease outbreaks in a population?[1,2,3]

Necessary and Sufficient as Concepts of Disease Causality

Causality assessment uses some critical thinking approaches. To determine cause-effect relationships certain elements must be present for a disease to occur. One causality element that is needed is termed *necessary*. "Necessary" refers to the idea that a certain variable (pathogen or event) must always be present and precede an effect, producing a cause-effect association. The *effect* part is not limited to the *cause* of one event or variable.

A second causality term is *sufficient*. "Sufficient" refers to the idea that a certain variable inevitably produces an effect or at least initiates the effect. A pathogen may be necessary to cause a disease but has to be present in sufficient amounts to do so. Two variables may be present, but only one actually causes the disease and therefore that pathogen is necessary to be present in order to establish the predictable cause-effect association. Pathogens may always be present in sufficient numbers to cause disease, but the conditions necessary may not be there. For example, bacteria are always present in the mouth but may not cause tooth decay unless the mouth's environment is right. If the medium necessary for bacteria growth is missing, the bacteria will not produce, grow, or cause decay. Toothbrushing removes the plaque which is the growth medium for the bacteria which cause caries and the element *necessary* is missing even though *sufficient* bacteria are present.[1,2,3,4,5]

Ten Causality Criteria

Sir Austin Bradford Hill in 1965 published nine factors that may be used to assess causality of disease and disease outbreaks.[6] Ten advanced and renewed concepts of causality are presented below.

    1. Consistency   When the same variable, factors, or events appear over and over in different circumstances, and have the same repeated association with disease. (In the Kuru disease in Papua New Guinea the natives regardless of male or female or age who always ate the brains of their dead relatives developed Kuru disease symptoms.)

    2. Strength   When the association shows that a given factor makes some disease or disease outbreaks more likely to be due to the presence of one factor more than to other factors or events and it occurs at a relatively high level or in high numbers. (Dr. John Snow, in the 1854 cholera epidemic, observed that the more of the cholera bacteria present the more severe the case of the disease and/or the more the likelihood of getting the disease.)

    3. Specificity   When the cause-effect association of a disease outbreak is specific to one or two connected diseases. The cause-effect relationship does have the ability to produce a true negative association. That is, in an outbreak the cause-effect assessment is focused on those who do not have the disease. The people in the population during an outbreak are shown to be the ones who do not have disease and are categorized as not having the disease. (In a lung cancer study most of all the nonsmokers are determined to not have lung cancer.)

    4. Time Relationship   When a cause-effect relationship event or exposure logically occurs before the development of the disease or condition, time factors are considered. (Mosquito bite occurs before and leads to malaria.)

    5. Congruence   When a cause-effect relationship is suspected, does the association fit within existing knowledge and do the observations and logical assessments make sense, scientifically? (*Coherence* was the term originally presented addressing association and how it should be in accordance with the natural history of the disease and known facts about the disease, i.e., eating uncooked chicken, which most often is naturally contaminated with the *salmonella* bacteria, leads to *salmonellosis* food poisoning.)

    6. Sensitivity   When an outbreak of disease occurs does the cause-effect analysis hold true and does the assessment have the ability to identify correctly that those who are ill from the disease are in fact, ill from the suspected cause? (For example, a group of blue-collar workers were screened for lung cancer. Fifty percent of the cases have the disease and it was concluded that the lung cancer was due to cigarette smoke. Further investigation revealed that 80% of the diseased group worked in insulating buildings with asbestos for 3 years. When tested for asbestosis, it was confirmed that the lung cancer was actually due to the asbestos exposure.)[1,2,3]

7. Biological/Medical   If the association is based on the virility of the pathogen or risk factor and its ability to cause a disease or condition (dose response relationship), and the level of susceptibility of the host, then the relationship is causal. (An unvaccinated person is exposed to the polio virus and then develops the initial symptoms of the disease.)

8. Plausibility   Association should be proved to be causal based on current biological, medical, epidemiological and scientific knowledge. Logical analysis based on new knowledge should not interfere with or restrict obvious and commonsense causal inferences. (The consumption of cholera infested water leads to the development of the disease.)

9. Experiments and Research   Knowledge and inferences of cause-effect associations based on research and experiments add substantial supporting evidence and weight of the causal nature of the association. (The experimental demonstration that chickenpox can be prevented by immunization.)

10. Analogy Factors   If associations that are similar have been shown to be causal and show a cause-effect association, then the transfer of knowledge should be useful and by analogy the association could be evaluated as being causal. (The historical observation that a vaccination with cowpox can prevent smallpox.)

Causality in disease transmission can be *direct* or it can be *indirect*. **Direct causes** are the clear and obvious ones. That is, if a person at a picnic eats potato salad that sat in a warm room for a few hours and is contaminated with staphylococcal pathogens, the chance of getting food poisoning directly from the potato salad is quite good. However, in a lung cancer case with the asbestos workers, the direct cause is not quite so clear. **Indirect causes** are often much more complicated in their transmission and recognition. In the cases of bladder cancer, the cause is not clear and obvious. Cancer of the bladder has been attributed to many sources, from drinking too much coffee, to high levels of chlorine in the drinking water from surface water sources, to taking excessive amounts of vitamin C. In paraplegics confined to a wheelchair, the rate for cancer of the bladder is higher than the normal population. Some urologists suggest that the bladder cancer is due to the paraplegic person having to hold the urine for long periods of time, causing the urine to become concentrated. The **indirect cause** of the bladder cancer might be the paraplegia handicap and being confined to a wheelchair. Or it might be a combination of excessive coffee drinking and not being able to drain the bladder frequently or the coffee being made too strong, or the simple strong concentration of the substance sitting in the bladder for prolonged time periods. The epidemiologist must be careful to assess all variables in the causality of disease and look for both direct and indirect causes of a disease.[1,2,3,4,5]

Causation of Disease and Epidemiological Study

Epidemiological causal associations or cause-effect associations are used to study and determine how different events, exposures, or disease-causing situations relate to each other. *Association* is used to ascertain if events or exposures have a cause-effect relation, such as a pathogen causing a communicable disease or a chemical serving as a carcinogen in the cause of a certain type of cancer. In the early investigations of causality by Louis Pasteur and Robert Koch, both taught their colleagues to seek the microbe as a single cause of disease. In chronic diseases, conditions, and disorders, a single cause or agent is rarely responsible for disease. Multiple causes or risk factors are often present in chronic diseases and that is why the concept of *webs of causation* has been found useful in epidemiological studies of complex conditions such as occupational, environmental, behavioral, or lifestyle caused diseases.

In Chapter 3 several events and studies are presented about scientists in historical times who attempted to determine cause-effect relationships between certain diseases and pathogens related to disease causation. In the study of causation of disease, it was found that a single agent often was responsible for a certain disease. Dr. Robert Koch established the relationship between the tubercule bacillus and tuberculosis. From the work of Koch and his teacher Jacob Henle, three postulates or guidelines of causation were developed and are referred to as the **Koch Postulates**. Through his studies and development of hypotheses about various pathogens, Koch derived the postulates from his observations. Using the original terminology, the three postulates state that

1. The parasite occurs in every case of the disease in question and under circumstances that can account for the pathologic changes and clinical courses of the disease.

2. It occurs in no other disease as a fortuitous and nonpathogenic parasite.

3. After being fully isolated from the body and repeatedly grown in pure culture, it can induce the disease anew.[5,7,8,9,10]

Even though the postulates were derived in the late 1880s, and with all of their limitations, due to lack of knowledge at the time, Koch provides the epidemiologist with a sense of importance for developing good observational skills and applying them to causation in the investigation of an epidemic.

Kelsey, Thompson and Evans[5] and Evans[10] have suggested criteria for causation that epidemiologists should consider when setting up an epidemiological investigation. Adapted from Kelsey et al. and Evans, the following list presents the 12 criteria for causation.

Twelve Criteria for Causation to Consider in an Epidemiological Investigation

1. The cause of a disease or condition should be distributed in a population at the same level as the disease if no interventions or prevention measures exist.

2. The incidence of a disease should be much higher in those exposed to the cause of the disease than those not exposed.

3. Exposure to the cause of the disease should be more frequent among those with the disease than those without the disease.

4. A case of the disease should follow an exposure to the cause of the disease.

5. The larger the dose and/or the longer the exposure to the cause, the greater the likelihood of getting the disease.

6. For some diseases and conditions, the host should respond after exposure to the cause within expected scientific, medical and biological parameters, ranging from mild to severe.

7. The association between the cause and disease should be found in the same populations when different study methods are used or in various populations when proved study methods are used consistently.

8. Other possibilities for the cause-effect association should be ruled out.

9. Control methods used to eliminate or modify the cause of the disease or to change or control the vector (or vehicle) carrying the disease should decrease the incidence of the disease.

10. Prevention, control, or modification of the individual's reaction to a disease by reducing the cause's ability to produce the disease should decrease or eliminate the disease in populations (for example, immunization of a population against the disease).

11. The disease should occur at higher rates in subjects in experimental settings (animal experiments) when purposely exposed to the cause than in similar subjects not exposed.

12. All cause-effect relationships and findings and associations should make scientific, medical, biological and epidemiological sense.[5,10]

PREVENTION AND CONTROL APPROACHES DERIVED FROM CAUSATION

One aspect of the chain of events of disease causation is that the body must acquire some diseased state and have immune responses with the protective mechanisms within the body responding. Sometimes the response to disease causes protective and preventive changes, i.e., developing immunity to a certain bacteria. When the human body is at risk of death or disability, for example, by getting the disease poliomyelitis, external protective measures are taken such as an immunization. In the 1700s Benjamin Jesty gave his family what appeared to be a mild case of smallpox by exposing them to cowpox in order to protect them from death. Jesty did what he saw as a preventive measure that would help control the effects of the more serious form of the disease, by giving them a milder form of the disease cowpox. When exposed to smallpox the family did not get the disease.

Epidemiology exists as a part of public health for the primary reason of assisting in disease control, protection, and prevention activities. The study of causation, association and related concepts is done, not as an entity in and of itself, but to help discover the cause and spread of diseases in individuals as it affects populations. Biostatistics are useful in developing associations and showing the significance and probability of causality. The epidemiologist must not lose sight of the fact that if biostatistical analysis does not contribute to prevention and control measures needed in public health in order to stop disease or control disease outbreaks, it is of limited public health value. Thus, the focus of any epidemiology study of association and disease causality must be for the purpose of learning more about cause-effect relationships so that public health officials can utilize the knowledge gained for the protection of the public's health through disease control and prevention.

FACTORS IN CAUSATION OF DISEASE

Many factors have been found useful in assessing the causation of disease at the community level. The assessment of causation of disease in populations is one approach found effective in recent times in two key areas of public health activities, health education and health promotion.

Green et al. developed several factors and criteria to conduct community health diagnoses for health promotion and health education. In the PRECEDE Model, Green et al. suggest risk factors to health status that can be intervened into with health education and health promotion approaches. Six phases of assessment are suggested. Phase 1 and 2: epidemiological and social diagnosis, Phase 3: behavioral diagnosis, Phases 4 and 5: educational diagnosis, Phase 6: administrative diagnosis. Under the educational diagnosis, Green et al. adapted the three disease causation factors of epidemiology and applied them to health educational assessments. The three educational diagnosis factors are (1) predisposing factors, (2) enabling factors, and (3) reinforcing factors.[11]

The assessment of the *causation of disease factors* in populations has previously been used in epidemiology in a more complex approach and more factors have been used than were suggested by Green et al. The causation of disease factors common to epidemiology investigations occur in a step by step process and are (1) predisposing factors, (2) enabling factors, (3) precipitating factors, and (4) reinforcing factors. Each factor has certain identifying activities and characteristics and a summary of each is presented below.

1. **Predisposing Factors**   These are the factors or conditions already present that cause the host to respond to pathogens or agents in a certain fashion. If the host is immunized against the disease or if the host has a natural resistance to the disease, it will respond accordingly by not getting the disease. If not protected, the host will respond accordingly by getting the disease, as it is predisposed to that circumstance when exposed to the pathogen or agent. If sensitized to a condition the host will respond accordingly. For example, if the host has an allergic sensitization to a substance and then is exposed to the substance, an allergic reaction will follow.

2. **Enabling Factors**   These are the factors or conditions allowing or assisting the disease, condition, injury, disability, or death to begin and to be able to run its course of events. Some of the factors that can enable a disease to spread can be the lack of public health and medical care services. Conversely, the availability of and access to public health and medical care services can prevent, control, intervene into, treat, and facilitate recovery from diseases and conditions, while improving the health status of the population. The obvious disease causation concern and epidemiological approach is to enable health services and halt the promotion and production of disease.

3. **Precipitating Factors**   These are the factors essential to the development of disease, conditions, injuries, disability and death. In the causation of disease, the cause of the disease, condition or injury may be fairly obvious, while in other cases it may not be so obvious. Many times several risk factors may be present in the cause, especially in the chronic diseases or those caused by lifestyle and behavior. A communicable disease may have precipitating factors of poor sanitation, no immunizations, high levels of susceptibles in the community with only one pathogen causing the disease. In chronic disease or behaviorally related conditions a multitude of factors can contribute to a condition. Automobile and traffic related deaths have affected the health status of the population of the United States in a detrimental manner. The automobile accident problem was studied. It was found that lack of seat belt use, drinking and driving, and lack of helmet use by motorcycle riders all were precipitating factors to the high levels of traffic deaths. Thus, laws have been passed to prevent deaths by requiring the citizens to buckle-up, not drink and drive, and wear helmets while riding motorcycles.[1,5,10] (See the concepts of *necessary* and *sufficient* as presented earlier in this chapter.)

4. **Reinforcing Factors**   Like enabling factors, reinforcing factors have the ability to support the production of and transmission of disease or conditions or support and improve a population's health status as well as help control diseases and conditions. The factors that help aggravate and perpetuate disease, conditions, disability, or death are negative reinforcing factors. Negative reinforcing factors are those which are repetitive patterns of

behavior and are recurrent in the perpetuation and support of a disease spreading and running its course in a population. Positive reinforcing factors are those that support, enhance, and improve the control and prevention of the causation of disease.[1,4,5,11]

WEBS OF CAUSATION

Epidemiologic investigation of causation and association in disease began historically with communicable disease epidemics (Figure 10.1). Communicable diseases are relatively easy to investigate, as compared to chronic diseases and conditions, because they often have only one cause: a pathogen. Chronic diseases and conditions are often caused by multiple risk factors,

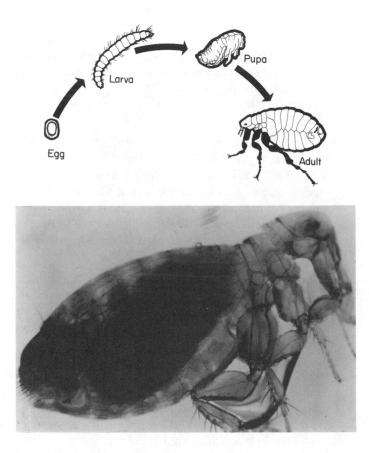

FIGURE 10.1 The top picture is the life cycle of the flea. The bottom picture is an actual microscopic photograph of a flea. Fleas, as hosts and vectors of disease, historically have been implicated in *causation* of disease in worldwide plagues such as the bubonic plague that killed up to one-fifth of the population of England in 1655. Rats and other rodents serve as hosts to fleas and as vectors of this same disease, and have been implicated in *causation* of the spread of bubonic plague each year in the southwestern United States. (Picture courtesy of Centers for Disease Control and Prevention, Atlanta, Georgia)

often associated with occupation, environment, behaviors, and lifestyle. The variety of factors leading to chronic disease are not easy to investigate nor are they simple to study. Because of the complexity of risk factors and variables contributing to occupational, environmental, chronic, and lifestyle diseases, a method of study is needed that is effective in the assessment of complex factors of causation and that can account for all possible factors of causation.

Webs are graphic, pictorial, or paradigm representations of complex sets of events or conditions caused by an array of activities connected to a common core or common experience or event. In **webs of causation** the core or final outcome is the disease or condition. Webs have many arms, branches, sources, inputs, causes, etc., that are somehow interconnected or interrelated to the core. Webs can also have a chain-of-events effect, that is, some events must occur before others can happen. The concepts of *necessary* and *sufficient* as presented earlier in this chapter also apply. An example of the chain of events is seen in the condition of lead poisoning from paint chips. The chain of events may include the following: the lead must be in the paint and the paint applied and time has to pass for the paint to dry into chips. Poverty often has to exist so that substandard housing is lived in. Children have to live in housing that has paint chips in it, have a lack of education about paint chips and lead and the health implications, be unsupervised, and have the opportunity to ingest the dried paint chips (see Figure 10.4 on page 344). To be effective in understanding noncommunicable disease epidemiological phenomena, webs of causation must be presented graphically.

Web of Causation and Lifestyle Diseases, Behavior Induced Diseases and Chronic Disease

In modern society a single isolated cause or factor does not cause all diseases or conditions as in the past. One microbe cannot be singled out as the cause of diseases in behaviorally, occupationally or environmentally caused chronic conditions or disorders. What does occur in lifestyle, work related and behaviorally induced disease states is that individuals take risk factors in small doses, sometimes in many doses and from many sources, all resulting in a chain of causation. The many risk factors and their various sources make for a complex web of causations of a chronic disease that may involve several organ systems within the body and possibly several sites of a single organ system. Single line chain of events may be found in parts of or within phases of a web of causation. Single chain of events can be seen in some chronic, behavioral, or environmentally caused diseases or conditions. The complexity of behavioral or lifestyle caused conditions or environmentally caused diseases requires that all facets, risk factors, exposure, or contributing causes be understood and shown in order for understanding and an investigation to be thorough. Cardiovascular disease and heart disease are good examples. Many factors contribute to coronary heart disease, the same factors can also lead to a stroke (cerebral vascular accident). All risk-factors impact the health status (or lack of) of the cardiovascular system. Figure 10.2 is one example of a web of causation for coronary heart disease, and Figure 10.3 is a second web of causation for myocardial infarction. Both webs are slightly different but are also similar and illustrate the complexity of a chronic disease and the multitude of causes that the epidemiologist needs to consider.[1,2]

A web of causation is useful in identifying the risk factors of the disease, the chain of events and exposures *necessary* and *sufficient* to cause the disease. Even though webs of causation are complex, two concepts universally apply. *First*, a complete understanding of the

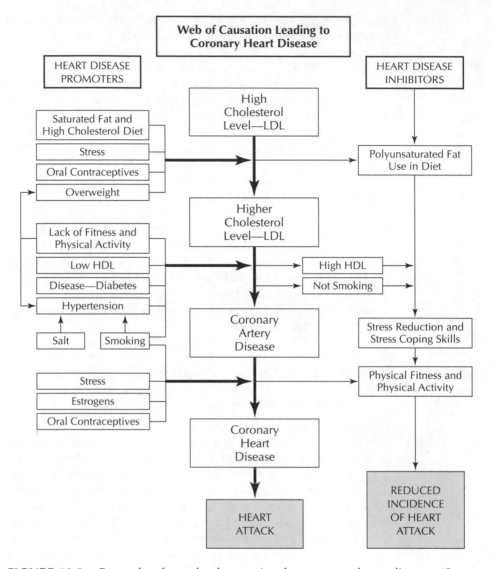

FIGURE 10.2   Example of a web of causation for coronary heart disease. (Source: Adapted from R. Sherwin, in Mausner, J.S., and Kramer, S. *Epidemiology: An Introductory Text*, W.B. Saunders, Philadelphia, 1985)

causal factors and mechanisms is not required or necessary for the development of effective prevention and control measures. *Second*, it is possible to interrupt the production of a disease by cutting the chains of occurrences of the various factors at strategic points that will stop the chain of events in the causation of the disease.

Webs of causation are enhanced by identifying and ascertaining the specific details of the various factors leading to disease, disability, injury, or death. Two approaches to enhancing webs of causation are decision trees and fish bone cause-effect analysis diagrams. The decision tree is a flow chart that visually presents a process through which lines and

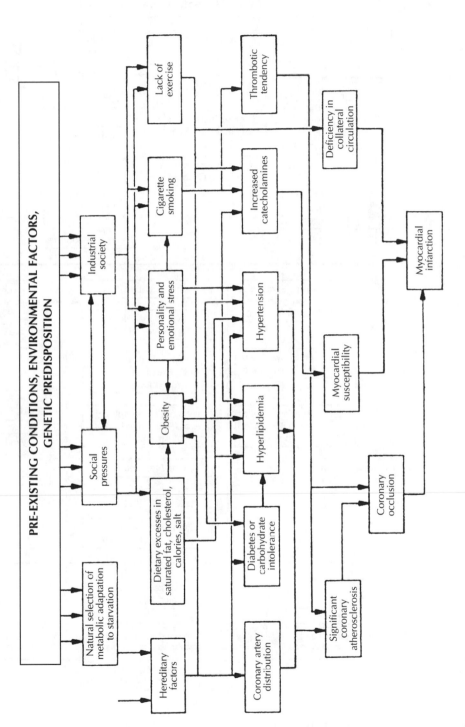

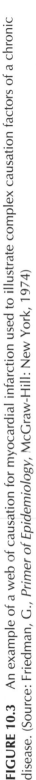

FIGURE 10.3 An example of a web of causation for myocardial infarction used to illustrate complex causation factors of a chronic disease. (Source: Friedman, G., *Primer of Epidemiology*, McGraw-Hill: New York, 1974)

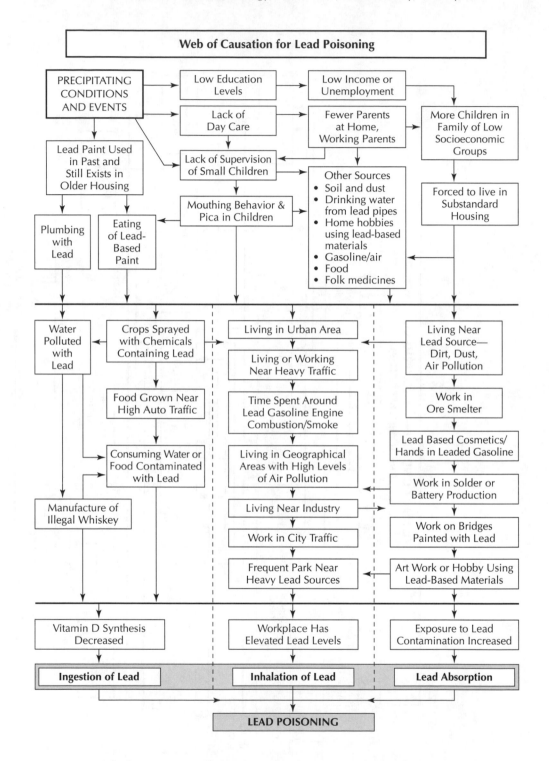

FIGURE 10.4   Example of a web of causation for lead poisoning.

symbols lead to proper decisions and understanding of the role of certain risk factors in webs of causation. Fish bone diagrams provide a visual display of all possible causes that could potentially be contributing to the disease, disorder, or condition under study. (See Chapter 12.)

Environmental Causes of Disease

Conditions caused by environmental factors are complex making it difficult to identify causal factors, as causation usually is from an array of sources and risk factors. An example of an environmentally caused disease is lead poisoning; a condition that can be precipitated by a multitude of events and sources. For example, child lead poisoning is one of the most common pediatric health problems in the United States and is entirely preventable. Children are particularly susceptible to lead's toxic effects. Lead poisoning, unlike other childhood diseases, produces no symptoms early in the disease, the child has no reaction to the exposure and does not appear ill at first, thus most cases go undiagnosed and untreated. Over the years, the Centers for Disease Control and Prevention have set the safe lead exposure levels lower and lower. Scientific studies and clinical observation in children continue to show that even the smallest amount of lead exposure in children can have detrimental effects. In screening of children to determine levels of lead in the body the test of choice is now blood lead measurements. The primary control of lead poisoning is prevention measures, especially if targeted at high risk populations. Screening and medical treatment of lead poisoned children remains important until the sources of lead in the environment are eliminated.[12] Figure 10.4 is an example of the web of causation showing the complexity of environmentally caused diseases—in this case lead poisoning.

EPIDEMIOLOGICAL ASSOCIATION IN CAUSATION OF DISEASE

The concept of association does not mean that the relationship is causal (Figure 10.5). Causation of disease can rely on understanding the association of events, variables and exposures to disease onset, severity, course, etc. Thus, at the beginning of the chapter causality is presented separately. However, because certain factors are present at the same time as others does not mean they are a cause of a disease. For example, an epidemiologist might investigate the factors present in cancer of the prostate in men. It is discovered that all men had drunk cow's milk. This does not mean that milk is the cause of the cancer.

It has been shown over and over that, when people have particular exposures or characteristics, they are more likely to develop certain diseases than those without those exposures or characteristics. When a person has the disease *and* the particular exposure or characteristic, the characteristic is said to be *associated* with the disease. For example, if a person who has smoked for 25 years develops lung cancer, and this is seen over and over in thousands of cases, cigarette smoking is the identified exposure *associated* with the disease. A strong *association* between the exposure and the disease is scientifically observed. A cause-effect relationship is observable, as is an *association*. If you smoke for 25 years, you may get lung cancer; but if you do not smoke at all, the chances of getting lung cancer are very small. When coal miners smoke and are exposed to coal dust, they are more likely to develop lung

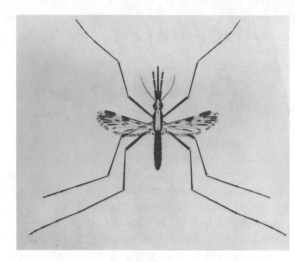

FIGURE 10.5   The mosquito has been implicated in massive worldwide epidemics of yellow fever, malaria, and encephalitis, especially in the tropics. However, it was not until the early 1900s that these diseases were associated with the mosquito. Many times it is difficult for epidemiologists to draw *association* with cause of a disease and its mode of transmission, especially when host and vector mask the cause-effect relationship, as in malaria. The mere name *malaria* ("bad air," usually thought to occur around dusk) shows the difficulty of drawing *association* of the mosquito to *causation* of malaria. (Picture courtesy of Centers for Disease Control and Prevention, Atlanta, Georgia)

cancer than coal miners who do not smoke, yet both may get "black lung." Thus, coal dust is ruled out as the cause of cancer, but a strong association with cigarette smoking and lung cancer is observed. It has been shown that men in their late sixties or seventies are more likely to develop prostate cancer than men in their twenties or thirties. Thus, an *association* between age and the disease is drawn. (See Person in Chapter 9.) One goal of analytical epidemiology is to search for and show cause-effect relationships; determine *how* and *why* various diseases have certain relationships to particular characteristics or exposures; and discover whether such a relationship exists at all. All coal miners might have drunk coffee, but coffee is not exposed to the lungs, nor has it been shown to cause lung cancer. Thus, just because a person is exposed to some agent or element does not mean that an *association* exists, nor is a cause-effect relationship established.

Association deals with how different events or circumstances are related to each other or how a cause-effect association exists in causing a disease, condition, injury, illness, disability, or death. A strong cause-effect association that makes biomedical and scientific sense must be established not by chance, but by strong evidence and with a high level of assurance. For example, it has been discovered that most fatal automobile accidents involved the presence of alcohol in the blood of the driver who caused the accident. Thus, most every state in the United States now has passed laws against drinking and driving. (The chance of causality has been presented earlier in this chapter.)

Association as it relates to causation of diseases and conditions is concerned with how groups of events that are scientifically understood to cause disease, disorders, conditions, injury, disability, or death connect, how the cause-effect association leads to these maladies, and how the causative factors impact populations or groups of people.

Association is also the degree of statistical relationship existing between two or more disease events or occurrences. When disease-related events occur more closely together in *time* and *place* or with a greater frequency than usual in the general population, the greater the chance of the events being associated. The epidemiologist must assure that the frequency of events occurring together is at a high enough level and that the relationship of events is stronger than the epidemiologist would accept by chance. The testing of association by inferential statistics can assist in ascertaining how likely observations and relationships are to occur by chance, what level of statistical relationship exists, or determine if no association exists at all. The statistical chance of events connecting and how statistically significant the cause-effect relationship is can be of value to the epidemiological study; however, the assessment of probabilities and levels of significance provided by inferential statistics or biostatistics is one example of how biostatistics does merge somewhat with epidemiology. Biostatistics can be of assistance in the analysis of data at the end of epidemiological studies.

Association does have to be scientifically proved. A group of people with different customs comes down with a unique disease and other groups are not coming down with the disease; when such events occur, this suggests some common factors, behaviors, traditions, and customs among the first group may create an association possibility within the group. Such circumstances are used as trigger points in deciding whether or not to do an epidemiological investigation. For example it was discovered that women and children in the Papua New Guinea, Fore Tribe had a shaking disease with neurological conditions leading to death (Kuru). No other tribe or group had such a disease. The investigation within the tribe included an analysis of all possible infectious diseases, foods, water, plants, environmental factors, and treatment with antibiotics. It was discovered that customs and traditions were the factors that led to disease causation. While preparing dead family members for burial the women and children would occasionally consume the brains of the dead relatives. Such an association and causality is difficult to develop.[1,2]

A continuum is used as a progressive assessment of proof that association and causation exist. The continuum of association presented in Figure 10.6 can be used to determine

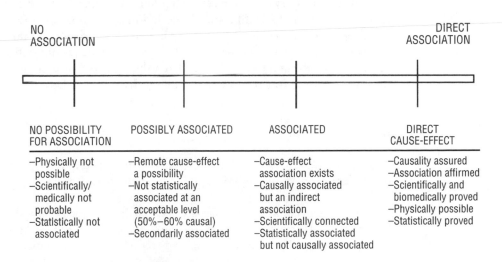

FIGURE 10.6   Continuum of association.

the potential of association, its strength, or how closely the possibility of association and cause-effect factors may be related.[1,2]

In developing an association in epidemiology, populations and categories of people are used, not individuals. In a group of people, some individuals who have been vaccinated become ill, and others who are not vaccinated do not get the disease. Some people may have even contracted disease from the vaccine, yet overall the majority of the people within the group are protected from the disease. (See Herd Immunity, Chapter 2.) The occurrence and distribution of a disease in the population or a group should follow a natural distribution and should be consistent with identified cause-effect relationships.[1,2]

Strength of Association

The stronger the association, the more likely it is that the relationship between events or exposures is due to cause-effect variables. When the frequency or intensity of the event or exposure increases, and the effects from the exposure also increase, then a causal relationship possibility increases and an association would exist. That is, if exposure increases and then the disease incidence and severity increase, the association possibility also increases. Strength of the association also increases when time factors are right, as well.[1,2]

Time Factors in Association

Causation factors possibilities increase as time sequences or key time related elements increase. When a series of events occurs in proper sequence, has the right duration, and has proper timing, then the strength of the association increases.[1,2]

Scientific Congruence in Association

Any disease or injury causation association must be congruent and compatible with current biomedical and scientific knowledge and information. Causation must be based on and supported with epidemiological and biomedical evidence and information. Proof of causation can include responses of control groups, evidence of reactions from those not getting the illness and those excluded from the exposure or event as well as proof from those exposed and who become cases with the disease or malady.[1,2]

Direct and Indirect Association

At least two levels of association are considered, *direct* and *indirect*. Additionally, two types of association are studied by epidemiologists, *asymmetrical* and *symmetrical*.

Direct Association   The difference between direct association and indirect association is best seen in the continuum of association in Figure 10.5, as there is a gray area between the two extremes. The difference between direct association and indirect association is more relative than concrete. Direct association relies on the limitation of current scientific knowledge and the amount of knowledge known about the cause-effect relationship at the time,

As knowledge advances and as information is gathered about a particular disease, the more the epidemiologist will know about the direct association and indirect association aspects of the disease. *Direct association* has the inference that the causality is based on congruence of scientific knowledge, is directly related to the event or exposure, and that the relationship is obvious and clear in both strength and time factors. Direct association generally confirms causality of disease, but must be affirmed scientifically.

Indirect Association   Indirect association, also referred to as indirect causal association, assists with the deductive reasoning aspects of association, while searching for solid proof of causality. Two types of indirect association are commonly presented as useful to epidemiology.

1. *Common factor indirect association:*   Disease event or risk factor B (Figure 10.7) is the common underlying factor. Disease event A may be related to risk factor C only because both are connected to risk factor B. Changes in risk factor C will not cause a change in the frequency of disease A unless a change in C affects B. Event B has to be altered or changed in order for either A or C to be affected.

2. *Intervening indirect causal association:*   Event B (Figure 10.8) is an intervening or intermediate factor in causality. A change in risk factor C could produce a change or response in the frequency of disease in both B and A. A change in C will produce a change in B, which in turn can produce a change in A.

Symmetrical Association   Some extraneous events or risk factors not clear and obvious may be viewed as unimportant in the causality of disease due to the lack of a clearly seen direct cause-effect relationship. When a relationship between events, risk factors, and disease lacks a clear and obvious association, these events have a **symmetrical association**. At least four different conditions affect or at least influence symmetrical associations in the causality of disease. Due to the indirect nature and distant association of symmetrical factors, any observed association may lack the elements of being causal (have a cause-effect response or function). Four symmetrical association factors can be observed.

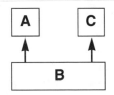

FIGURE 10.7   Common factor indirect association.

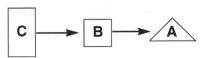

FIGURE 10.8   Intervening indirect causal association.

1. *Functional interdependence:*   One event or risk factor cannot occur without the presence of the other or the activity of the other factor occurring first.

2. *Common complexity:*   Two or more events or risk factors arise together and are not interdependent upon each other nor is one needed for the other to occur or function.

3. *Alternative factors in the same source:*   That is, one broad-spectrum antibiotic that affects several pathogens, conversely several strains of gonorrhea that respond to the same antibiotic.

4. *Common cause response:*   Certain carcinogens can cause different types of cancer.

Asymmetrical Association   Asymmetrical events have direct association to disease and are of greater use to the epidemiologist than the counterpart of symmetrical. When two factors of disease causation are known, the third can be found mathematically. When new cases occur in a population and when the time element is known, then other factors such as prevalence can be determined.

HYPOTHESIS DEVELOPMENT FOR EPIDEMIOLOGY

What is a hypothesis and what value is it to epidemiological investigations? A **hypothesis** is an inference used to explain a general principle. A hypothesis suggests the relation of certain variables to other phenomena; a tentative suggestion that certain relationships exist in certain activities or in a chain of events. A *hypothesis* is a suggestion or supposition made by learned and scientific observation from which theories or predictions are made. A *hypothesis* is also a statement explaining the relationship of facts and is used to predict future trends or possibilities.[13]

Hypotheses, as used in epidemiology, are used to make suggestions of possible events, cause-effect relationships, associations of events to disease, and to ask questions that go beyond simple observations, direct or indirect. Possible suggestions are made, which are used to develop, plan, and guide epidemiological investigations. Upon completion of an epidemiological investigation, hypotheses can serve as a guide to answering research questions and for making learned scientific predictions.[13]

Hypothesis Development

Fundamental to the development of hypotheses are scientific reasoning approaches. Inductive reasoning, the process leading from a set of specific facts to general statements that explain those facts, is used in epidemiology.

Inductive reasoning relies on several concepts.

1. Exact and correct observation,

2. Accurate and correct interpretation of the facts in order to understand findings and their relationship to each other and to causality,

3. Clear, accurate, and rational explanations of findings, information, and facts, in reference to causality,

4. Development based on scientific approaches, using facts in the analysis and in a manner that makes common sense, based on rational scientific knowledge.[13]

Four different approaches can be used in the formulation of hypotheses: method of difference, method of agreement, accompanying/co-joint variation and method of analogy.

Approach 1 **Method of Difference:**   The frequency of a disease occurrence is extremely different under different situations or conditions. If a risk factor or event can be identified in one condition and not in a second, it may be that factor, or the absence of it, that may be the cause of the disease. For example, valley fever (Coccsi) occurs only in the deserts of the Southwest United States.

Approach 2 **Method of Agreement:**   If events or risk factors are common to a variety of different circumstances and the events or risk factors have been positively associated with a disease, then the probability of that factor being the cause is extremely high. Cigarette smoking in males caused an increased rate of lung cancer in males. Females followed the pattern and now have lung cancer rates higher than males.

Approach 3 **Accompanying/Co-joint Variation:**   The frequency or strength of an event or risk factor varies with the frequency of the disease or condition. Increased numbers of children not immunized against measles causes the incidence rate for measles to go up.

Approach 4 **Method of Analogy:**   One disease and its pathogen may be similar to another established disease, in growth process, mode of transmission, appearance, symptoms, etc. Cowpox is similar to and prevents smallpox.[13]

Hypothesis Assessment

Using the *method of difference* and the *method of agreement*, the epidemiologist can ascertain more clearly these situations in which places, events or suspected risk factors are present or absent. The more circumstances in which the disease frequency is increased or decreased, the fewer acceptable alternatives there are.

When two events, exposures, or risk factors are associated with a disease or condition, the closer the cause-effect relationship is between the two events, exposures, or risk factors. The less importance the cause-effect relationship has toward a disease, the less the *association*.

Disease association may be more significant for certain factors or variables than for others. The variables of age and sex may be more important to consider in developing disease associations than other variables. In the discussion of the *person* in Chapter 9 it was pointed out that age will show more variation and different results in disease or epidemiological investigations than any other single variable.

To find value or importance in the hypotheses and research findings, it may not always be necessary that all variables and circumstances show the complete cause-effect mechanism. If information is missing or gaps in the findings are seen, several factors could be the reason. The epidemiologist or assistants could have made observation errors in conducting screening or tests or interpreting the results. Multiple causes or sources of the disease are possible and not all of them are seen or recognized. The knowledge about the disease and its classification may be lacking.

The evaluation of the hypotheses should be congruent with and correlate with scientific and biomedical research findings and other related observations from similar experiences or sources. The epidemiologist must be knowledgeable enough about the field to know if the observations are similar or relate to other findings.

As the strength of statistical associations increases, the more useful the hypotheses are. Increases in strength and time factors help validate the hypothesis. Inferential statistics can be used to verify hypotheses once the epidemiological investigation is completed.

Observable changes over time also help validate the hypotheses. If the disease is of short duration and the changes occur in shorter time spans, the changes are more easily observed. Chronic disease and associated risk factors are much more difficult to observe as the chronic diseases develop over time and time span of disease development is long.[13]

Any substantial set of hypotheses rarely is derived from one research question or one theoretical speculation. If association with two or three variables is found and each has a number of commonly understood explanations, then a good hypothesis may be achieved. Before making a hypothesis consider this checklist. Are there

- errors of measurement or judgment?
- differences in closely associated variables?
- differences in behavior and environment?
- differences in physiological constitution, immunity, etc.?
- differences in genetic make-up, heredity, and familial tendencies?

ANALYTICAL EPIDEMIOLOGY

Analytical epidemiology (also referred to as analytic epidemiology), like descriptive epidemiology, has the main purpose of investigating the causes of disease. Analytical epidemiology uses scientific study methodologies and has included the experimental design. In fact, analytical epidemiology is a term that confuses true epidemiological investigations with traditional research designs, including those employed in biomedical empirical research endeavors. It is through this confusion that biostatistics is implied to be epidemiology.

Analytical epidemiology is a hypothesis-testing approach used in assessing the association between disease events or exposures and risk factors. Groups or populations are classified and evaluated according to characteristics that influence disease rates.

True analytical epidemiology uses questions, such as: What is the difference in disease frequencies between two or more populations with one common disease factor among the two populations, and should not the frequency of that factor appear more often in those populations with the disease than in those without the disease?

Analytical epidemiology uses a rational study approach, incorporating an analytical matrix design. A 2×2 matrix of four cells is used to assist the epidemiologist in analyzing a population experiencing a disease outbreak. Figure 10.9 is the standard 2×2 matrix with four cells as commonly used in epidemiological studies to compare exposed groups or populations to unexposed groups.[1,2,3,4,13]

The epidemiological matrix analytical approach (Figure 10.9) encourages good research design. Those individuals in the group with the disease and those exposed to the disease but not yet ill can be compared to a control group (controls—those without the disease and those not exposed to the disease). Association and causality of disease in populations can better be determined when both ill and well groups are studied, compared, and analyzed. The epidemiological matrix can be used in a variety of different studies: retrospective, case control, cross-sectional, longitudinal, etc.

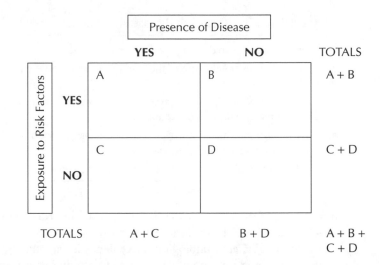

FIGURE 10.9 2 × 2 four-celled epidemiological matrix used to analyze findings of epidemiology studies.

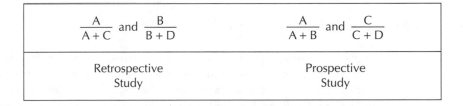

FIGURE 10.10 Different comparisons available from the 2 × 2 four-celled matrix.

Using the epidemiological matrix, subjects can be studied based on the presence or absence of the disease (A + C and B + D). The controls are those without the disease (B + D). Data and findings are determined by selecting the groups that were or were not exposed to the risk factors (A + B and C + D) with the focus of the analysis being on comparison between the groups with frequencies of exposure. From the analysis using the matrix, the *incidence* of a disease can be obtained.[1,2,3,4]

There is an array of approaches in the comparison of the four different cells within the epidemiological matrix. Figure 10.10 shows the different approaches.

Surveillance in Epidemiology

Surveillance is a general term referring to the ongoing observation, persistent watching over, scrutiny, constant monitoring, and assessment of changes in populations related to disease, conditions, injuries, disabilities, or death trends. In epidemiology the continual *watching over* is aimed at the occurrence or incidence of diseases or conditions in a population, making this a key public health activity. In epidemiology, surveillance, or the

TABLE 10.1   Five factors of disease surveillance

1. Mortality and morbidity data collection and analysis
2. Assessment and evaluation of the findings of individual cases and field investigations of outbreaks of diseases
3. Assessment of data on the natural, active, acquired, and passive immunity levels in groups or segments of the population
4. Reports and information furnished by agencies and laboratories on their findings about the disease causing the epidemic
5. Epidemiological data from general and routine sources

monitoring of trends in diseases, is done mostly in order to initiate investigations and to develop public health prevention and control programs.[2,13,14,15]

Additionally, **epidemiological surveillance** is the ongoing and systematic collection, analysis, and interpretation of data related to health, disease, and conditions. The findings of epidemiological surveillance activities are used to plan, assess, evaluate, and implement prevention and control programs for public health.[14] See Table 10.1 for five factors the epidemiologist must consider in any investigation.

Surveillance in Public Health: Healthy People 2000

Public health surveillance is a health data collecting process which includes not only the systematic collection of information, but also involves the analysis, interpretation, dissemination, and use of health information. In the health objectives for the United States as set forth in *Healthy People 2000*, surveillance and data systems made one of the five major areas of focus. Public health surveillance and data systems provide information on morbidity, mortality, and disability from acute and chronic conditions; injuries; personal, behavioral, occupational, and environmental risk factors. Such factors are associated with illness, premature death, morbidity and mortality prevention, control and treatment services, and costs. Results of the surveillance and data collection and analysis are used to better understand the health status of the population in order to plan, implement, describe, and evaluate public health programs that control and prevent adverse health events. Thus, for the data to be useful they must be accurate, timely, and available in a usable form.[16]

Four areas of surveillance and data collection system activities are used by the U.S. Public Health Service:

1. Collecting and analyzing health information at the national, regional, and to an extent at the state and local levels
2. Providing data to federal, state, private, and local agencies for analysis and use
3. Assisting states and private and local agencies in conducting health surveillance, collection and evaluation of data through providing standards, definitions, methods, computer software, training, and coordination
4. A federal, state, and local network of public health surveillance of diseases of importance to public health is coordinated[16]

Healthy People 2000 health objectives were determined for the most part from information gained from the national surveillance and data systems of the federal government.

Healthy People 2010 is under development and is to come out in the year 2000. The various surveillance and data collection systems are presented with some explanation, at the ends of Chapters 5 and 6.

With the use of computers, surveillance and data collection have become quite efficient and effective. However, even if data exist, not all potential users can have ready access to the data in a timely manner. Some of the data files are too large and complex for easy use and others are not available for public use. Other concerns include a lack of comparability in collection and use and a lack of agreement on what variables or indicators are the best measures of health status.[16]

Disease surveillance, being a constant and persistent watching over of all facets of disease, can help discover and control the transmission of infectious diseases. The list of notifiable diseases as well as other diseases or conditions of concern are monitored, so that prevention and control programs can be planned and implemented.[2,14,15]

A facet of disease surveillance is the systematic surveying, collecting, and analysis of morbidity and mortality data. The most common approach to surveillance is the survey. The federal government early on recognized the survey approach was very important, thus the U.S. Congress approved the National Health Survey in 1935. The National Center for Health Statistics continues many surveys in order to continue surveillance at the national level. Chapters 5 and 6 present most of the national health surveys conducted on a regular and ongoing basis.[15,17,18]

Morbidity Surveillance

Surveillance has been used in infectious disease in a most effective manner. Cross-sectional studies have helped to establish prevalence rates for infectious diseases. Chronic disease control and prevention using longitudinal studies have assisted surveillance activities, even though some studies have taken years to complete.[2,15,17]

Occupational Disease Surveillance

In 1970 the National Institute for Occupational Safety and Health (NIOSH) was formed and set forth the task of carrying out surveillance projects aimed at specific occupational health problems. In the beginning these surveillance activities used existing data banks and sources, with limited internal data collecting activities taking place. In the 1980s, NIOSH supported and encouraged state health departments to establish surveillance for occupational health related injuries and illnesses. From this effort SCANS (Surveillance Cooperative Agreement between NIOSH and States) was developed and implemented. The outcome was that state health departments and related data sources improved their capabilities for tapping into death and birth certificates and other data gathering sources. Additional efforts in the late 1980s and into the 1990s (for example, Sentinel Event Notification System for Occupational Risks—SENSOR) have been continually developed and have assisted states in expanding their surveillance efforts.[14]

Data have been routinely collected on occupational diseases, providing surveillance of occupationally induced and related diseases for many years. Many of the sources of data presented in Chapters 5 and 6 have been used in surveillance and range from death certificates to birth certificates to health survey reports. All sources are used not only in general public health surveillance, but in occupational health and environmental health surveillance as well.[2,14,15,19]

A comprehensive occupational health surveillance system at the worksite by the epidemiologist or industrial hygienist would include sampling and surveying for risk factors in the work place. Periodic multiphasic health screening, direct environmental health and safety monitoring, and close observation of events, activities, and exposures that can affect the health of workers on the short term and over time should be done. Hospital, HMO, clinic, and workman's compensation treatment/medical records are also good sources for gathering occupational health surveillance data. Insurance data bases as well as medical records and accident records from within the company, including the company medical clinic as well as direct health surveys of the workers, all provide surveillance data and insights for control and prevention of work related injuries and illnesses.[14,19]

Surveillance is used in communicable disease, chronic disease, occupational health, environmental health, and with various events affecting the control, prevention, treatment of diseases, injuries, conditions, disabilities, and death. Surveillance information is used by health service administrators, health planners, public health departments, and other government agencies to monitor prevalence, incidence, and unusual events, including how these events affect the cost of health care and the health status of a population. Infant mortality and mortality rates in hospitals are monitored by the Health Care Financing Administration of the U.S. Social Security Administration, the agency that funds Medicare, as a barometer of quality of care in hospitals. The Chronic Disease Surveillance Branch conducts surveillance of a variety of health related events and occurrences.

One ambitious surveillance system that was developed in 1973 and which still continues is the Cancer Surveillance, Epidemiology and End Result (SEER) program. The SEER program was developed by the National Cancer Institute. Eleven population-based cancer registries were established in the United States and Puerto Rico. The SEER network geographic areas were selected to represent various regions and ethnic groups in the United States. The National Cancer Institute receives reports from the various SEER registries where they are analyzed, compiled, and published. The SEER program has eight surveillance goals covering all the usual aspects of surveillance but with a special focus on cancer.[5]

Case Example of Surveillance

The following is a summary of the Surveillance of Major Causes of Hospitalization Among the Elderly for the year 1988, using Medicare records as the source of information for the surveillance, and is presented as an example of surveillance activities.

Surveillance of Major Causes of Hospitalization Among the Elderly 1988

Using Medicare records as a source of data for surveillance of elderly persons hospitalized in 1988, major diseases that contribute to hospitalization were evaluated. Each Medicare record has a unique personal identifier which allows the differentiation of different hospitalizations and permits public health researchers to generate both counts and rates of hospitalizations by person and event. In 1988, approximately 9.1 million hospitalizations covered by Medicare occurred among person 65 years old and older. The major disease categories were for circulatory disease (7,448 per 100,000) and blood diseases (247 per 100,000).

Among persons 65 years and older, many diseases and injuries are more prevalent than among younger groups. Medicare covers hospitalization expenses for about 95% of the elderly population and is a useful source of information for monitoring hospitalizations in the elderly. Records were selected from 14 major disease categories and within these, 49 conditions listed in ICD-9-CM (International Classification of Diseases-9 Revision-Clinical

Modification) were used. The frequency of conditions varied markedly by age, race and gender. Among men bladder and lung cancers, abdominal hernia and aneurysms were more frequent than in women. Hip fractures, intestinal obstructions and diverticula and affective psychoses ranked higher among women than men. Hip fractures and osteoarthritis were more frequent among whites than blacks. Diabetes, renal failure and hypertension ranked higher among blacks than whites. Chronic ischemic heart disease, hyperplasia of the prostate, and asthma were less common in the oldest age group than in the youngest of the elderly. Hip fractures, gastrointestinal hemorrhage and septicemia accounted for proportionately more hospitalizations for the oldest age group. Table 10.2 lists the 14 categories and the 49 different diseases listed as principal diagnosis as the major cause of hospitalization among the elderly in 1988.[20]

RISK IN ASSOCIATION AND CAUSALITY

When discussing association and causality of disease, the concept of risk must be considered and evaluated. Risk is closely related to incidence. The concern for the epidemiologist is that of the probability of developing a disease over a period of time. Because of the closer relationship of risk to morbidity rates, risk and related formulas were presented in Chapter 5.

Risk is the chance that an event or exposure will lead to some disease, condition, disability, or even death. Risk has also been used to describe the probability of some unfavorable outcome of a health or medically related event or experience. Association and risk can be measured statistically and statistical probabilities can be generated regarding the chance of risk.

The probability of developing a disease during a specific time period can be predicted mathematically and can be observed generally from practical experience with a given disease. An experienced epidemiologist can easily estimate the effect of a measles outbreak in an elementary school where the level of immunity is very low. Herd immunity can be evaluated and predictions made from herd immunity level assessments. (See Chapter 2 for herd immunity information.) The estimate of risk is the proportion of the population developing the disease over (divided by) the period of time under study. Risk must take into account those persons who die or who are lost to follow-up. The epidemiologist must take into account the fact that the occurrence of disease in some members of a population group under study removes them from the population at risk and from newly developing disease in the future. When the time period of observation is short and the incidence rate is low, the association between risk and getting the disease is fairly high and the loss of cases in the assessment of risk will be low.[5]

Risk factor exposure can help determine risk as well. **Risk factors** are those behaviors, events, experiences, or exposures associated with the chance of disease, condition, injury, disability, or death occurring. The more exposure to risk factors, the greater the probability of a specific disease or other negative result occurring. Risk factors are often taken by individuals in small doses, a little at a time. A person only smokes one cigarette at a time, but it is a risk factor each time which can lead to a whole array of diseases ranging from heart disease, to lung cancer, to chronic obstructive pulmonary disease. Once risk factors are identified, they can be intervened into, modified, controlled, and prevented through health education, health promotion, and preventive measures. Those risk factors that can be changed or prevented are often referred to as *modifiable risk factors*.

Risk ratio, risk difference, attributable risk, attack rates, and relative risk have all been presented in detail in Chapter 5.

TABLE 10.2 Categories and forty-nine different diseases as principal diagnosis as the major cause of hospitalization among the elderly in the United States—1988

Condition	No. of Persons	All Bene-ficiaries	Gender		Race		Age Group (years)		
			Male	Female	White	Black	65–74	75–84	>85
Infectious/parasitic									
Septicemia	98,537	360.8	370.3	354.5	348.5	530.0	198.6	460.1	942.9
Neoplasms									
Oral cancer	9,240	33.8	49.4	23.4	34.2	31.5	34.3	35.1	27.5
Colorectal cancer	89,909	329.2	380.4	294.9	333.0	313.6	252.1	425.3	460.4
Lung cancer	71,834	263.0	417.2	159.7	261.5	300.1	284.8	270.2	124.2
Breast cancer	64,678	236.8		395.3	243.0	181.0	231.1	261.4	194.9
Cervical cancer	3,217	11.8		19.7	9.9	33.2	11.8	11.5	12.8
Prostate cancer	74,838	274.0	682.9		267.9	379.2	220.0	361.9	304.5
Bladder cancer	38,291	140.2	256.3	62.4	147.5	80.6	105.4	183.6	199.6
Endocrine/metabolic									
Diabetes mellitus	107,880	395.0	364.0	415.8	352.0	874.2	370.5	444.7	379.8
Fluid/electrolyte	177,546	650.1	533.6	728.2	617.9	1093.4	339.2	838.8	1770.5
Blood diseases									
Anemias	30,723	112.5	109.3	114.7	107.8	179.4	73.0	144.2	231.9
Mental disorders									
Pre/senile dementia	24,079	88.2	85.0	90.3	85.7	131.8	38.3	140.8	201.6
Affective psychoses	61,698	225.9	161.2	269.3	237.8	114.0	227.4	252.1	139.8
Nervous system									
Alzheimers	3,262	11.9	11.6	12.2	11.8	15.2	5.2	20.0	24.4
Cataracts	23,906	87.5	66.1	101.9	85.8	107.7	50.3	129.3	164.6
Circulatory diseases									
Hypertension	32,257	118.1	86.0	139.6	104.9	276.0	108.4	136.2	116.8
Hypertensive H.D.	32,769	120.0	101.5	132.4	101.9	335.6	84.3	158.1	199.7
Acute ischemic H.D.	499,820	1830.2	2148.2	1617.0	1877.2	1432.4	1566.8	2212.5	2116.5
Chronic ischemic H.D.	259,886	951.6	1244.3	755.5	983.4	647.2	1038.2	915.5	590.7
Cardiac dysrhythmias	248,797	911.0	992.0	856.7	925.2	857.9	669.3	1190.1	1387.7
Congestive heart failure	388,308	1421.8	1514.6	1359.7	1401.8	1798.9	826.9	1882.3	3269.4
Cerebrovascular disease	490,269	1795.2	1862.9	1749.8	1773.0	2216.3	1150.3	2405.5	3466.5
Atherosclerosis	31,667	116.0	147.5	94.8	107.8	222.4	98.6	129.6	169.2
Aneurysms	43,107	157.8	285.0	72.7	165.4	84.5	149.5	187.1	115.6
Embolism/thrombosis	46,205	169.2	205.4	144.9	169.2	188.3	145.3	193.8	225.2
Thrombo/phlebitis	33,146	121.4	104.9	132.4	125.2	89.8	103.0	146.6	145.7
Respiratory diseases									
Acute bronchitis	119,171	436.4	490.7	400.0	452.8	292.4	365.9	522.2	562.0
Pneumonia	413,741	1515.0	1785.7	1333.6	1539.8	1361.2	862.0	1907.4	3879.3
COPD	68,120	249.4	334.6	192.4	253.1	227.1	236.6	294.7	184.2
Asthma	64,741	237.1	199.9	262.0	230.5	312.3	236.8	253.8	188.7
Pneumonitis	37,267	136.5	168.1	115.3	135.6	154.9	48.6	178.9	485.8
Digestive diseases									
Ulcers	110,982	406.4	449.8	377.3	409.7	389.5	300.2	515.8	655.1
Gastritis/duodenitis	43,506	159.3	144.0	169.6	157.7	187.8	128.4	192.0	229.3
Abdominal hernia	122,511	448.6	720.1	266.6	463.8	312.5	414.5	515.8	432.9
Gastroent/colitis	53,224	194.9	137.4	233.4	198.4	166.8	145.3	240.7	327.0
Intestinal obstruct	96,141	352.0	323.0	371.5	352.4	383.4	233.5	448.5	706.3
Intestinal diverticula	88,011	322.3	242.1	376.0	327.1	303.4	234.6	407.3	543.5
Chronic liver/cirrhosis	13,812	50.6	65.1	40.9	51.2	42.9	58.3	45.8	23.1
Cholelithiasis	134,811	493.6	458.1	517.5	508.8	319.9	468.5	528.6	525.4
G.I. hemorrhage	86,421	316.4	326.0	310.0	311.6	393.7	186.9	404.6	754.9
Genitourinary diseases									
Renal failure	41,589	152.3	189.8	127.2	135.8	347.7	101.4	193.7	304.2
Kidney/ureter stones	51,418	188.3	288.1	121.4	194.6	127.9	207.0	179.5	113.2
Hyperplasia of prostate	172,900	633.1	1577.8		646.1	53.9	614.6	732.7	436.7
Genital prolapse	42,992	157.4		262.9	166.8	51.1	186.2	142.5	45.9
Musculoskeletal/connective									
Osteoarthritis	117,132	428.9	364.6	472.0	446.8	263.2	418.9	510.8	239.1
Intervertebral disc	38,285	140.2	139.3	140.8	145.3	87.2	163.8	123.9	60.9
Osteoporosis	2,517	9.2	2.3	13.9	9.9	2.1	4.7	13.2	21.7
Injuries/poisoning									
Hip fracture	194,270	711.4	369.4	940.5	754.9	327.9	238.0	966.5	2512.5
Complications	150,006	549.3	669.6	468.6	549.5	586.0	505.8	623.6	563.2

(Source: Centers for Disease Control and Prevention, "Surveillance of Major Causes of Hospitalization Among the Elderly, United States, 1988, *Morbidity and Mortality Weekly Report*, Vol. 40, SS-1, pp. 7–21, April 1991)

SCREENING AND DISEASE DETECTION IN POPULATIONS

The mission of epidemiology is to support public health programs. The epidemiologist's goal is to understand the causality and association of disease so that disease control, prevention, and protection programs can be developed and implemented in order to protect a population. Screening programs are one tool used to meet the mission and goals of epidemiology. Screening programs can be as basic as eye exams in elementary schools or as ambitious as multiphasic screening in shopping malls or health fairs. **Screening** is defined as the use of quick and simple testing procedures to identify and separate persons who are apparently well, but who may be at risk of a disease, from those who probably do not have the disease. Screening is used to identify those persons suspected of having a disease so they may be sent for more definitive diagnostic studies and medical exams. **Multiphasic screening** is the use of a combination of tests and diagnostics performed in a battery by technicians under medical direction on large groups of apparently well persons. Multiphasic screening uses this battery of screening tests as a preventive measure in order to attempt to identify any of several diseases or conditions being screened for in an apparently healthy population.[21]

Screening is sometimes confused with diagnosis, but is a precursor to diagnosis. Screening tests, such as vision tests, blood pressure, pap smears, blood tests, and chest x-rays are all given to and applied to large groups or populations. Screening tests have cutoff points which are used to determine which persons are not diseased and which are diseased (or sometimes borderline). Diagnosis is applied to a patient on a one-on-one basis by a physician or other qualified health care provider in a medical setting. Diagnosis, in addition to using the results of tests, involves the evaluation of signs and symptoms, and may involve subjective judgment based on the experience of the physician. Diagnosis is a prerogative of the physician. Screening tests can be conducted by medical technicians under the supervision of a physician. Screening is not meant to compete with diagnosis, but is a process used to detect the possibility of a diseased state so that it may be referred for diagnosis. Diagnosis cannot only confirm or disprove a screening test, but can also help establish validity, sensitivity, and specificity of the tests.[1,2,3,4,5,15]

Screening Program Considerations

Wilson and Junger set forth several items that epidemiologists should consider when planning and implementing a screening program. From a public health perspective, screening is most effective when it can reach a large percentage of the population.[22]

Below are 10 factors that need to be considered when planning a screening program for large population groups:

1. The disease or condition being screened for should be a major medical problem.
2. Acceptable treatment should be available for individuals with diseases discovered in the screening process.
3. Access to health care facilities and services for follow-up diagnosis and treatment for the discovered disease should be available.
4. The disease should have a recognizable course, with early and latent states of the disease being identifiable.
5. A suitable and effective test or examination for the disease(s) should be available.

6. The test and the testing process should be acceptable to the general population.

7. The natural history of the disease or condition should be adequately understood, including the regular phases and course of the disease, with an early period identifiable through testing.

8. Policies, procedures, and levels on tests should be determined in order to establish who should be referred for further testing, diagnostics, and possible treatment.

9. The process should be simple enough to encourage large groups of persons to participate.

10. Screening should not be an occasional activity, but should be done on a regular and ongoing process.[22]

Screening Tests

Screening relies on tests, not just one test but batteries of tests. Thus, screening activities are only as effective as the tests and examinations used. Therefore, each screening test needs to have strong *validity* and *reliability*. **Validity** of test is shown by how well the test actually measures what it is supposed to measure. If it is a cholesterol screening test, the question is: can it give accurate enough readings so that the individual actually knows how high or low his or her cholesterol really is? Validity is determined by the *sensitivity* and *specificity* of the test. **Reliability** is based on how well the test does in use over time—in its repeatability. Can the test produce reliable results each time it is used and in different locations or populations? *Yield* is another term sometimes used in reference to screening tests. **Yield** is the numbers or amount of screening the test can do in a time period—how much disease it can detect in the screening process. The validity of a test can be affected by the limitations of the test and the traits of the individuals being tested. The state of the disease, the severity of it, the level and amount of exposure, nutritional health, physical fitness, and other factors influencing the health status of the individual also influence and affect test responses and findings.[1,2,3,4,5,15]

SENSITIVITY AND SPECIFICITY: TESTS OF VALIDITY

Sensitivity is the ability of a test to correctly identify those who *have* the disease—the percentage of those who have the disease and are proven to have the disease as demonstrated by a test. Sensitivity shows the proportion of truly diseased persons in a population who underwent screening and who are correctly identified as being diseased by the screening test.[1,2,3,4,5,15]

$$\text{Sensitivity} = \frac{\text{True positives}}{\text{True positive} + \text{false negatives}} = \frac{\text{True positives}}{\text{All persons with the disease}} \times 100 \text{ (stated as \%)}$$

Specificity is the ability of a test to correctly identify the percentage of those who *do not* have the disease—those who do not have the disease and are proved to not have the disease as demonstrated by a test. Specificity shows that proportion of nondiseased persons in a population who underwent screening and who are correctly identified as not being diseased by the screening test.[1,2,3,4,5,15]

$$\text{Specificity} = \frac{\text{True negatives}}{\text{True negatives} + \text{false positives}} = \frac{\text{True negatives}}{\text{All persons without the disease}} \times 100 \text{ (stated as \%)}$$

Sensitivity and specificity are not absolute values, as each individual test will produce a slightly different response. Sensitivity and specificity are developed for each test by use over and over throughout a span of time. The long term use of a test establishes reliability, validity, and reveals the shortcomings of the test. The epidemiologist must know how well the test works and if it will effectively screen sick people from well people in a general population. The epidemiologist also wants to know of the test's ability to produce *false positives* and to produce *false negatives*. How sensitive is the test? The results of a screening test could be compared to a diagnosis made by a physician, which would help establish validity, sensitivity, and specificity of the test as well as help standardize the test.[1,2,3,4,5,15]

A **false positive** is when a screening test indicates that the individual has a disease but the person does not have disease. The test was wrong in indicating that the person had the disease when the person was in fact well and not diseased. The test *wrongly said yes* to being diseased, labeling a healthy person as diseased.[1,2,3,4,5,15]

A false negative is the opposite of false positive. A **false negative** is when a screening test indicates that the individual does not have a disease but the person in fact does have the disease. The test was wrong in indicating that the person is well when the person will get sick or is diseased. The test *wrongly said no* to being diseased, labeling a diseased person as healthy.[1,2,3,4,5,15]

True positive is when the test says the person has a disease and the person indeed has the disease. **True negative** is when the test says the person is healthy and has no disease and the person in fact is healthy and disease free.

Standardization of tests is the term used to show that a test has been used over a long period of time, has had widespread use, the cutoff levels/values have been well established, and the test has a proven track record over time with normative data. Screening programs should use standardized tests as it is important to have tests with high predictability, reliability, validity, and long term use. This usually means that the test has been refined and retested in order to make it as effective and accurate as possible.

Understanding the Results of Screening, Sensitivity, and Specificity

From each screening program, individuals are classified as either negative (those without the disease) or positive (those with the disease). However, because the sensitivity and specificity of a test is often less than 100%, false negatives and false positives occur. Thus, the epidemiologist classifies the individual participants into four categories.

False Negatives (FN)	True Negatives (TN)
False Positives (FP)	True Positives (TP)

These four categories are used to understand and evaluate the results of screening programs. These categories are also used to assess test results and for data analysis of a study

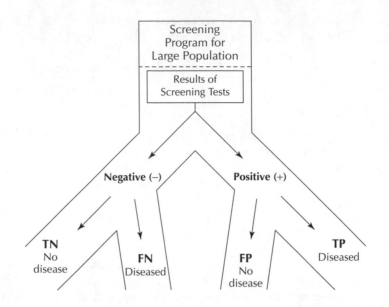

FIGURE 10.11   A decision tree used to assist in the understanding of the effects of screening tests through a pictorial comparison.

population. To more easily understand the role of the four categories, it is helpful to use a graphic presentation of the screening process and where each of the four possible outcomes of a test fits. Figure 10.11 is a decision tree presenting visually the placement of the four possible outcomes (FN, TN, FP, TP).

The information in the decision tree is used in combination with the 2 × 2 four-celled matrix, so that the epidemiologist can determine the place and effects of the four possible outcomes of screening tests. Both the decision tree and the matrix allow a pictorial presentation of the four effects and help in understanding an analysis.

Below are the various arrangements that can be derived from the matrix in Figure 10.12 and the percentage of each. Sensitivity and specificity are proportionate and therefore expressed in percentages. Ideally, the epidemiologist would like to see a test that works so well that both sensitivity and specificity are at 100%.

Percent sensitivity = % of people **with** the disease who are detected by the test $\dfrac{TP}{TP + FN} \times 100$

Percent false negatives = % of people **with** the disease who were **not** detected by the test $\dfrac{FN}{FN + TP} \times 100$

Percent specificity = % of people **without** the disease who were correctly labeled by the test as **not** diseased $\dfrac{TN}{TN + FP} \times 100$

Percent false positives = % of people **without** the disease who were incorrectly labeled by the test as **diseased** $\dfrac{FP}{FP + TN} \times 100$

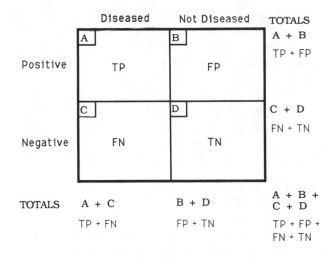

FIGURE 10.12   2 × 2 four-celled epidemiological matrix used to analyze findings of epidemiology studies.

To help in the analysis, some observations about sensitivity and specificity will be helpful. As the percentage of true negatives (TN) and true positives (TP) goes up, sensitivity and specificity go up. As the percentage of false negatives (FN) and false positives (FP) goes up, sensitivity and specificity go down. In summary, sensitivity is the ability to identify correctly those with the disease. Specificity is the ability to identify correctly those without the disease.

An inverse relationship exists between true positives and false positives (Figure 10.13). Conversely an inverse relationship exists between false negatives and true negatives (Figure 10.14).

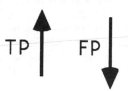

FIGURE 10.13   True positives are inversely related to false positives.

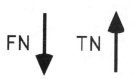

FIGURE 10.14   False negatives are inversely related to true negatives.

The percentage of false negatives is the complement of sensitivity. Conversely, the percentages of false positives is the complement of specificity. The epidemiologist wants a sensitive test so that the test will identify a high proportion of those who have the disease and a test that will generate few false negatives. Conversely the epidemiologist wants the test to be specific enough to detect the disease, so that responses are limited to the study group who are truly diseased and few false positives are produced. Once a screening process is complete, a diagnosis is needed to establish the disease in those who are suspected of having it and rule out those persons screened who are suspected of being diseased but are not.[1,2,3,4,5,15]

Below is an example of a case showing the use of screening test activities used to evaluate suspected sexual abuse that showed false positive results from testing methods.

False-Positive Screening Test Results in Chlamydia Tests Used in Evaluation of Suspected Sexual Abuse in Ohio—1990

On June 21, 1990, a commercial laboratory reported to a private residential care facility for profoundly retarded persons in Ohio that rectal cultures from 10 residents tested positive for Chlamydia trachomatis. A patient presented herself at the emergency room of a hospital with vaginal bleeding. Upon suspecting sexual abuse, Chlamydia trachomatis and other STD testing was done and came up positive. The facility's medical staff collected multiple specimens with swabs from 25 of the remaining 26 residents. The specimens were sent to a commercial laboratory for analysis. The lab reported that the rectal cultures were positive for chlamydia in 10 residents, 6 females and 4 males, age range 10 to 25 years. All other specimens were negative. Pharyngeal swabs for chlamydia culture were obtained from the 10 residents with the positive rectal cultures. The 10 pharyngeal cultures were reported as positive for Chlamydia trachomatis. Being alerted to the possibility of an outbreak of Chlamydia trachomatis, rectal, pharyngeal and urethral and cervical swabs for chlamydia culture and rectal swabs for gonorrhea culture were obtained from 75 residents of the remaining three units in the facility, as well as the 15 original cases. All staff members were asked to undergo similar testing.

On June 22 and 25, the laboratory reported that it had used the immunofluorescence (IF) staining method to identify chlamydia. The testing and report implied the true presence of chlamydia in the rectal specimens. The lab indicated that 9 months before, it had changed from the IF method to a new EIA method for detecting the chlamydial antigen in cell culture and only the EIA confirmation method had been used to identify the 10 rectal and four pharyngeal specimens as positive, as well as the specimens from the three residents of the week of June 25.

On July 6, the EIA and IF methods were compared with duplicate rectal and pharyngeal specimens from the residents identified as infected. Tests were also sent to CDC's Division of Sexually Transmitted Disease Laboratory Research Center for Infectious Diseases which used the IF culture confirmation only. None of the specimens from the residents were positive by IF culture confirmation at either lab. Those specimens tested by the EIA culture were reported positive. CDC detected no chlamydia in any of the specimens that it tested.

It was concluded that the initial reports from the commercial lab using the EIA method for positive chlamydia represented false positive reports. No sexual abuse was found nor proved. CDC reports that when done by experienced technologists, cell culture isolation of Chlamydia trachomatis is the most sensitive and specific test. The EIA test has a history of false-positive findings and is less sensitive than the cell culture test.[23]

Predictive Value of a Test

The **predictive value** of a screening test is the most important aspect of a test. The ability of a test to predict the presence or absence of a disease is a determinant of the test's worth. The higher the prevalence of a disease in a population, the more the sensitivity and specificity of a test affects the predictive value of a test. The higher the prevalence of a disease in a population, the more likely it is that high numbers of true positives should occur. The more sensitive the test, the higher the predictive value and the lower the numbers of false positives and false negatives the test should produce, which are also measures of predictive value. When conducting a negative test, the predictive value is the percentage of nondiseased persons among all participants with negative test results.[1,2,3,4,5,15]

The *predictive value* of a *positive* test is the percentage of true positives among those individuals with positive results from the test. The predictive value of a *negative* test is the percentage of nondiseased persons among those having negative results from the test. A disease has to reach a level of 15 to 20 percent in a population before a useful predictive value is achieved. Prevalence information is used to calculate and separate the study group into diseased and nondiseased individuals.

The formula for the predictive value of a positive test

$$\text{Predictive value of a positive test} = \frac{\text{True positives}}{\text{True positives} + \text{False positives}} \times 100 = \%$$

The formula for the predictive value of a negative test

$$\text{Predictive value of a negative test} = \frac{\text{True negatives}}{\text{True negatives} + \text{False negatives}} \times 100 = \%$$

The example in Figure 10.15 is used to demonstrate how to determine the predictive value of a hypothetical test. A screening test for TB in a small private college was conducted. The findings of the screening test were as follows:

New screening test done on 1,850 students.
Diseased and positive on the test   =   50
Diseased and negative on the test   =   15
No disease and positive on the test   =   75
No disease and negative on the test   =   1,710

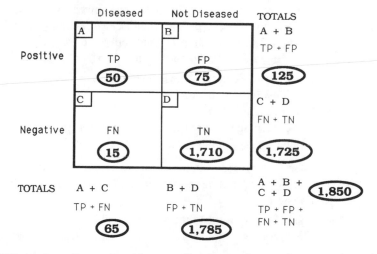

FIGURE 10.15   Example of how to determine the predictive value of a test.

$$\text{Predictive value of a positive test} = \frac{50}{50 + 75} = \frac{50}{125} \times 100 = 40\%$$

$$\text{Predictive value of a negative test} = \frac{1,710}{1,725} \times 100 = 99\%$$

EXERCISES

Key Terms

Define and explain the following terms.

analytical epidemiology	predictive value
association	reliability
asymmetrical association	risk
causality	risk factors
causation of disease	scientific congruence
congruence	screening
direct cause	sensitivity
disease surveillance	specificity
epidemiological surveillance	standardization
false negative	surveillance
false positive	symmetrical association
hypothesis	true negative
indirect cause	true positive
Koch Postulates	validity
multiphasic screening	web of causation
observational study	yield

Study Questions

10.1   A screening test for a newly discovered disease is being evaluated for its effectiveness and sensitivity as a screening test in industry. In order to determine the effectiveness of the new test, it was administered to 880 workers; 120 of the individuals diagnosed with the disease tested positive for it. Results from the test showed a negative test finding for 50 people with the disease. A total of 40 persons not diseased tested positive for it.

From the information presented above and from this chapter, including the use of the epidemiology 2×2 matrix, determine and calculate the following:

a. The prevalence of the disease (expressed as a rate)
b. The sensitivity of the test
c. The specificity of the test
d. The percentage of false negatives (of sensitivity)
e. The percentage of false positives (of specificity)

10.2   Calculate and provide an analysis of the predictive value of tests. To do this analysis complete the following using the data above in Question 10.1. Use Figure 10.15 to assist you in your answer.

a. The predictive value of the test as a positive test
b. The predictive value of the test as a negative test

10.3   As an occupational health epidemiologist you are required to measure the effect of stress on your workers in your manufacturing plant. Two different tests previously developed to measure stress in industrial workers are selected: Stress Test Alpha and Stress Test Delta. The sensitivity and specificity of each test are shown below. This exercise is aimed at showing the inverse relationship of sensitivity and specificity.

Stress Test Alpha	Stress Test Delta
Sensitivity = 60%	75%
Specificity = 95%	90%

From the above information, determine which test will generate the greatest proportion of false negatives. Next, determine which test will generate the greatest proportion of false positives. Which test will produce the greatest number of true positives? Which test will produce the greatest number of false negatives?

10.4   Define and explain the concept of hypothesis. Four approaches to hypothesis development are presented. Explain and discuss each approach and give an example of a disease or condition of each approach and explain why it is a good example.

10.5   Explain and discuss the basic concepts of *association* in causation of disease. Compare and contrast *direct association* with *indirect association, symmetrical association* with *asymmetrical association.*

10.6   a. From information on pages 361–362, identify the various aspects of testing and screening presented in this case and then explain the significance of each aspect.
       b. Explain the personal, psychological, social, and economical aspects of the importance of having highly specific and sensitive tests. Use the case on page 364 as an example to support your explanation.

10.7   An array of possibilities and outcomes exists in the 2 × 2 epidemiological matrix used to analyze findings of epidemiology studies. List and explain all possible arrangements found in Figure 10.9. Compare the arrangements of a retrospective study to that of a prospective study.

REFERENCES

1. MacMahon, B., and T.F. Pugh. 1970. *Epidemiology: Principles and Methods.* Boston: Little, Brown and Company.
2. Mausner, J.S., and S. Kramer. 1985. *Epidemiology: An Introductory Text.* Philadelphia: W.B. Saunders.
3. Lilienfeld, A.M., and D.E. Lilienfeld. 1980. *Foundations of Epidemiology.* New York: Oxford University Press.
4. Friedman, G.D. 1978. *Primer of Epidemiology.* New York: McGraw-Hill.
5. Kelsey, J.L., W.D. Thompson, and A.S. Evans. 1986. *Methods in Observational Epidemiology.* New York: Oxford University Press.
6. Hill, A.B. 1965. "The Environment and Disease: Association or Causation?" *Proceedings of the Royal Society of Medicine*, Vol. 58, pp. 295–300.
7. Slome, C., D.R. Brogan, S.J. Eyres, and J. Lednar. 1982. *Basic Epidemiological Methods and Biostatistics.* Monterey, CA: Wadsworth.
8. Buck, C., A. Llopis, E. Najera, and M. Terris. 1988. *The Challenge of Epidemiology: Issues and Selected Readings.* Washington, D.C.: Pan American Health Organization, Pan American Sanitary Bureau.
9. Rivers, T.M. 1937. "Viruses and Koch's Postulates," *Journal of Bacteriology*, Vol. 33, pp. 1–12.

10. Evans, A.S. 1976. "Causation and Disease: The Henle-Koch Postulates Revisited," *Yale Journal of Biological Medicine*, Vol. 49, pp. 175–95.
11. Green, L., and M. Krueter. 1991. *Health Promotion Planning*, 2nd edition. Mayfield Publishing Company.
12. Centers for Disease Control and Prevention. October 1991. *Preventing Lead Poisoning in Young Children*. Public Health Service, U.S. Department of Health and Human Services.
13. Shindell, S., J.C. Salloway, and C.M. Oberembt. 1976. *A Coursebook in Health Care Delivery*. New York: Appleton-Century-Crofts.
14. Baker, E.L. (Editor). 1989. "Surveillance in Occupational Health and Safety," *American Journal of Public Health. Supplement*, Vol. 79, December.
15. Fox, J.P., C.E. Hall, and L.R. Elveback. 1970. *Epidemiology: Man and Disease*. New York: Macmillan.
16. Public Health Service. 1992. *Healthy People 2000*, U.S. Department of Health and Human Services. Boston: Jones and Bartlett Publishers Inc.
17. National Center for Health Statistics. October, 1990. *Vital and Health Statistics: Current Estimates from the National Health Interview Survey, 1989*. Centers for Disease Control and Prevention, Public Health Service, U.S. Department of Health and Human Services.
18. National Center for Health Statistics. 1991. *Health in the United States 1990*. Hyattville, Maryland: U.S. Department of Health and Human Services, Public Health Service, Centers for Disease Control and Prevention.
19. Monson, R.R. 1990. *Occupational Epidemiology*, 2nd edition. Boca Raton, Florida: CRC Press.
20. Centers for Disease Control and Prevention. April 1991. "Surveillance of Major Causes of Hospitalization Among the Elderly, United States, 1988," *Morbidity and Mortality Weekly Report*, Vol. 40, SS-1, pp. 7–21.
21. Timmreck, T.C. 1987. *Dictionary of Health Services Management*. Owings Mills, MD: National Health Publishing.
22. Wilson, J.M.G., and F. Jungner. 1968. *Principles and Practice of Screening for Disease, Paper No. 34*. Geneva, Switzerland: World Health Organization.
23. Centers for Disease Control and Prevention. January 4, 1991. "False-Positive Results with the Use of Chlamydia Tests in the Evaluation of Suspected Sexual Abuse—Ohio, 1990. *Morbidity and Mortality Weekly Report*, Vol. 39, Nos. 51 & 52, pp. 932–935.

CHAPTER

11

Developing and Conducting Investigations and Studies

CHAPTER OBJECTIVES

This chapter on developing and conducting investigations and studies

- addresses the methods used in setting up and conducting epidemiological studies and analysis in populations at risk of or experiencing outbreaks of disease and disorders;

- reviews the role of the epidemiologist in planning and establishing an epidemiological study used to study epidemics in groups and populations;

- presents the key and important facets of planning an epidemiological study program;

- presents the step-by-step process of conducting several types of epidemiological studies;

- helps understand the various facets and aspects of establishing that an epidemic has occurred and study is needed;

- presents the various administrative measures to treat the ill person, make referrals for definitive diagnosis and treatment, develop prevention and control measures;

- helps understand the importance of searching for every possible source of infection or every risk factor;

- presents epidemiological questions that may assist the epidemiologist in an investigation;

- presents and defines key terms and outlines the principles of epidemiological investigations through study questions.

369

INTRODUCTION

The more interesting, exciting, and challenging part of the work of the epidemiologist is the work in the field doing epidemiological investigations of an epidemic. In the field is where the chain of infection can be studied, understood and broken. In the field is where the prevention and control measures are planned and implemented. In the field is where public health measures save lives and increase health status of the community. Epidemiologists have been called disease detectives, and what makes the field of epidemiology exciting is the detective work in the field.[1]

Even though the work is exciting and interesting, it is also very challenging, as successful epidemiological investigations require much painstakingly gathered information and data. Collecting samples, interviewing people, tracing the chain reaction of the transmission of disease, gathering information and data on all aspects of person, place, and time elements of the epidemic, the analysis of findings, and producing reports are but a few of the chores to be completed. Much rational assessment and commonsense evaluation of the events related to the outbreak are serious tasks of the epidemiologist. Tools range from maps and water testing equipment to paper and pencil tests and computers.

The steps set forth in this chapter are not totally comprehensive as the type of disease or condition being investigated will dictate to an extent the approaches and steps needed. Chronic diseases, lifestyle diseases, behaviorally caused diseases and conditions have different risk factors and multiple causes as compared to one communicable disease caused by one infectious pathogen. The steps are not always accomplished in the order presented. It is not uncommon to simultaneously set into motion several investigative actions at once, as long as the diagnosis has been established or the condition verified when the level of the outbreak is of concern and that an epidemic is imminent.[2,3]

An **epidemiological field study** involves several major activities. In a study of individual cases, specimens for laboratory tests are often needed, clinical exams are required to verify a diagnosis, understanding the course of the disease, knowledge of the usual sources of infection or risk factors, using computers to plot clustering, plotting maps, plotting graphs of epidemic curves, careful observation and data recording and collection, and related activity.[2,3]

PLANNING AND ADMINISTRATION OF EPIDEMIOLOGICAL STUDIES

An epidemiological study, like any public health program requires good administration. Good administration requires sound program planning and program development. For the epidemiological study to be effective, the epidemiologist must not only understand behavioral and biomedical science and epidemiological methodology, but must also be knowledgeable about the basics of program development and planning. Organization and planning, or the lack of it, can determine success or a questionable outcome of a study. The fundamentals of planning and program development, like an epidemiological study, have certain steps and activities that need to be completed. Following is a list of steps to program development and planning. However, this list presents only the most basic information for each step, with each one having many complex concepts and activities required for each step. The list is provided here only as a guide. The epidemiologist in charge of organizing and developing an epidemiology study is encouraged to consult resources on program planning and use general administration concepts in order to assure good success.

Ten Steps to Program Planning and Development

1. Statement of overall purpose based on an obvious need.
2. Organizational assessment: Done in order to assure that the epidemiologist has the support of the organization, has the support of the community and the resources necessary to carry out the epidemiological study.
3. Write goals and objectives of the epidemiological study. **Goals** are general; **objectives** set forth the detailed specific activities and responsibilities of each activity.
4. Population assessment. Evaluate the study group and approaches to assessing the cases individually and as a group.
5. Determine priorities and the focus of the study.
6. Set forth the step-by-step activities and procedures of the epidemiological study.
7. Develop timelines for activities of the study.
8. Implement the study.
9. Evaluation and **feedback**.
10. Intervention, control and prevention methods implemented.

WORKING UP AN EPIDEMIOLOGY STUDY

When an investigation of a disease outbreak is necessary the results must be rational, have an element of commonsense, be scientifically sound and proved, be clear in the findings, and be of value to those affected by the results—the population group. The population group to be subjected to disease or injury prevention control methods may not always readily accept governmental intervention into risk factors. In 1992 in California, a helmet law was passed requiring motorcyclists to wear helmets while riding a motorcycle. However, the law has not been well received, protests were launched, and the statistics used to justify the law have been discounted by those who were affected by the law. Some segments of the medical and public health community have used epidemiological studies to show the effect of helmet use and nonuse on mortality and morbidity rates. The helmet debate is based on freedom of choice as American citizens vs. forced compliance done through laws based on the health care concern of reducing fatalities from motorcycle crashes. The results of an epidemiology study should be of value to the group and to the general population, be accepted by them and most of all enhance the public's health. Political, economical and health concerns for the individuals of the society are all factors affecting public health and epidemiological investigations.

STEPS IN AN EPIDEMIOLOGY INVESTIGATION

1. Establish the Existence of an Outbreak.   First the epidemiologist must verify an epidemic is occurring. Incidence levels and prevalence rates of the past need to be compared to current statistics for the disease to verify the level of occurrence of new cases of the disease.

2. Confirm and Verify the Diagnosis or the Existence of the Medical or Health Problem.   Medical evaluations, clinical testing, and laboratory studies by medical personnel are usually necessary to confirm the diagnosis. Input from environmental health specialists and other health care providers may be required to confirm the existence of a health problem. Assessment of the clinical findings should be done to assure correctness and reliability of the findings. In the case study in Chapter 10, a false positive from a laboratory caused much concern and gave false information in a disease investigation. Some conditions, injuries, or behaviorally caused occurrences have no clinical tests nor laboratory tests that are applicable. It is easier to diagnose a bacteria-caused disease, while an occupational or environmental disorder or condition is not easily diagnosed but still must be verified to exist. On the other hand, some diseases or conditions are only verifiable by laboratory findings and some exotic or unique diseases are determined only by a limited number of specialized labs, including the Centers for Disease Control and Prevention.

3. Establish Criteria for Identifying Individuals as Cases.   The identifying features will depend upon the condition and disease under investigation. Identifying features will rely on signs, symptoms, course of the disease, place and type of exposure, lab findings and clinical exams in identifying cases.

4. Search for Missed Cases.   The epidemiologist must search for cases that may have slipped through the cracks, not recognized as cases, that have not been reported or were not recognized as being a possible case. Physicians, clinics, HMOs, hospital emergency rooms, public health clinics, migrant health clinics, and related facilities should be canvassed to ascertain if other cases might have the disease or condition under investigation. Asymptomatic persons or mild cases and their contacts should be evaluated. Individuals of the group are placed into appropriate categories, initially separating the suspected cases from probable cases.

5. Rough Case Count Using Standard Approaches, References, Methods, and Systems.   The number of individuals who have been exposed as well as the number of ill persons need to be determined. The index case as well as all cases with disease are accounted for and a diagnosis confirmed by standard medical assessments, tests, and procedures. The study population (population at risk) is determined. All persons who are at risk, close or distant, must also be accounted for.

6. Orient the Study and Data to *Time*, *Place*, and *Person*.
Time: Determine each case by time of onset using an *epidemic curve*. Be knowledgeable about incubation periods, time's effect on modes and vehicles of transmission. Chronological events, step-by-step occurrences, chains of events tied to time, and time distribution of the onset of cases must be determined and plotted on charts and graphs. From the epidemic curve information, determine the nature of the course of the disease, ascertain if the group of people were exposed and infected at about the same time or at different times. Look for clustering of disease by both *time* and *place*. Determine and fix the time of the index case and the time of onset of the outbreak. Use the information from incubation periods to determine time factors in the course of the disease peaks and valleys in the epidemic curve.

Place: Using dot or spot maps, plot the location of the cases. If possible and useful, the epidemiologist might also plot on a map the location of exposures or location of each case at the time of the event or exposure. Possible sources of the disease, climatic, and topographic factors need to be assessed. Concentration of events needs to be determined with regard to place of residence and work and possibly recreation of all cases. Was each case present at the time of exposure? Location of sources of chemicals, pollutants, reservoirs of infection, etc., need to be ascertained. (*Place* was covered in Chapter 9.)

Person: The epidemiologist should quickly become acquainted with the person-related issues and characteristics related to the disease under investigation. All cases need to be tabulated by age, sex, race, education, occupation, religion, and other pertinent traits. The interactions of family, friends, fellow workers, and relatives need to be considered. Certain characteristics of the person will have more relevance to some diseases or conditions than others. For example, if diabetes is discovered to be occurring in epidemic proportions, the epidemiologist should want to include the characteristics of race in the analysis, as certain races have higher rates of some diseases than others: e.g., Native Americans have high rates of diabetes; blacks have higher rates of hypertension; Asians have lower rates of cardiovascular diseases.

Attack Rates in the Person: From the assessment of person characteristics, the epidemiologist can discover what group of persons or populations will be most likely to be or have been attacked by the disease, exposure or event. Analysis of factors related to the person should include attack rates if appropriate.

7. Classifying the Epidemic. Based on the case identification, the rough case counts, information gathered on time, place, and person and the tabulation of the data and information an initial epidemic type is determined. The mode of transmission is assessed and a determination is made as to it being a **common source epidemic** or a **propagated epidemic.**

Epidemic Sources—Questions to Ask!

Common Source or Common Vehicle Epidemic

- Is the outbreak from a single source or a single point exposure?
- Is disease spread from person to person?
- Is there continued exposure to a single source?

Propagated or Progressive Epidemic

- Is the outbreak from multiple sources and/or exposures?
- Is the outbreak airborne, behaviorally or chemically caused, and does it involve multiple events or exposures?
- Are the sources of infection from inapparent sources?
- Is there a vector involved in the transmission?
- Is there an animal reservoir of infection?

8. Determine Who Is at Risk. The epidemiologist must determine and classify the ill people from the well people. Who are the ill persons in the group? Who are the well persons in the group? The people in the group can be classified by their individual disease and exposure histories. Clinical, medical and lab findings need to be confirmed, evaluated and analyzed for all cases to substantiate the diagnosis. Asymptomatic individuals or mildly ill persons should be medically evaluated. Search for human and animal sources of infection in those at risk. Those people "exposed" are separated from the "not exposed." The "ill" are separated from the "well." The status of the health of each case needs to be determined by

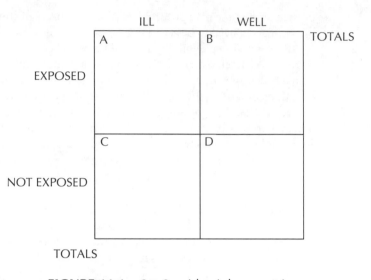

FIGURE 11.1 2 × 2 epidemiology matrix.

exposure. Thus, the four-celled 2 × 2 epidemiological matrix (Figure 11.1) is used to help the epidemiologist classify cases and understand counts, data and develop epidemic information.

9. Analyze the Findings and Data.   The epidemiologist gathers, compiles, tabulates, analyzes, and interprets the findings. Data analysis and the results of the findings assist in making decisions about hypotheses and those at risk. Computers can be used to assist in analysis and making graphics. All the findings and analysis should be consistent across all of the sources and all of the analysis. Findings should support the hypotheses, if not, new hypotheses should be considered.

10. Develop Hypotheses.   Firmly establish the source and type of epidemic. Is the outbreak from a common source or a propagated one? Identify the most probable source for the epidemic—the event, infection, or exposure source. Establish the mode of transmission. Use and analyze the information acquired earlier in the investigation, including but not limited to case counts, assessing those at risk, the sources of the epidemics, time, place or person, and attack rates. For example, if it is a foodborne epidemic, the source of food must be investigated, as should the food handling, preparation, production, and preservation approaches as well as those ill from the exposure. If the outbreak is environmentally caused, the conditions of the environment in which the individuals spent time must be investigated, i.e., the air within the worksite, skin exposure to chemicals, etc. Also under consideration should be the water supply, milk and food sources, sanitary methods, etc. Consider all possible sources from which the disease may be contracted—milk supplies, water supplies, seafood sources, food packing houses, imported foods, etc. (See Figure 11.2.)

Animal sources of infection as well as humans should be considered. Attack rates for the well/unexposed and the ill/exposed should be studied. All suspected vehicles of transmission should be evaluated. Frequency and levels of exposures should also be assessed. Variations in prevalence and incidence should be evaluated. As information comes in it

Life Cycle of *Giardia lambliaprotozoana*

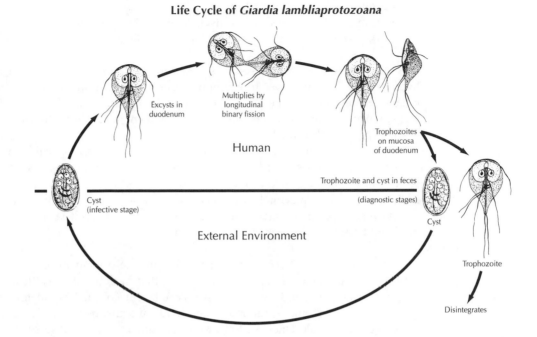

FIGURE 11.2   Giardiasis (*Giardia lambliprotozoana*) is a waterborne disease caused by ingestion of protozoan cysts in fecally contaminated, unfiltered water. Outbreaks have occurred in a variety of places, ranging from mountain streams to day care centers. Waterborne disease outbreaks like foodborne epidemics, require all the steps of an epidemic investigation. (Picture courtesy of Centers for Disease Control and Prevention, Atlanta, Georgia)

should be evaluated and data assembled. Pertinent grouping of data based on time, place, and person characteristics and attack rates needs to be completed. Findings of collateral investigators and personnel, such as physicians, laboratory personnel, and hospital health care providers, need to be gathered and assessed. Overall the epidemiologist should develop hypotheses concerning the source of the outbreak as well as the mode of transmission (if an infectious disease).

Hypotheses need to be developed for all aspects of the investigation. For example, in a foodborne outbreak, hypotheses should be developed for the following:

- the source of infection
- the vehicle of infection
- the suspect foods
- mode of transmission
- type of pathogen (based on clinical symptoms, incubation periods)
- time factors in the outbreak and course of the disease
- place factors in the outbreak
- person characteristics and factors in the outbreak

- outside sources of the infection
- transmission of the disease outside of the study population
- the exposed, unexposed, well and ill cases/individuals

11. Testing the Hypotheses.   As data and information are acquired, the various hypotheses need to be proved true or untrue. The various hypotheses need to be tested and established and shown to be consistent or inconsistent with established facts. If facts or information are lacking to substantiate a hypothesis, then more information must be gathered or the hypothesis discarded.

For each hypothesis, facts and information must match the speculations and deductions for that hypothesis and be inconsistent for all other hypotheses. Assure the hypotheses are consistent with all known facts and with scientific and biomedical knowledge and understanding. The epidemiologist should not rely on any single finding, fact, circumstance, or data analysis. Conclusions about and acceptance of the hypotheses must be based on all pertinent findings, facts, evidence, and analysis.

12. Control and Prevention.   The main purpose of epidemiology and its investigations is to understand disease outbreaks so that basic public health morbidity and mortality prevention and control measures can be employed. An epidemiological investigation not only identifies the source and mode of transmission, but also identifies the links in the outbreak. Once the links to the continuance of the disease are understood, then intervention can occur, the link(s) can be broken and the course of the disease outbreak stopped. The aim of public health **disease control** programs and epidemiology is to stop the spread of disease, stop epidemics, and prevent them from starting. Immunization programs are the first line of defense in prevention and control of some communicable diseases. Risk factor prevention and health protection programs are the first line of defense in behaviorally caused, environmentally founded, and chronic diseases. Epidemiological investigations are conducted if prevention and control measures have failed or were never adequately implemented.

13. Developing Reports and Informing Those Who Need to Know.   The epidemiologist must use the results of an investigation and the overall outcome of the study to develop written reports. The report typically presents a narrative of the investigation and review of the course of the epidemic in the form of a case study. Tables, graphs, charts, dot maps, or any useful and helpful illustrations are presented as well as any pertinent epidemiological data, tests, lab reports, information, and characteristics. A good epidemiological report addresses the information presented under hypothesis ranging from source or mode of transmission and any suggested control and prevention measures.

One purpose of the development of a report is the process of communication and information dissemination. The list of those who need to know would depend upon the type of disease: communicable vs. chronic. Those who need to know about chronic disease would be policy makers, medical insurance companies, hospital officials, government health care officials, and health care agencies, and most of all, those exposed to or with a potential for exposure to the risk factors.

Communicable diseases pose a more urgent need to inform those who need to know. When a disease poses a risk or danger to the public, then those who are in a position to intervene and **control** the **epidemic** need to be informed first. Public health officials, related government agencies, physicians, hospitals, HMOs, medical clinics, schools, universities, and any group of people who are at risk are among those who need to be informed. Unfortunately, many times public health officials know of a health concern, but fail to inform those who most need to know—the population at risk. Public health officials have a responsibility to warn the public and the population at risk, and should not hesitate to do so. Sometimes officials are fearful that upon informing the population at risk, a panic will occur, but this should not be a reason to not inform the public or a least those who are at risk. Individuals should have a choice to leave the area or take protective measures to protect their families and themselves, and epidemiologists should be supportive of this position.

14. Administration and Planning Activities.   Public health measures are accomplished only through an organized effort under government assistance and administration. Organization, coordination, communication, planning, and funding assistance is necessary for epidemiological activities to occur and be successful. Immunization clinics and programs must be established and implemented. In the case of an epidemic, administrative plans and measures to provide treatment and care for the victims of the epidemic must be attended to. Unbiased investigations are best handled by an agency without vested interests. Government agencies often have the experts and professionals to carry out appropriate investigations of diseases, conditions, and disorders. Specialized investigations often require assistance from special laboratory facilities, cooperation with private physicians, hospitals, HMOs and clinics, and individuals, all of which are more likely to cooperate with the administration of a public health department. Financial support to protect the public's health is provided through the administrative activities of government agencies and entities.[2,3,4]

Quick Checklist and Summary of Steps in an Epidemiological Investigation

- Establish the existence of an outbreak.
- Confirm and verify the diagnosis or the existence of the medical or health problem.
- Establish criteria for identifying individuals as cases.
- Search for missed cases.
- Rough case count using standard approaches, references, methods, and systems.
- Orient the study and data to *Time, Place,* and *Person.*
- Classify the epidemic.
- Determine who is at risk.
- Analyze the findings and data.
- Develop hypotheses.
- Test the hypotheses.
- Control the epidemic and prevent future outbreaks.
- Develop reports and inform those who need to know.
- Develop administration and plan activities.

Disease Investigation and Control

Disease Control Measures for Tuberculosis Resurgence

Tuberculosis (TB), thought to be under control in the mid-1980s, has had an alarming resurgence. From 1985 through 1991, cases of TB increased 18%, reversing a 5% decline in the preceding 30 years. In 1991, 26,283 new active cases of TB were reported, with 14% of the cases involving the TB organism most resistant to at least one of the drugs most commonly used to treat this disease. With the onset of AIDS/HIV, many cases of TB occurred in immune system–compromised persons and needle-using illegal drug users. Multiple drug-resistant organism outbreaks have occurred in prisons and hospitals, with not only inmates catching the disease, but with health care workers also being exposed. Refugees, both illegal and legal, have also had a high incidence of TB.

Severely reduced federal, state, and local budgets, combined with complacency about the danger of TB, its control, and spread, made certain special populations vulnerable to TB epidemics. Since 1991, outbreaks of TB have been reported in high school populations, passengers and flight crews on commercial aircraft, and children infected by their parents. The usual isolation and quarantine measures to control TB have been employed, including lock-up hospitals for noncompliant patients. Homeless and street people pose a big threat—the spread of TB within their own groups and to others who interact with them. The greatest threat is that this group of people being IV drug users are not responsible for taking their treatment medications; thus, the lock-up therapy.

Another option has been "Direct Observed Therapy" (DOT). Drug-resistant strains of TB require the patient to take many different drugs daily. The initial treatment of TB includes at least 4 drugs. DOT is carried out in the field by public health workers, including culturally and linguistically competent outreach workers, to make sure that every patient takes all of his or her drugs every day. In some cases, the workers have gone to the person's place of residence or work to assure that they take all of their drugs every time. Physicians are advised to have all TB patients receive early and appropriate treatment and that they complete it. By law, all household contacts are examined. Reporting TB cases in penal institutions to the public health department is required by law. In some states, all hospital cases of TB must have public health approval prior to release.

(Sources: Morbidity Mortality Weekly Report *41, 1992; 42, 1993;* California Morbidity, *November, 1994)*

SETTING UP A COHORT OCCUPATIONAL EPIDEMIOLOGY STUDY

Presented above is the traditional approach to an epidemiological investigation, based mostly on a communicable disease model using cross-sectional (prevalence) or prospective (incidence) studies. Epidemiologists also spend much time conducting cohort studies. A fairly new area of epidemiological interest is that of occupational health, as some occupational diseases are related to substance, chemical, or toxic exposures. Long-term effects of low-level occupational exposures have to be studied over time. Cohort studies were presented in Chapter 8 and are valuable and effective in occupational health settings. Cohort studies often are retrospective studies. Retrospective studies have many advantages, but the major advantage is that medical records, employee personnel records, union records, public health mortality and morbidity records, and other documents containing regularly recorded information can be tapped into in order to gain a great deal of information. Death certificates can provide some data on causes of death as well as related diseases and conditions.[1,5,6]

The most important concern for cohort occupational epidemiology is that of worksite health and medical matters. Basic to worksite and job related health factors are the work history and worksite clinical records. A work history may or may not be available from the department of human resources/personnel. Work history documents relating to health status at the worksite are not always routinely kept as part of personnel records. Most large industries have their own on-site medical clinics, and medical records from such clinics are valuable in cohort epidemiology studies. For those companies without clinics, the job of the epidemiologist is much more difficult, as the work health history must be compiled by the epidemiologist.[1,6]

Steps in Cohort Occupational Epidemiology Investigations

The fundamentals of a cohort **occupational epidemiological study** are provided below. This is more of an outline than a comprehensive review of all facets of the study. **Cohort studies**, being studies of groups of persons of the same birth year and same or similar characteristics, have a unique interest in deaths of the people within the cohort. Thus, the tracking and studying of mortality of cohorts is a major focus. If more information is needed on the detailed complexities of cohort study methodologies, cohort studies are covered in Chapter 8 or further library research may be warranted.

1. Establishing the study rationale, goals and objectives
2. Selecting the study population and issues and areas of concern
3. Developing the hypotheses
4. Defining the cohort
5. Following up the mortality status at the end of the study period
6. Dividing the cohort into exposure level groups and gathering exposure data as they occur over time
7. Analyzing the data, including mortality issues (modified life tables allow people to enter and exit the study; develop person years at risk; Standard Mortality Ratios [SMR] or Proportionate Mortality Ratios [PMR] are usually calculated, see Chapter 4)
8. Developing final reports
9. Developing prevention and intervention procedures

STEPS IN WORKING UP A FOODBORNE ILLNESS INVESTIGATION

Food poisoning, foodborne illness, and food-caused epidemics are quite common, but most are not serious and people rarely see their physicians unless it is serious, thus little public health attention is paid to such occurrences. However, the 1993 Jack-In-The-Box epidemic caused by *E. coli*, which received national media attention, brought the concern of food protection and preparation into the living rooms of families across America. Hamburger meat contaminated in meat processing plants was identified as the possible source of infection.

Even if an epidemic of staphylococcal food poisoning is occurring (for example, being acquired from a fast-food restaurant), most people simply take care of the matter at home, have a bout of diarrhea, take some over-the-counter antidiarrheal drugs, and feel better the next day. Hundreds of persons could be involved, but the medical and public health community never knows, as the outbreak is short, individuals recover quickly, and the family doctor is rarely seen, let alone the outbreak being reported to the epidemiologist at the public health department. In more serious foodborne and waterborne illnesses such as salmonella, giardia, amoebic dysentery, and shigella, people do not recover so quickly, the symptoms are stronger, last longer, and medical intervention is usually needed. These diseases are serious and sometimes cause death, thus are most likely to be reported.

Illnesses arising from consumption of contaminated or spoiled foodstuffs and liquids, i.e., solid foods, liquid foods, milk, water, and beverages are classified as **foodborne illnesses**. Foodborne illness are usually of three classifications: (1) food infections, (2) food poisoning, and (3) chemical poisoning.

Food infections are a result of the ingestion of disease-causing organisms (pathogens), such as bacteria, and microscopic plants and animals. Examples of food infections are salomonellosis, giardiasis, amoebiasis, shigellosis, brucellosis, diphtheria, tuberculosis, scarlet fever, typhoid fever, and tularemia.

Food poisoning is the result of preformed toxins in foods prior to consumption, often the waste products of bacteria. The two most common forms are staphylococcus food poisoning, which produces cramps and a short bout of diarrhea about 6 hours after consumption, being a milder form of food poisoning. The most serious and deadly form of food poisoning is that of botulism. It is said that the amount of botulism that will fit on the head of pin will cause death in humans. Obviously this toxin is extremely poisonous.

Chemical poisoning from foodstuffs is caused by poisonous chemicals from plants and animals.

Public health and medical personnel, as in any disease investigation, must work together as a team. Personnel involved in a major disease investigation could possibly include epidemiologists, sanitarians, physicians, nurses, and laboratory personnel such as microbiologists, medical technologists, medical lab techs, and chemists.

The epidemiology team interviews, if possible, all persons who were present at the time of the ingestion of suspect foodstuffs. When large groups or populations are involved in an outbreak, it may not be feasible to interview all suspected cases. It has been suggested that in groups of over 50, half be interviewed and in groups over 100, 25% be interviewed. The use of random sampling techniques should be used to select persons to be interviewed and tested. Standardized interviewing procedures should be used. Standardized questions and information should be collected on a standardized form, which all interviewers should use.

Any good epidemiological investigation should interview both ill and well persons. Half of the study population should come from each category. Tabulation and analysis of the data should be completed as presented in earlier chapters of this book. In foodborne disease outbreaks, certain rates should always be included in the analysis and reports. Those factors necessary to a good investigation will identify and include

- who ate the food
- who did not eat the food
- calculating attack rates for each food
- for each food calculating the attack rates among those who ate the food
- for each food calculating the attack rates among those who did not eat the food
- computing the relative risk (the ratio of the attack rate of those eating the food to those who did not eat the food (relative risk is covered in Chapter 4)

Steps in Investigating a Foodborne Disease Epidemic

1. Obtain a diagnosis and disease determination.
2. Establish that an outbreak has or is taking place.
3. Determine which foods are contaminated and which are suspect.
4. Determine if toxigenic organisms, infectious organisms, or chemical toxins are involved.
5. Ascertain the source of contamination. How did the foodstuff become contaminated? Who contaminated it? Where was it contaminated? Contaminated by direct or indirect sources?
6. From determining the source of poison and contamination, ascertain how much growth or the extent of contamination that could occur.
7. Identify foods and people implicated in the contamination and intervene to stop further spread of the disease.
8. Assure medical treatment.
9. Exercise intervention, prevention, and control measures.
10. Inform those who need to know—private citizens, appropriate leaders, and public officials.
11. Develop and distribute reports.

BASIC EPIDEMIOLOGICAL QUESTIONS

A basic investigative approach used by most epidemiologists is that of asking **epidemiological questions**. The epidemiological question approach and questions asked are commonly known among practicing epidemiologists. Rarely is a list of epidemiological questions ever written out, let alone published in a textbook. The reasons for this are many and some unknown. One reason is that each case or epidemic poses a new and different set of questions to be asked. However, some commonality does exist among the many epidemiological questions that can be asked. Below are some epidemiological questions that the beginning epidemiologist can refer to, if for no other reason than to stimulate thought and possibly stimulate new and different questions about the investigation. The 2 × 2 epidemiological matrix may be a tool of value to the epidemiologist in asking and answering investigative questions.

Some Investigative Epidemiological Questions to Consider

- In whom (which groups) is the disease present?
- In whom (which groups) is the disease absent?
- What are the sick people doing that the healthy people are not?
- What are the healthy people doing that the sick people are not?
- What are the healthy people not doing that the sick people are?
- What are the sick people not doing that the healthy people are?
- Can you determine whether certain cause-effect relationships are present in individuals with the condition, disease, or characteristics of interest?
- Can you determine whether certain cause-effect relationships are blocked or not present in individuals with the condition, disease, or characteristics of interest?
- What are the common experiences among all of the ill persons? Common food? Common water? Common exposure to the disease? Common housing? Common clothing? Common use of fomites? Common exposure to animals/vectors? Frequenting the same places? Common behavior? Common lifestyle?
- What are the common experiences among the well persons? Common food? Common water? Common immunity to the disease? Common housing? Common use of sanitation? Common control of animals/vectors? Frequenting the same places? Common behavior? Common lifestyle?
- Does the disease cluster by *time* and *place*?
- What risk factors are present in persons with the condition?
- Are risk factors present in persons without the condition?
- What risk factors are absent in persons who do not have the condition (healthy people)?
- What risk factors are absent in persons with the condition?
- What exposures to the disease exist in the sick population?
- What exposures to the disease are lacking in the healthy population?
- *Vehicles of Transmission* (Some of the questions above may be useful in reviewing the questions below.)
- *Vectors* What vectors can be implicated in the disease exposure and outbreak?
- How have the cases been exposed to the vectors?
- *Fomites* What fomites can be implicated in the disease exposure and outbreak?
- *Waterborne Transmission* What waterborne activities and exposures are implicated in the disease outbreak?

TICK-BORNE ENCEPHALITIS

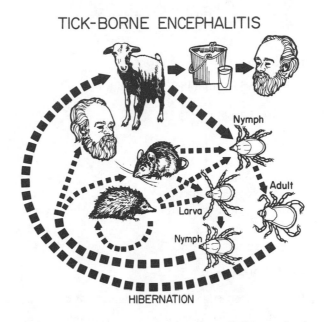

FIGURE 11.3   Epidemic investigations require that all disease harborages, carriers, modes of transmission, zoonotic implications, hosts, reservoirs, vectors, and related causation factors be considered. (Picture courtesy of Centers for Disease Control and Prevention, Atlanta, Georgia)

- *Foodborne transmission* What foodborne activities and exposures are implicated in the disease outbreak?
- *Airborne transmission* What airborne activities and exposures are implicated in the disease outbreak?
- *Risk factors* What risk factor activities and exposures are implicated in the disease outbreak? (See Figure 11.3.)

In summary, if a disease occurs only in the summer, the epidemiologist searches for the causative factors that would be available only in that time period. Is the increase in the disease due to the exposure of new water sources? For example, drinking from a stream in the mountains, swimming in a contaminated public swimming pool or a lake. Is it a vectorborne disease? What vectors are available for disease transmission in the given time period and are missing at other times of the year or seasons? Are vehicles of transmission present during the time period that are not present during other time periods? Are the cases/subjects exposing themselves during this time period to environments, situations, places, or circumstances not available at other times of the year or in other seasons, such as hiking or camping in the woods in the summer when insects are present that are implicated in vectorborne diseases? Are certain fomites used during a certain time period that might not be used during other seasons, such as shared drinking glasses or containers? Are risk factors only seen in certain locations or places? Do they occur only at work or only at home or at the site of recreation (mountains, beaches, public swimming pool, etc.)?

EXERCISES

Key Terms

Define and explain the following terms.

chemical poisoning
cohort study
common source epidemic
control (disease)
control (epidemic)
epidemiological field study
epidemiological questions
feedback

foodborne illnesses
foodborne infection
food poisoning
goal
objective
occupational epidemiological study
prevention activities
propagated epidemic

Study Questions

11.1   Figure 11.4 presents an AIDS epidemic and the numbers of cases and categories.

    a. What can the epidemiologist learn from this data?
    b. What can be predicted about this epidemic of AIDS?
    c. Why?
    d. Given the data in Figure 11.4 what prevention and control measure can the epidemiologist recommend to the Director of Public Health for the county?
    e. Which steps are necessary for working up an epidemiological investigation in this AIDS epidemic and why?

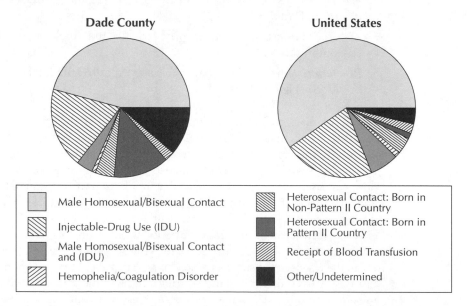

FIGURE 11.4   AIDS epidemic for Dade County and United States, 1981–1990. (Source: Centers for Disease Control and Prevention, "Acquired Immune Deficiency Syndrome—Dade County, Florida, 1981–1990," *Morbidity and Mortality Weekly Report*, July 26, 1991, Vol. 40, No. 29, pp. 489–493)

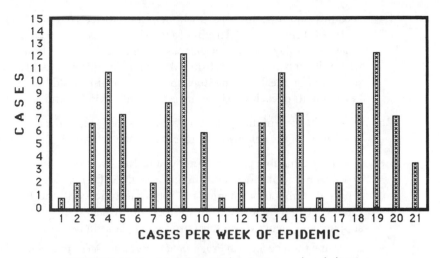

FIGURE 11.5 Measles epidemic in a school district.

11.2 Figure 11.5 shows a hypothetical measles epidemic in a school district, the epidemic curve, and the numbers of cases per week for the district.

    a. What type of epidemic is this?

    b. Why?

    c. What *time* factors are of concern to the epidemiologist in this case?

11.3 Figure 11.6 shows a hypothetical measles epidemic in an elementary school and the epidemic curve shows the numbers of cases per week for the school.

    a. What type of epidemic is this?

    b. Why?

    c. What *place* and *time* factors are important to this investigation? Why?

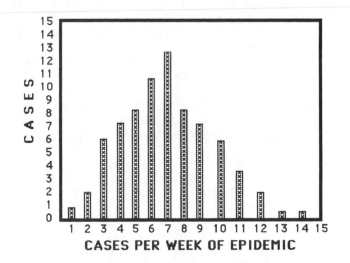

FIGURE 11.6 Measles epidemic in an elementary school.

11.4   A county public health department in a large city received physician reports from 5 private practices, 4 clinics, and 2 HMOs of a total of 22 cases of tuberculosis in patients 60 years and older in a 30-day period. The city has six senior citizen large housing apartment complexes, where all but two cases were from. Most all senior citizens attend a local senior center, which serves a noon meal. List the steps an epidemiologist would have to take and briefly explain key elements of each step in an investigation of this epidemic.

11.5   Make a list of all of the epidemiological questions you can derive for an epidemiological investigation of the chlamydia outbreak in Chapter 10.

11.6   A fast-food hamburger restaurant chain, *Fast-Food Joints of America*, has been named as possible source of a food-poisoning outbreak. So far 140 cases of bloody diarrhea have been reported from various clinics and physician offices and the *E. coli* bacteria is suspected. Cases have been reported from 15 stores in two states. All of the meat was supplied by one supplier and involved two meat processing plants in two counties.

     a.   Using the *Ten Steps to Program Planning and Development* listed in this chapter, present all administrative and planning activities necessary for successfully developing a full-blown epidemiological investigation of this foodborne epidemic.

11.7   A fast-food hamburger restaurant chain, *Fast-Food Joints of America*, has been named as possible source of a food poisoning outbreak. So far 140 cases of bloody diarrhea have been reported from various clinics and physician offices and the *E. coli* bacteria is suspected. Cases have been reported from 15 stores in two states. All of the meat was supplied by one supplier and involved two meat processing plants in two counties.

     a.   Using the 11 steps to working up an epidemiological investigation of a foodborne disease epidemic presented in Chapter 11, outline in detail all of the activities necessary to complete an investigation of the foodborne epidemic in the fast-food restaurant.

REFERENCES

1. Jaret, P. January, 1991. "Stalking the World's Epidemics: The Disease Detectives," *National Geographic*, Vol. 179, No. 1, pp. 114–140.
2. Mausner, J.S., and S. Kramer. 1985. *Epidemiology: An Introductory Text*. Philadelphia: W.B. Saunders.
3. Friedman, G.D. 1978. *Primer of Epidemiology*. New York: McGraw-Hill.
4. Lilienfeld, A.M., and D.E. Lilienfeld. 1980. *Foundations of Epidemiology*. New York: Oxford University Press.
5. Timmreck, T.C. 1991. *Handbook of Planning and Program Development for Health and Social Services*. San Bernardino, CA: Health Care Management Development Associates.
6. Monson, R.R. 1990. *Occupational Epidemiology*, 2nd edition. Boca Raton, FL: CRC Press.

CHAPTER

12

Behavioral and Chronic Disease Epidemiology

CHAPTER OBJECTIVES

*This chapter on the elements of chronic disease, behavioral,
and noncommunicable disease epidemiology*

- addresses the methods used in chronic disease, behavioral and noncommunicable disease epidemiological analysis of populations at risk for outbreaks of disease, disability and conditions;
- reviews the role of chronic disease, behavioral and noncommunicable disease causation in groups and populations;
- presents the importance of the various facets of chronic disease, behavioral and noncommunicable disease development in epidemiological studies and analysis;
- presents the role of webs of causation as tools of assessment and analysis in chronic disease, behavioral and noncommunicable disease epidemiology;
- presents the various aspects of risk measurement and assessment analysis in chronic disease, behavioral and noncommunicable disease epidemiology;
- presents several examples and cases of chronic disease, behavioral and noncommunicable disease epidemiology;
- presents several approaches to control and prevention and health protection in chronic disease, behaviorally caused and noncommunicable diseases;
- presents terms and study questions for study and review of chapter concepts.

INTRODUCTION

Epidemiology's roots lie in studying the cause and control of communicable disease epidemics. Historically, the main causes of death in the United States and industrialized nations were due to infectious diseases. In its infancy, epidemiology focused on a single pathogen, a single cause of disease. The epidemiologist's challenge was to isolate the single bacteria, virus, or parasite. Only in the last two or three decades have chronic diseases, behavioral and lifestyle caused diseases, disorders, and conditions become a concern to public health. Cardiovascular diseases, heart disease, cancer, accidents, diabetes, suicide, cirrhosis of the liver, and homicide are among the top leading causes of death in industrialized nations and are chronic diseases or behaviorally caused noncommunicable diseases. (See Chapter 1.)

Chronic diseases and behaviorally caused diseases and conditions are multifaceted in cause and source. Moreover, these modern diseases are mostly preventable and are taken in small doses; one cigarette at a time, one drink at a time; one high-fat, high-cholesterol food at a time. Like infectious diseases, chronic diseases have acts of omission as much as acts of commission. Failure to wash disease-contaminated hands is an act of omission and negligence in the communicable disease arena. Failure to make proper food choices and to exercise are acts of omission in the chronic disease areas of heart and cardiovascular disease.

CHRONIC DISEASE EPIDEMIOLOGY

Chronic diseases generally occur in those persons who have been alive long enough to acquire them. However, age alone is not always a determiner of acquiring a chronic disease. In fact, most chronic diseases have occurred at most any age, though most do occur in the later years in life. Since most infectious diseases have been fairly well controlled, **chronic disease epidemiology** has the challenge of conquering chronic and lifestyle forged diseases, many of which are associated with the aging process.

America is experiencing an increase of persons growing into old age. In 1990, more persons age 85 years and older were alive than had ever been age 85 or older up to that point in time in the history of the earth. The life expectancy of a 65-year-old in 1988 was 18.6 years for females and 14.8 years for males. Average life expectancy for all persons in 1992 was an average of about 75 years. As the population of America ages, more chronic diseases appear in individuals and thus, in population groups. The older population, 65 years and older, numbered about 31 to 32 million in 1992 and made up about 12.5% of the total U.S. population. One in every 8 persons is over age 65. In 1988, there were 18 million females and 12 million males over age 65. Since 1900, the percentage of persons over age 65 has tripled. The older population expects to continue to grow to about 35% of the population by the year 2000 and will represent more than 14% of the total population.[1,2]

The diseases of the 20th century mostly exist because of the lifestyles modern populations choose to lead. Experiences faced now are beyond the comprehension of past generations. Stress, career pressures, sedentary lifestyles, high density population living, poor diet, crime, drugs, gangs, poverty, pollution, fear, and economic struggles are much more common and more intense in modern times, many of which lead to chronic diseases.[1,2]

The national health promotion and disease prevention objectives for the year 2000 as set forth in *Healthy People 2000*, are aimed at reducing coronary heart disease deaths, cancer deaths, (especially lung cancer), the prevalence of mental disorders, work related injuries, and diabetes. The noncommunicable disease objectives targeted for older adults are aimed at reducing suicides, deaths from motor vehicle crashes, deaths from falls, deaths from fires, hip fractures, and tooth loss.[3]

The list of all chronic diseases known to occur to mankind is quite extensive. Additional information on noncommunicable and chronic diseases is presented in Chapter 2. The most common chronic diseases seen in modern times affecting those over age 65 are listed below:

- Alzheimer's disease
- Arrhythmia
- Atherosclerosis
- Cancer
- Cardiovascular diseases
- Congestive heart failure
- Coronary artery disease
- Depression
- Diabetes
- Glaucoma
- Gout
- Heart attack
- Osteoarthritis
- Osteoporosis
- Parkinson's disease
- Peripheral vascular disease
- Rheumatoid arthritis
- Stroke (cerebral vascular accident)

In general, the incidence of chronic disease increases with age and causes the majority of visits to health care providers, mostly in the older population group. Most of these disease are due to lifestyle and behavioral causes, and the aging process. Few visits are due to infectious diseases as the source of illness. Lifestyle and behavior are the key risk factors.

Postulates on Chronic Diseases

Dr. Robert Koch developed several guidelines for etiological and **chronic disease causation** factors. Below are the postulates and causation factors.[4]

Postulates on Chronic Disease Causation

1. The suspected characteristics of a chronic disease must be found more frequently in persons with the diseases in question than in persons without the diseases.

2. Individuals possessing the chronic disease characteristic must develop the disease more frequently than do persons not possessing the characteristic.

3. Any observed association between a risk factor characteristic and the chronic disease must have the relationship between the risk factor characteristic and disease tested, as well as any similar related risk factor characteristic that could cause the disease under study.

4. The incidence of the chronic disease should increase in relation to the duration and intensity of the risk factor.

5. The distribution of a risk factor should parallel that of the chronic disease in all factors.

6. All facets of a chronic disease illness should be related to the level of exposure to the risk factor.

7. The reduction or removal of the risk factor exposure should reduce or halt the disease.

8. Populations of people exposed to the risk factors in controlled studies should develop the chronic disease more often than those not exposed.[4]

Five Elements of Causation in Chronic Diseases   A set of elements relating the association between a suspected cause and the development of a chronic disease have also been developed. Below are the five elements associated with causation in chronic disease.

1. Consistency of the cause-effect association.

2. The strength of the cause-effect association.

3. The specificity of the association.

4. The time factor aspects of the association.

5. The coherence of the cause-effect association.[4]

RISK FACTORS IN CHRONIC DISEASES AND BEHAVIORALLY CAUSED DISEASES

The source of risk factors for noncommunicable diseases and chronic diseases are behavioral, physiological/genetic, environmental and social. **Risk factors** are those experiences, behaviors, acts or aspects of lifestyle, that increase the chances of acquiring or developing a disease, condition, injury, disorder, disability, or death. Risk factors can be due to predisposing conditions, attributes, or risk exposures. Increased risk factor exposure increases the probability of disease occurrence, and an epidemiological association of getting the disease. One way risk factors are determined is by reducing or modifying the exposure to the risk and observing the results. For example, when exposure to smoking is reduced, rates for lung cancer decrease.[5,6,7,8]

Risk factors are also referred to as at-risk behavior, predisposing conditions, or predisposing factors. **At-risk behaviors** are those activities done by persons, who are healthy, but see themselves at greater risk of developing a particular disease, condition, or disorder. **Predisposing factors** are those factors or circumstances existing which influence behavior by providing a motivation for the health behavior to happen. For example, the fact that a school-age child's parents smoke is a predisposing factor influencing the possibility of the child also smoking.[5,6,7,8]

Many lifestyle, work-related, environmentally, and behaviorally caused risk factors come from an array of influences and sources that are not always well defined, including choices in lifestyle, living conditions, social influences, and environmental exposures. Using the top eight causes of death that are chronic disease related, or behaviorally caused, a table comparing risk factors is presented in Table 12.1.[5,6,7,8]

In addition to the leading causes of death and the related risk factors, epidemiologists are concerned with additional noninfectious factors which affect the health status of populations.

TABLE 12.1   Risk factors compared to leading causes of death and related chronic diseases

	Top 8 Causes of Death by Chronic Diseases Compared to Risk Factors							
	Causes of Death/Chronic Diseases							
Risk Factors	*Heart Disease*	*Cancer*	*(CVA) Stroke*	*Accidents*	*Diabetes*	*Cirrhosis*	*Suicide*	*Homicide*
Behaviorally Related								
Smoking/Tobacco Use	X	X		X				
Alcohol Use/Abuse		X		X		X	X	X
Nutrition/Diet	X	X	X		X	X		
Lack of Exercise/Fitness	X	X	X		X			
High Blood Pressure	X		X					
Cholesterol Levels	X		X					
Overweight/Obesity	X	X			X			
Stress	X		X	X			X	X
Drug Use/Abuse	X		X	X			X	X
Lack of Seat Belt Use				X				
Environmentally Related								
Worksite Risks/Exposures		X		X				
Environmental Hazards		X		X				
Vehicular Hazards				X				
Household Hazards				X				
Medical Care Risks	X	X	X	X	X	X	X	
Radiation Exposures				X				
Infectious Pathogens	X	X						
Engineering/Design Hazards				X				
Biological/Genetic Related								
Chromosome/genetic defects	X	X	X		X	X	X	
Congenital anomalies	X	X	X		X	X	X	
Developmental defects	X	X	X		X	X	X	
Socially Related								
Poverty	X	X	X	X	X	X	X	X
Low Educational Level	X	X	X	X	X	X	X	X
Lack of Work Skills	X	X	X	X	X	X	X	X
Disrupted Families	X	X	X	X	X	X	X	X

(Sources: Centers for Disease Control and Prevention, *Chronic Disease and Health Promotion Reprints From MMWR, 1985–1989*, Public Health Services, U.S. Department of Health and Human Services, 1992; National Centers for Health Statistics, Health In The United States—1990, Public Health Services, U.S. Department of Health and Human Services, 1991; National Cancer Institute, *Strategies to Control Tobacco Use in the United States*, Public Health Services, U.S. Department of Health and Human Services, 1992; Green, L.W., and Krueter, M.W. *Health Promotion Planning*, Mayfield Publishing: Mountain View, CA 1991)

Such diverse and varied factors include but are not limited to gunshot wounds, suicide without use of firearms, drug abuse, pedestrian death due to hypothermia, carbon monoxide poisoning, drinking and driving fatalities, effect of drought on nutritional status of children in underdeveloped countries, seat belt use, auto fatalities, etc. For example, heart disease risk factors can be prevented if health education, health promotion, and disease prevention efforts are undertaken within a population.

In heart disease, seven behaviors can be undertaken to reduce risk factors. The seven include

1. Attain and maintain desirable weight.
2. Check for high blood pressure regularly.
3. Stop smoking and tobacco use.
4. Avoid drinking alcohol, especially heavy drinking.
5. Begin and participate in regular exercise.
6. Maintain a good diet low in saturated fats.
7. Develop a low stress lifestyle and good coping skills.

NEWS FILE

Teenage Smoking (Behavioral Epidemiology)

Teen Smoking Continues to Rise

While tobacco companies are being sued for disease and related costs of smoking, and while the government continues stepped-up legal efforts against tobacco companies, teenage smoking continues to rise. Federal reports say that 3 million or more teenagers now smoke, with up to one-third eventually dying from diseases caused by smoking.

Teenagers start smoking for the same reasons today as they did 25 years ago—peer pressures, curiosity, to be cool, to look grown up, and because they think only of what is happening today. Most teens start smoking to look cool to their friends. Soon they find that they are lighting up alone and that smoking is no longer a social event but an addictive need. In one study, 6% of eighth graders said they needed to have a smoke. Nicotine in cigarettes is an addiction teens cannot escape if they start smoking. Some studies show that teens think they will not be smoking 5 years from now, but facts show they will be lighting up 16 years later, long enough for cancer to affect some. If they quit smoking by age 30, the negative effects of smoking often reverse themselves, and the chances of dying of a smoking-related disease are greatly reduced. Studies show that the later teens start to smoke, the more likely they are to quit.

Newer and tougher laws are being passed in every state, and old ones are now being strictly enforced. Some cities are arresting teens and are strictly enforcing the existing laws. Many teenagers say they buy their own smokes illegally, instead of getting them from others. A Centers for Disease Control and Prevention report states that teens buy their own cigarettes 62% of the time. Selling tobacco to teenagers is illegal in all states, yet four-fifths of them say they bought their smokes at a small store.

ODDS RATIO IN CHRONIC DISEASES

The ratio of the chance of the occurrence of a chronic disease or condition compared to the chance of a nonoccurrence is referred to as **odds ratio**. Odds ratio or odds risk ratio is the ratio of the odds of the probability of getting a chronic disease to the odds of the probability of not getting the disease once exposed to risk factors. Odds ratio has been presented in detail in Chapter 5.

DEVELOPING WEBS OF CAUSATION FOR CHRONIC DISEASES OR BEHAVIORALLY CAUSED DISORDERS

Since multifaceted behavioral, environmental, physiological/genetic, and lifestyle choices all contribute to causation risk factors of chronic diseases, a methodology for their assessment is needed. Some infectious disease outbreaks have been easy to investigate, as sources of causation are based on one agent or pathogen. Even when it may come from multiple sources, limitations are placed on the transmission of the disease.

Some behaviorally founded chronic diseases are developed from a single source and single agent from **multiple exposures**, one dose at time. Smokeless tobacco makes a good case. Cancer of the lip, gums, mouth, and throat from chewing tobacco is a good example. The chewing tobacco is the single agent and single source used in multiple exposures. The *person, place*, and *time* elements are quite limited yet identifiable, as smokeless tobacco use is growing in some segments of the population, especially younger males in certain places in the United States, especially rural areas with the "cowboy," image, trends, and social influences. A **web of causation** for cancer of the mouth with smokeless tobacco would be fairly simple and would include factors such as tobacco companies giving free samples to teens with hopes of hooking the youth on the habit, social influences, sex, age, place, parental influences, physiological factors, addiction factors, etc.[7]

When obvious cause-effect associations are seen as in the smokeless tobacco and cancer of the mouth, then investigations are easy to accomplish. However, when a population group comes down with a single disease or several related diseases with a single clear and obviously identifiable source lacking, a web of causation can be of value. For example, if a high rate of pancreatic cancer occurs in a group of children within a limited geographical area, the search for the source and the actual cause is not a simple task. If cancer of the pancreas, kidneys, and liver are seen in the same population group, the investigation becomes even more complicated. Even though all three organs are located within the abdominal cavity, the functions of each and chance for exposure for each vary as each has totally different physiological processes. Questions about causation are not easily answered. In the case of pancreatic cancer, the epidemiologist might ask, What are the sources or type of carcinogen? Radiation? Chemical? Is there some genetic predisposition in the population group? When lacking a common and clear source of disease, citizens have looked at all kinds of possibilities. For example, high tension powerlines in the area, such as in a case in Denver, Colorado, have been suspected in certain types of cancer and genetic diseases. The possibility of hazardous waste dumps under the homes, food, water, the surface soil, pesticides, and herbicides, air pollution, gases, living close to chemical plants or other industries, and other sources are considered when the cause of disease is not clear. Thus a web of causation could be constructed to help solve the mystery of sources and causation.

Constructing Webs of Causation and Causation Decision Trees

Webs of causation have limitations in that they may not directly lead the epidemiologist investigator right to the cause. Decision trees, used with webs of causation, are the suggested approach. When constructing a web of causation, a separate decision tree would be developed for each aspect, factor, and causation element. The yes-no response of decision trees leads the epidemiologist closer to discovering the cause than a web of causation alone. **Decision trees**, as used in disease diagnosis, can ask leading questions that are answered either yes or no, thus eliminating possibilities of causation while leading the investigator down the correct path toward discovery, assuming the questions are answered correctly.

Some branches of a web of causation may require second level assessments as secondary levels of causation or risk factors may have to be taken into account. A second level set of webs may be required to be developed. In some cases a third level of assessment may be required which includes a third level set of webs. The second level and third level of webs feed into the appropriate branches of the main web, accounting for all possible risk factors or factors that contribute to the disease, directly and indirectly.

Web construction approaches have been developed several ways; flow charts starting from the top moving to the disease diagnosis at the bottom in a step-by-step fashion; a central downward flowing core with branches from each side. (See Figures 10.2 and 10.4 in Chapter 10.) In the case of lead poisoning, the mode of entry into the body influenced a three-channel flow toward the cause of the disease. (See Figure 10.4 in Chapter 10.) In the spirit of a true web approach, Figure 12.1 presents a spiderweb configuration to illustrate in a general fashion the elements of a web of causation with the disease as the focus. Figure 12.2 presents a second web of causation with a focus on the causes of the disease/risk factors. Figure 12.3 presents an example of a decision tree that must be adapted for each situation and element under consideration in the investigation. In summary, a web of causation is a quasi-flow chart that identifies every remote possible risk factor from every dimension of living, leading eventually to the diagnosed disease. At each step and for each element, a decision tree is established and worked through in order to assure the correct decision is being made leading to *causation* of the disease.

Construction of a Web of Causation and Decision Trees

1. Identify the problem, affirm the condition, obtain an accurate diagnosis of the disease.
2. Place the diagnosis at the center or bottom of the web.
3. Brainstorm and list all possible sources for the disease.
4. Brainstorm and list all risk factors and predisposing factors of the disease.
5. Develop sub-webs and tertiary level sub-webs for the various branches of the webs if needed.
6. Organize and arrange lists of sources and risk factors from general and most distant from the disease, in steps, being more specific and focused as the steps move closer toward the diagnosis of the disease.
7. Develop and work through causation decision trees for each element under consideration on the way toward the diagnosed disease.

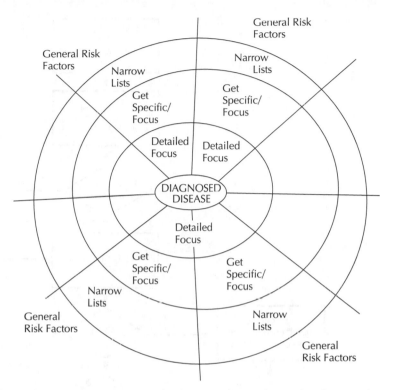

FIGURE 12.1   Basic concepts in the construction of a web of causation with the disease as the focus.

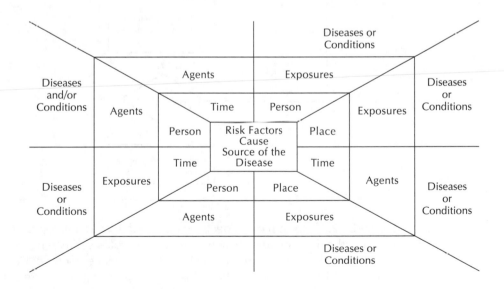

FIGURE 12.2   Web of causation with risk factors, cause and source of disease as the focus of the investigation.

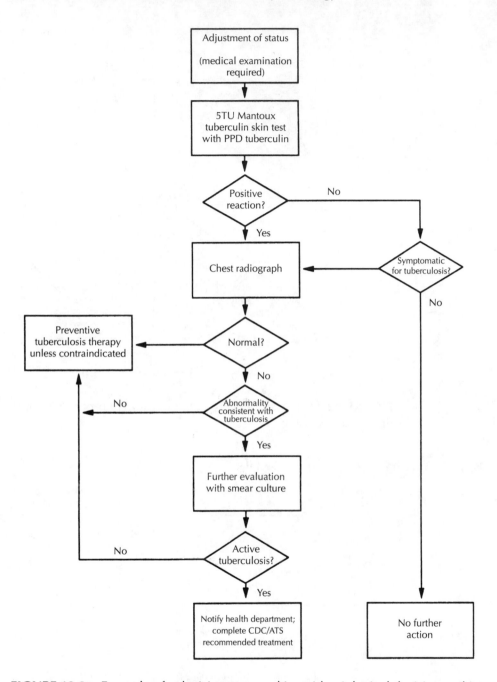

FIGURE 12.3 Example of a decision tree used in epidemiological decision making, showing the decision making activities for tuberculosis screening for non-immigrants in the United States who request permanent residence. (Source: Centers for Disease Control and Prevention, "Tuberculosis Among Foreign-Born Persons Entering the United States," *Morbidity and Mortality Weekly Report*, Public Health Services, U.S. Department of Health and Human Services, Vol. 39, No. RR-18, December 28, 1990)

Decision Trees in Webs of Causation

Decision trees have been used as decision making tools with regard to administration of pharmaceuticals, medical diagnoses, emergency care decision making, health screening, communicable disease investigation, and other related activities. In chronic disease and behaviorally caused diseases and disorder investigations, decision trees are supportive to the web investigation process. In webs of causation, decision trees are not techniques in and of themselves, but assist the web investigation method. Multiple decisions may be used in complex disorders with multiple risk factors, multiple exposures and agents, such as found in heart disease, stroke and cancer.

In order to understand how decision trees work, Figure 12.3 is provided. Diamond shaped boxes represent decision points. Rectangular boxes represent activities; "yes" and "no" decision points are indicated and arrows show the direction to the next activity or decision point. Decision trees can reroute activities back toward the beginning if certain criteria are not met or the decision falls short of meeting expectations. Decision trees are followed until the final step is met, in the case of Figure 12.3, "No further action is the final result."[7]

Using the decision tree technique within the web of causation may be less complex in some cases and may not require extensive decision trees for all risk factors. On the other hand, other certain risk factors may be quite complex and thus, the decision trees must also be complex. For example, in a hypothetical case of an outbreak of increased heart attacks in air traffic controllers, all risk factors would be listed and then decision trees would be developed for each risk factor or sub-element of the risk factor. For example, the risk factors considered might be stress, smoking or tobacco use, drug use, illicit drug use, alcohol use, age, hours worked, years in profession, emotional stability, personal problems, social problems, sleep habits, physical fitness, and diet and nutrition. Using diet and nutrition as an example, a decision tree could be constructed on eating habits and food selection, vitamin and nutrient intake, fat consumption and cholesterol levels, salt intake, sugar and caffeine consumption.

Fish Bone Diagrams (Cause-Effect Diagrams)

Fish bone diagrams (Figure 12.4) are also referred to as **cause-and-effect diagrams** and are developed to provide a visual presentation of all possible factors that could contribute to a disease, disability, or death. Fish bone diagrams assist the epidemiologist when trying to define, determine, uncover, or eliminate possible causes.

The first step in the fish bone diagram activity is to brainstorm lists of all potential causes or contributing risk factors. The fish bone diagram is then constructed by placing the categories of causes on the "bones" of the diagrams, making it a visual display for easy study and analysis. The second step is to develop subcategories of all specific causes for each of the major category areas. Each branch of the fish bone is given a label or becomes a category and subcategories are placed on the lines that make up the bones. A third level of cause or tertiary level is possible to add to the bones of the diagram. The head of the fish bone is a box that contains the *effect* or outcome which is the disease, disability, condition, injury or death. The diagram is finished when all possible risk factors or causes have been properly placed

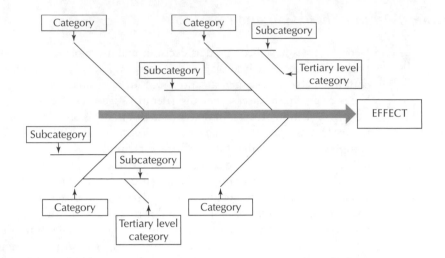

FIGURE 12.4   Example of construction of fish bone diagram.

within the categories and subcategories in the diagram on the lines that create the fish bone effect. An outline of the categories, subcategories, and tertiary levels can be developed and presented as well. An assessment of the cause-effect relationship statements of facts of occurrence at the tertiary, subcategory, and category levels are made for each and every one. The statements are answered *yes* or *no*, or are answered *true* or *not true*.

CHRONIC DISEASE, BEHAVIORALLY CAUSED, AND NONCOMMUNICABLE DISEASE EPIDEMIOLOGICAL STUDIES (SOME EXAMPLES)

Chronic disease epidemiology and studies of disorders caused by occupation, environmental agents, lifestyle, behavior, and other noncommunicable disease factors have surfaced as the new epidemiology of the future. Epidemiology has been used in a variety of noninfectious disease situations and in many unusual circumstances found to be detrimental to the health status of selected groups and populations. Below are several examples of chronic disease (see also Figure 12.5), behaviorally caused and noncommunicable disease epidemiological studies.

Pedestrian Deaths in New Mexico—Retrospective Study

Pedestrian fatalities constitute approximately one seventh of all traffic-related deaths in the United States. In New Mexico, approximately half of the population are minorities, mostly Hispanics and Native Americans. Death rates due to injury for these groups are substantially higher than national rates, especially for Native Americans.[8]

Vital records on pedestrian fatalities for 1958–1987 were analyzed. Cases met the International Classification of Disease definitions for motor vehicle traffic-related deaths.

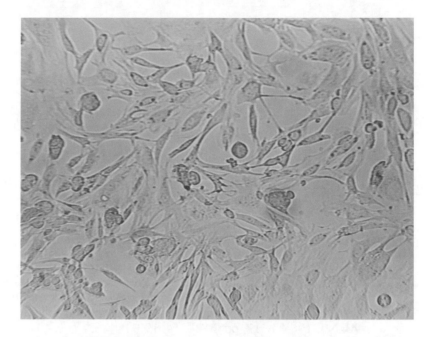

FIGURE 12.5   This is a picture of the enteroviruses that cause infectious hepatitis or viral hepatitis A. Chronic diseases can be caused by certain infections. If victims of hepatitis A do not recover, they may get chronic liver disease. Cirrhosis of the liver can result if persons who acquire hepatitis remain untreated. In hepatitis C, chronic liver disease is most certain. (Picture courtesy of Centers for Disease Control and Prevention, Atlanta, Georgia)

Ethnic classification came from information from death certificates. Denominators were obtained from U.S. Census Data from 1960, 1970, 1980, and were age-adjusted for the 1970 population. Most (87.4%) of the pedestrian fatalities were attributed to motor vehicle traffic; 7.7% were motor vehicle but nontraffic-related, 4.6% were train-related, and .03% were due to other vehicles, such as horse-drawn wagons. The rates were highest for Native American men age 35–44 years. Injury burden is disproportionally greater for minority groups. Rural living, lack of access to emergency transportation (lack of personal transportation for many Native Americans), and being struck at high speeds while walking increases likelihood of death. The implication of alcohol in the New Mexico study was not done. However, in the United States, 32.7% of the fatal pedestrian crashes involved pedestrians who were legally intoxicated. Figure 12.6 presents the age-specific pedestrian fatality rates for males by age group and race in New Mexico for years 1983–1987.[8]

In 1992, M.M. Gallaher, D.W. Fleming et al. completed a similar **retrospective study**. The Gallaher, Fleming et al. study was on pedestrian and hypothermia deaths among Native Americans in New Mexico. The study covered the dates of January 1–December 21, 1989, and added the element of hypothermia. This study reported that Native Americans were 8 times more likely to die in pedestrian motor vehicle accidents and were 30 times more likely to die of hypothermia compared to other New Mexico residents. Alcohol issues were also

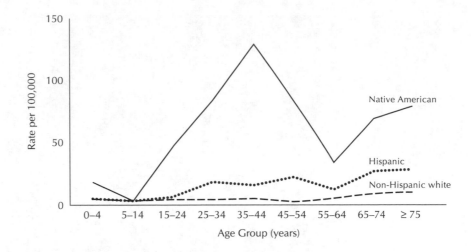

FIGURE 12.6   Age-specific pedestrian death rates for males, by age group and race for New Mexico, 1983–87. (Source: Centers for Disease Control and Prevention, "Pedestrian Fatalities—New Mexico, 1958–1987." *Morbidity and Mortality Weekly Report,* Public Health Service, U.S. Department of Health and Human Services, Vol. 40, No. 19, May 17, pp. 312–314, 1991)

included in this investigation. It was reported that at the time of death, 90% of those who were tested were highly intoxicated.[9]

A risk factor for pedestrian and hypothermia deaths for Native Americans is that of lack of transportation. Most Native Americans live on reservations, and most deaths occurred off the reservations in border towns or on roads connecting the communities to the reservations. Another risk factor, that would not obviously be regarded as one, is that of prohibition on the reservations. This forces Native Americans to travel to neighboring communities off the reservation, located long distances away, to drink alcohol. Native Americans also travel these distances to shop, visit family, attend college, seek entertainment, etc. All these factors, in the context of this study, become risk factors. Figure 12.7 is a dot map showing the deaths of Native Americans from pedestrian and hypothermia accidents.[9]

Death from Carbon Monoxide Gas Poisoning—Retrospective Investigation

During the Hippie Era of the late 1960s and 1970s, it was not uncommon to read a report of one or more persons dying in a micro-bus from trying to cook with charcoal briquettes within the confined space of the closed van. Burning charcoal briquettes produces almost pure carbon monoxide and makes for a serious and most always fatal result.

In December of 1990, three children, ages 6, 10, and 11 died from carbon monoxide (CO) poisoning from inhalation of this gas while riding under a camper shell in the back of their parents' pickup truck. Death from CO poisoning is preventable. At various stops the children appeared to be healthy. At 50 miles the children were fine and had no complaints. At 250 and 550 miles they appeared to be sleeping. Upon arrival at their destination, the children could not be aroused. Resuscitation attempts were unsuccessful. Passengers in

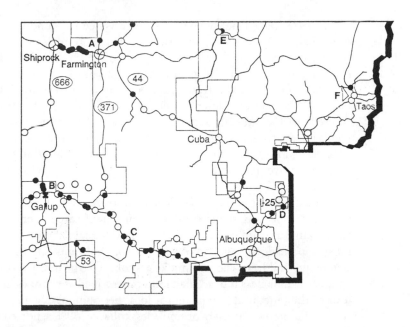

FIGURE 12.7   Dot map of deaths of Native Americans due to pedestrian accidents and hypothermia accidents in northwest New Mexico. (Source: Gallaher, M.M., Flemming, D.W., Berger, L.R., and Sewell, C.M. "Pedestrian and Hypothermia Deaths Among Native Americans in New Mexico," *Journal of the American Medical Association*, Vol. 267, No. 10, March 11, 1992, pp. 1345–1349)

the cab of the truck were asymptomatic. Autopsy examinations revealed lethal carboxyhemoglobin levels. An inspection of the 1970 model pickup showed that the muffler had been replaced but was not securely joined and several holes in the wall of the truck bed allowed the fumes to enter the enclosed bed. Negative pressure allowed a vacuum to form and the CO gases were sucked into the back of the pickup.[11]

Of 68 deaths attributed to CO poisoning in vehicles in Maryland, 1966–1971, older vehicles were implicated; 51 out of the 68 were older and had defective exhaust systems and holes in the vehicle.

Since 1968 the average quantity of CO produced by new cars has been reduced by more than 90%. Compliance with the Clean Air Act and improved engineering has helped reduce the risks. Preventive maintenance also is important in reducing the risk.[12]

Use of Smokeless Tobacco—Cross-Sectional Study

Increases in smokeless tobacco use by pre-adolescent and adolescent males is of national concern. Smokeless tobacco products have become more popular among students in schools across the United States. National data indicate that 8–36% of male high school- and college age- students use smokeless tobacco products regularly. An 11% usage rate among 8- to 9-year-olds and an overall average age of first use of 10.4 years of age (5th graders) was seen in the United States in 1986.

In 1985, Dane County Youth Survey in Wisconsin conducted a cross-sectional survey of students in grades 7–12 and showed that more males used smokeless tobacco than smoked cigarettes. Some of the findings included 45% of 8th grade boys had tried smokeless tobacco at least once. Regular use of smokeless tobacco products increased from 9% of 7th grade boys to 22% of 12th grade boys. Fifteen percent of 12th grade boys were daily users. Wisconsin's Division of Health's Project Model Health for Rural Wisconsin Schools showed that 12 years (7th grade) is the mean age of initiating smokeless tobacco use. Among regular users, students chew or dip smokeless tobacco an average of 6 times per day, with 25% partaking over 10 times per day, for an average duration of one hour. It is projected that one in five pre-adolescent and adolescent males in Wisconsin are regular smokeless tobacco users.[13]

The disease effects of smokeless tobacco are not well recognized. Smokeless tobacco products, especially moist snuff, contain potent carcinogens. A strong association between snuff use and oral cancer has been well established. Carcinogens are found in the most popular forms of smokeless tobacco. Oral tissue changes have been reported for school age children who use smokeless tobacco. In rural Colorado, 62.5% of teenagers who used smokeless tobacco had lesions described as changes in texture, color, and contour of the mucousal lining, and/or local periodontal degeneration. Other studies have shown that in regular users of smokeless tobacco, 39% reported white, wrinkled patches (Leukoplakia) and 37% reported a sore, ulcer, blister, or lesion of the gums, lips, or mouth. It has been estimated that 1–18% of leukoplakia transforms into malignancies. Nicotine has been associated with contributing to coronary artery and peripheral vascular disease, hypertension, peptic ulcer disease, and fetal morbidity and mortality.[13]

Regional Variation in Smoking Prevalence and Quit Ratios— Cross-Sectional Study

Smoking has reached its lowest level in 3 decades, with cigarette consumption as low as 24% in 1992. In 1986, it was found in the Behavior Risk Factor Surveillance System (BRFSS) survey that smoking rates varied from 18% to 35%. Geographical variation in smoking rates was studied and found to vary by region.

Health departments in 25 states and the District of Columbia collected data by random-digit dialing by telephone from persons 18 years and older, with an average of 1,200 (approximately 31,200 subjects) per year for each state for 1986. Every smoker (100 or more cigarettes in lifetime), current smokers and former smokers were determined. When ranked according to smoking rates and quit ratios for each state, it was found that the states with the highest smoking rates were all clustered east of the Mississippi River, primarily along the Ohio River Valley. When ranked according to quit ratios, states with the highest quit ratios were widely distributed geographically. States with the lowest quit ratios were clustered east of the Mississippi River. The western and northern states had the highest rates of persons quitting smoking. Figure 12.8 shows the geographic distribution of "current smoker" rates in the United States (selected states) for 1986. Figure 12.9 shows the geographic distribution of smoking quit ratios in the U.S. (selected states) for 1986.

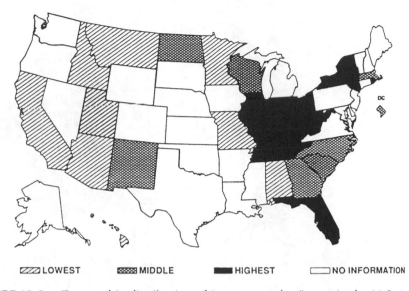

FIGURE 12.8 Geographic distribution of "current smoker" rates in the U.S. (selected states) for 1986. (Source: Centers for Disease Control and Prevention, "Regional Variation in Smoking Prevalence and Cessation: Behavioral Risk Factor Surveillance, 1986," *Chronic Disease and Health Promotion Reprints from the MMWR, 1985–1989, Vol. 2, Tobacco Topics*, Public Health Service, U.S. Department of Health and Human Services, pp. 36–38, 1991)

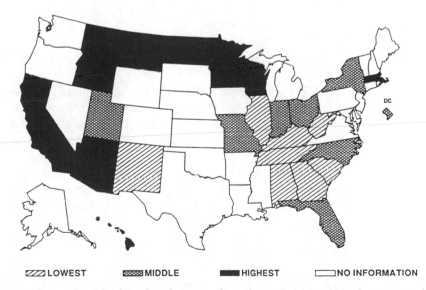

FIGURE 12.9 Geographic distribution of smoking quit ratios in the U.S. (selected states) for 1986. (Source: Centers for Disease Control and Prevention, "Regional Variation in Smoking Prevalence and Cessation: Behavioral Risk Factor Surveillance, 1986," *Chronic Disease and Health Promotion Reprints from the MMWR, 1985–1989, Vol. 2, Tobacco Topics*, Public Health Service, U.S. Department of Health and Human Services, pp. 36–38, 1991)

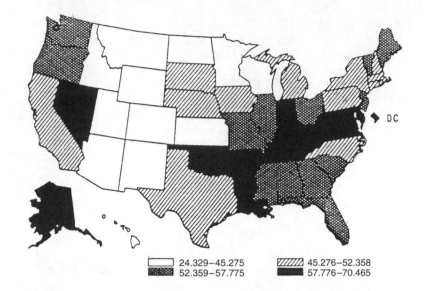

☐ 24.329–45.275		▨ 45.276–52.358	
▓ 52.359–57.775		■ 57.776–70.465	

FIGURE 12.10   Map of lung cancer mortality in the United States in 1986. (Rates are per 100,000 population.) (Source: Centers for Disease Control and Prevention, "Chronic Disease Reports: Deaths from Lung Cancer—United States, 1986," *Chronic Disease and Health Promotion Reprints from the MMWR, 1985–1989, Vol. 2, Tobacco Topics*, Public Health Service, U.S. Department of Health and Human Services, pp. 36–38, 1991)

Deaths from Lung Cancer in the United States—Prevalence Study

In the year 1986, 126,000 persons in the United States died from cancer of the trachea, bronchus, or lung. Lung cancer has increased by 15% overall from 1979 to 1986. Moreover, lung cancer has increased 7% among males and 44% among females. Lung cancer mortality rates increase with age, with 62% of lung cancer deaths occurring in persons age 65 and older.

Age-adjusted lung cancer mortality rates are higher in the southern and midwestern states. The highest age-adjusted lung cancer mortality is in Alaska (71 persons per 100,000 population). The lowest age-adjusted rates are in Utah (24 persons per 100,000 population).

The cause-effect relationships between cigarette smoking and lung cancer mortality have been extensively documented. Passive smoke has also been associated with increased risk for lung cancer. Numerous agents have been associated with lung cancer, radon case and asbestos fibers being the two most common factors. The risk associated with radon is estimated to be 6 to 11 times higher in smokers. Risk is also higher in asbestos workers who smoke, and higher for smokers who live in areas with high levels of air pollution.

The single most important means of controlling lung cancer in the United States is to eliminate cigarette smoking. Reduction of smoking would also decrease the numbers of smoking-related deaths, but a smoke-free population would be the best choice. Figure 12.10 presents a map of lung cancer mortality in the United States in 1986.

Occupational Lead Exposure and Strabismus in Offspring— Case Control Study

In the past, longitudinal studies have shown low-level lead exposure in children is a risk factor for cognitive, memory, perceptual, and motor impairment. One source of lead exposure for children is related to the occupation of the parents. Lead exposed mothers have shown high levels of umbilical cord blood lead levels and consequent elevated lead levels in children. Strabismus, or lazy eye, is when one eye fails in normal alignment, causing disruption in nervous system reflexes and visual images. In a **case-control study** in Maryland, 377 pediatric ophthalmology patients under age 7 were diagnosed with nonrestrictive strabismus. Mothers' worksites were assessed for lead exposure by industrial hygienists for the time period of conception through 9 months of age. Controls of 377 were established of similar race and sex distribution. The crude odds ratio for worksite lead exposure and esotropia was 2.6. Strabismus has been associated with neurological disturbance from exposures to cigarette smoking, and low birth weight. This study showed weak but positive association between maternal lead exposure and strabismus in offspring.[15]

Premature Births in California—Prevalence Study

Premature, preterm delivery is the greatest single cause of perinatal and neonatal morbidity in the United States and prematurity rates have increased during the last decade. Identified risk factors include mother's race, age, education, poor nutrition, weight gain during pregnancy, obstetric history, pre-existing diseases, complications, cigarette smoking, and drug use. Blacks have rates of prematurity double those of whites.

This **prevalence study** assessed 91% of all live births in California during 1989 and 1990. Excluded from analysis were multiple gestations, chromosomal abnormalities, and questionably long gestations. Preterm delivery was defined as a pregnancy with a gestation of less than 37 weeks. The Kessner index was used, which includes month of start of prenatal care, length of gestation, and total number of prenatal visits.

In California, Hispanic women had the largest number of preterm births, followed by white women. Table 12.2 presents preterm live births by race and ethnicity in California in 1989–1990.[16]

TABLE 12.2   Preterm births to females in California by race and ethnicity, 1989–1990[16]

% of Births by Race		Preterm Birth Rate (per 100 live births)	Relative Risk	% of Preterm Births
Total (100%)		9.55		100%
White	43%	7.55	1.00	34%
Hispanic	39	10.23	1.32	42
Black	8	16.41	2.01	14
Asians	6	9.34	1.22	6
Other	4	11.10	1.412	5

Epidemiology of Drug Use and Abuse—Cross-Sectional vs. Longitudinal Studies

Epidemiologists must recognize that using epidemiology to study chronic disorders necessitates a basic rethinking of approaches used in the past, while recognizing the limitations of **cross-sectional studies** in chronic disease investigations, especially if they do not include a range of age groups. The longitudinal study produces better results, though it is more difficult to do. Some factors to consider in drug use investigations include: When an attractive drug is readily available and is dependency-producing, one can assume it will be used in epidemic proportions; when a drug epidemic is recognized, it may be concentrated in one segment of the population, though not limited to any one social stratum or race; attractive drugs that cause dependence can be controlled by appropriate social effort and can be investigated epidemiologically; the epidemiologist must believe that abuse of any one drug may be checked and can be controlled, prevented and hopefully halted. Risk factors include: availability of the drug, lack of social controls and values, a market for the drug, severe population pressure, stress, social problems such as poverty and unemployment, societal values supportive of drug use, and drug-oriented mentality within society.[17]

Death Rates from Melanoma in White Men—Incidence and Retrospective Study

Deaths from malignant melanoma have increased in the United States disproportionally among white men. Incidence and death rates were obtained from the Surveillance, Epidemiology and End Results Program (SEER) of the National Cancer Institute and other databases.

From 1973 through 1988, the age-adjusted melanoma death rates for whites were higher for men than women. Among males, the death rate for malignant melanoma increased faster than any other cancer. The overall increase in the death rate was 50% for men and 21% for women. The greatest rise in deaths from melanoma occurred among men aged 50 years and older, with a peak increase of 78% for men aged 80–84 years. Incidence rates were nearly equal for white males and white females, age 40–44 years, but were higher for men age 50–54 than women. The incidence rates more than double for men age 65–69, than for women. The risk factors for malignant melanoma are unclear, but probably include sun exposure, presence of many and unusual moles, and a genetic predisposition. Figure 12.11 presents the melanoma death rates for white males and females by age group from years 1973 to 1988.

Diabetes Mellitus—Cross-Sectional Survey Study

From March of 1989 to 1990, an estimated 21.9 million people visited a physician, at which time the principal diagnosis was diabetes mellitus. Only 5% of the visits were made by new patients. The study is based on the National Ambulatory Medical Care Survey. More than half of the visits (57.5) were by females, 86.3% aged 45 years and over, with 79.3% being white. The visit rate to a physician for diabetes was 5.4 per 100 persons per year, and visit rates rose with age with significant increases seen in the 45–64 age group. Of all physician office visits in 1989, diabetes mellitus was the seventh most frequently reported principal

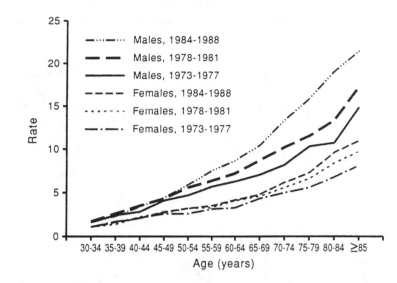

FIGURE 12.11   Melanoma of the skin death rates for white males and females in the United States, age-adjusted, 1973–1988. Per 100,000 population, adjusted to the 1970 U.S. standard population. (Source: Centers for Disease Control and Prevention, "Death Rates of Malignant Melanoma Among White Men—United States, 1973–1988," *Morbidity and Mortality Weekly Report,* Public Health Service, U.S. Department of Health and Human Services, Vol. 41, No. 2, January 17, pp. 20–21 and 27, 1992)

diagnosis and the fourth most frequently reported morbidity related principal diagnosis after essential hypertension, otitis media, and acute upper respiratory infections. (See Figure 12.12 and Figure 12.13.) General practice/family practice and internal medicine were the two most common types of physicians seen.[19]

Drinking and Driving and Binge Drinking—Cross-Sectional Prevalence Survey Study

Persons aged 18 and over in 12 states responded "one or more times," to two questions: (1) "During the past month, how many times have you driven when you've had perhaps too much to drink?" (2) "Considering all types of alcoholic beverages, that is, beer, wine, liquor as drinks, how many times during the past month did you have five or more drinks on one occasion?"

Data showed a decrease in drinking and driving among males 35 to 54 years of age between 1982–1985, but not among males 18–34 years of age, or males over age 55. Females show lower prevalence than males. A significant proportion of the 12 states reported a decrease in binge drinking among males 18 to 34 years of age and males 35 to 54 years of age as well as the 55 years and older group. A majority of statistics also showed a decrease in binge drinking for females, with a statistically significant decrease shown in the 18–34 years of age group.[20]

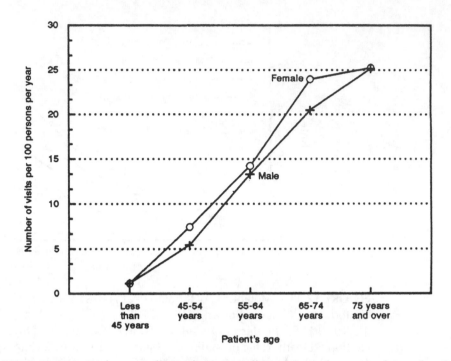

FIGURE 12.12   Diabetes mellitus physician office visit rate by age and sex of patients in the United States, 1989. (Source: Office of Vital and Health Statistics, "Office Visits for Diabetes Mellitus: United States, 1989," *Advanced Data*, Centers for Disease Control and Prevention, National Center for Health Statistics, Public Health Service, U.S. Department of Health and Human Services, No. 211, March 24, 1992)

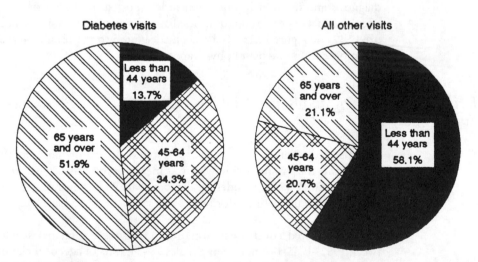

FIGURE 12.13   Percent of diabetes mellitus and all other diagnoses in physician office visits by age patients in the United States, 1989. (Source: Office of Vital and Health Statistics, "Office Visits for Diabetes Mellitus: United States, 1989," *Advanced Data*, Centers for Disease Control and Prevention, National Center for Health Statistics, Public Health Service, U.S. Department of Health and Human Services, No. 211, March 24, 1992)

PREVENTION AND CONTROL: A HALLMARK OF EPIDEMIOLOGY

The aim of epidemiology is in support of the major and key public health activities of prevention and control of diseases in populations. Epidemiology, being investigative in approach, must not lose sight of the reason for the investigations, that is, prevention and control. The future health status of the United States and other advanced societies must rely on prevention and abandon the past failures of trying to solve all health and medical problems by intervention after the disease, disorder, disability, or condition has occurred. The after-the-fact crisis intervention approach now used extensively is not only costly both financially and in human suffering terms, but makes little scientific or common sense. Prevention, health promotion, and protection against disease must be the approach of choice for government and political entities for populations and individuals.

The Institute of Medicine's Committee on the Study of the Future of Public Health recommended several functions for local public health units for the future:

- No citizen from any community, no matter how small or remote, should be without identifiable and realistic access to benefits of public health protection.

- Assessment, monitoring, and surveillance of local health problems and needs and resources for dealing with them.

- Policy development and leadership that foster local involvement and a sense of ownership, that emphasize local needs and that advocate equitable distribution of public resources and complementary private activities commensurate with community needs.

- Assurance that high quality services, including personal health services, needed for the protection of public health in the community are available and accessible to all persons; that the community receives proper consideration in the allocation of federal and state as well as local resources for public health and that the community is informed about how to obtain public health including personal health services and how to comply with public health requirements.[21]

The American Public Health Association, the national organization for state health officers, county health officials and local health officers and the U.S. Public Health Service developed what became known as the *Model Standards: A Guide for Community Preventive Health Services*, which has served as guide and a set of standards for organizing public health activities at the local level. The *Model Standards* lists 34 categories of public health services which should be available at the local level. In Table 12.3 is a list of the prevention, health promotion and protection services, from the list of 34 categories that should be found at the local public health department.

QUALITY OF ADJUSTED LIFE YEARS/*HEALTHY PEOPLE 2000*

Preventive services have played a key role in reducing preventable illness, injury, disability, and premature death. Considerable effort has been devoted to developing a comprehensive measure of the health of the nation that combines morbidity and mortality. The quality-adjusted life year (QALY) has emerged as one of the best measures of health status as it combines both mortality and morbidity. QALY is sensitive to changes in health among both the well and the ill.

TABLE 12.3   Model standards: A guide for community preventive health services, 34 areas in which to set standards for organizing public health activities at the local level

Model Standards: A Guide for Community Preventive Health Services	
Administration and Supporting Services	Maternal and Child Health
Aging and Dependent Populations	Mental Health
Air Quality	Noise Control
Alcohol and Drug Abuse and Addiction	Nutrition Services
Chronic Disease Control	Occupational Safety and Health
Communicable Disease Control	Primary Care
Immunizations	Radiological Health
Sexually Transmitted Diseases	Sanitation in Facilities
Tuberculosis	Child Care Facilities
Dental Health	All Public Buildings
Emergency Medical Services	Mobile Home Parks
Epidemiology and Surveillance	Recreational Areas
Family Planning	Schools
Food Protection	School Health
Genetic Disease Control	Solid Waste Management
Health Education	Tobacco Use and Addiction
Home Health Services	Toxic and Hazardous Substances
Housing Services	Vector and Animal Control
Injury Control	Violent and Abusive Behavior
Institutional Services	Water (Safe Drinking)
Laboratory Services	

(Source: American Public Health Association, the National Organizations for State Health Officers, County Health Officials and Local Health Officers and the U.S. Public Health Services)[20]

The calculation of the years of health life or quality-adjusted life years requires two sets of data. The first set of data is a life table of the population of people living and dying in age interval and secondly, the average number of years of life remaining at the beginning of each age interval. The measures of well-being include measures of mental, physical, and social functioning. By multiplying the measure of well-being by the number of years of life remaining at each age interval, an estimate of the years of healthy life is derived for a population group. The use of the years of health life indicator represents an innovation in the type of measures used to portray the health of the nation. As the life span expands the tradeoffs between quantity and quality of life are becoming more and more critical. The years of health life is an important indicator for populations and must be considered in policy and public health administration activities.[3]

PRIORITIES FOR PREVENTION AND HEALTH PROMOTION ACTIVITIES RELATED TO EPIDEMIOLOGY

Epidemiologists should understand and select priorities for projects based on factors that will affect the public's health status in a positive way. The prevailing health problems for a given population and how they affect the population group must be considered.

The following questions can be used in selecting prevention and health promotion activities.

1. Which disease, disorder, or condition has the greatest impact on illness, disability, injury, lost work time or school time, unnecessarily using up health resources, rehabilitation costs, causing family disruption, economic impact, and costs?

2. Are special populations or groups of people suffering from exposures to diseases, agents, risk factors, or hazards?

3. Which susceptible populations are most likely to respond to prevention, intervention, and control measures?

4. Which risk factors, diseases, agents, or hazards are most likely to respond to control measures?

5. Are there diseases, disabilities, injuries, disorders, or conditions that need to be investigated, that are being overlooked, that are not being responded to by other organizations or agencies?

6. Of the many risk factors, diseases, agents or hazards, which would yield the greatest improved health status, social impact, and economic benefit to the target population?

7. Of the many risk factors, diseases, agents, or hazards, which are of national, regional, state, or local concern and of major priority for an epidemiological investigation?[8]

Three Levels of Prevention and the Natural Course of Diseases

The three levels of prevention were presented and defined in Chapter 1. The three levels of prevention (**primary, secondary**, and **tertiary prevention**) are presented in the center of Figure 12.14, with the natural course (also referred to as the "natural history of disease") of the disease shown above and in relation to the three levels of prevention. Activities and elements of each of the 5 areas: (1) health promotion, (2) health protection, (3) early diagnosis and treatment, (4) limiting disabilities, and (5) rehabilitation are presented as they correspond to the three levels of prevention. Figure 12.14 portrays the interrelationships of prevention and the course of a disease.

HEALTH BELIEF MODEL IN CHRONIC DISEASE EPIDEMIOLOGY

The **health belief model** has been used for many years as a theoretical foundation of fields of disease prevention, health education, and health promotion. The health belief model is based on the construct that the convictions one holds about a health phenomenon is true for them, at least that individual will cling to the idea and do the resultant behavior. The health belief model is used by researchers, health promotion professionals, and in public health activities to predict health or disease related behavior based on belief patterns. Chronic diseases are often a result of individuals believing in a health related (actually disease related) behavior long enough to develop a disease. For example, a person finds more pleasure from smoking than they have concerns about the health consequences of the behavior, especially over the long term. Four basic premises have been developed about health

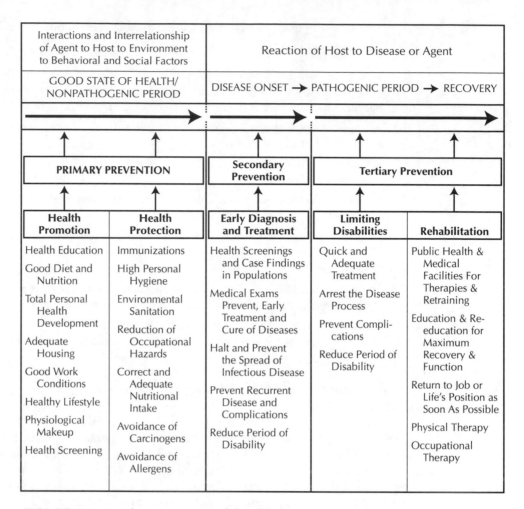

Interactions and Interrelationship of Agent to Host to Environment to Behavioral and Social Factors		Reaction of Host to Disease or Agent		
GOOD STATE OF HEALTH/ NONPATHOGENIC PERIOD		DISEASE ONSET → PATHOGENIC PERIOD → RECOVERY		
PRIMARY PREVENTION		**Secondary Prevention**	**Tertiary Prevention**	
Health Promotion	**Health Protection**	**Early Diagnosis and Treatment**	**Limiting Disabilities**	**Rehabilitation**
Health Education Good Diet and Nutrition Total Personal Health Development Adequate Housing Good Work Conditions Healthy Lifestyle Physiological Makeup Health Screening	Immunizations High Personal Hygiene Environmental Sanitation Reduction of Occupational Hazards Correct and Adequate Nutritional Intake Avoidance of Carcinogens Avoidance of Allergens	Health Screenings and Case Findings in Populations Medical Exams Prevent, Early Treatment and Cure of Diseases Halt and Prevent the Spread of Infectious Disease Prevent Recurrent Disease and Complications Reduce Period of Disability	Quick and Adequate Treatment Arrest the Disease Process Prevent Complications Reduce Period of Disability	Public Health & Medical Facilities For Therapies & Retraining Education & Re-education for Maximum Recovery & Function Return to Job or Life's Position as Soon As Possible Physical Therapy Occupational Therapy

FIGURE 12.14   The interaction of the three preventive measures of public health and the natural course of a disease.

and disease behavior patterns motivated by beliefs. Table 12.4 presents the four assumptions basic to the health belief model.[22]

Prevention is hard to measure and cannot always be demonstrated by empirical research, but, like quality, it is observable. Common sense dictates that prevention works and must be made the main focus of all health care and public health activity in order to maintain and improve the health status of populations. Fear and pain can be powerful motivational forces in changing behavior. However, to avoid chronic diseases, one must embrace healthy behaviors and lifestyles long before pain or fear occurs. Prevention and control of diseases, disorders, injuries, disabilities, and death in populations remains the primary purpose for the existence of epidemiology.

TABLE 12.4   Health belief model adapted for chronic disease epidemiology[22]

Four Premises of the Health Belief Model Applied to Chronic Disease Epidemiology

---

1. A person or population must believe that their health is at risk.

2. The person or population must sense the potential seriousness of the disease, condition or disorder, or the risk factors that contribute to it, in order to want it stopped.

3. The person or population must feel vulnerable to the disease, perceive themselves as having a susceptibility to it, and believe that the benefits from the change outweigh the costs, inconveniences and are within their grasp.

4. The individual or population must perceive a meaningful outcome and a cure for the action to happen must exist in order to motivate a response.

EXERCISES

Key Terms

Define and explain the following terms.

at-risk behavior

case-control study

cause and effect diagram

cross-sectional study

decision tree

fish bone diagram

health belief model

multiple exposures

odds ratio in chronic disease

predisposing factor

prevalence study

primary prevention

retrospective study

risk factor

secondary prevention

tertiary prevention

web of causation

Study Questions

12.1   Below is a study on assessment of overweight persons in the United States. Respond to the following questions.

a.   What type of study would this be classified as? Why?

b.   What are several limitations and problems with this study? Explain and discuss in detail.

c.   How could you improve this study and make it more valid?

An estimated 35 million adults are overweight in the United States. Being overweight increases the risk of chronic diseases such as diabetes, hypertension, and some types of cancer.

To examine patterns of overweight adults by geographic location, data were obtained from prevalence estimates from 32 states and the District of Columbia. Participating states were divided into four regions (West, Northeast, South, and Midwest) based on 1984 census divisions. State health departments collected data on behavioral risk factors using random-digit-dialed telephone interviews of adults 18 years of age and older. Prevalence estimates, obtained from self-reported weights and heights, were adjusted for age, sex, and race distribution of each state's population.

Overweight was defined as a body mass index (BMI = weight [kg]/height [m]), 27.8 or greater for males and 27.3 or greater for females. These values represent the sex-specific 85th percentile of BMI for U.S. adults age 20–29 years.

Overall, the prevalence of overweight ranged from a high of 25.7% in Wisconsin and Indiana to a low of 15.2% in New Mexico. Among men, the prevalence of overweight ranged from 26.9% in Wisconsin to 15.1% in Arizona. For women, the prevalence ranged from 25.8% in the District of Columbia to 13.7% in Hawaii. The median prevalence of overweight was 21.8% for men and 21.1% for women.

The median prevalence of overweight by region was lowest in the west (17%), followed by the Northeast (19.8%), the South (22.0%), and the Midwest (23.1%). Adjusting for regional population distribution by age, sex, and race did not change this pattern. Compared with the median prevalence of overweight for all 33 states (21.1%), the median prevalence by region is lower in the West and Northeast and higher in the South and Midwest. (Source: Centers for Disease Control and Prevention, "Prevalence of Overweight—Behavioral Risk Factor Surveillance System—1987," *Chronic Disease and Health Promotion Reprints from the MMWR, 1985–1989, Vol. 2, Tobacco Topics*, Public Health Service, U.S. Department of Health and Human Services, pp. 36–38, 1991).

12.2   Research, plan, develop, and construct a disease centered web of causation for the disease osteoporosis.

12.3   a.   Compare and contrast chronic disease with acute infectious disease with regards to time, place, and person issues, and disease clustering.

      b.   What is the relationship between chronic diseases and lifestyle and behaviors?

12.4   Research, develop, and construct a general problem centered web of causation for illicit drug abuse and for alcoholism.

12.5   Study the case and exhibits on pedestrian deaths in New Mexico (Figures 12.6 and 12.7) and develop a web of causation for this mortality problem.

12.6   a.   Review and study Table 12.1 and then explain the role of socially related factors on chronic disease and cause related risk factors.

      b.   Explain the role of behaviorally related factors on chronic disease and cause related risk factors.

12.7   Based on Figure 12.3 and the supportive concepts of decision trees as a part of a web of causation, develop and explain a decision tree supportive to a web of causation on alcoholism.

REFERENCES

1. *A Profile of Older Americans—1989*. Program Resources Department, American Association of Retired Persons and the Administration of Aging.
2. Porterfield, J.D., and R. St. Pierre. 1992. *Healthful Aging*. Guilford, CT: Dushkin Publishing.
3. Public Health Service. 1992. *Healthy People 2000: National Health Promotion and Disease Prevention Objectives*. U.S. Department of Health and Human Services. Boston: Jones and Bartlett Publishers Inc.
4. Evans, A.S. 1976. Causation and Disease: The Henle-Koch Postulates Revisited. *The Yale Journal of Biology and Medicine*, Vol. 49, No. 2, pp. 175–195.
5. Centers for Disease Control and Prevention. 1992. *Chronic Disease and Health Promotion Reprints from MMWR, 1985–1989*. Public Health Services, U.S. Department of Health and Human Services.

6. National Centers for Health Statistics. 1991. *Health in the United States—1990*. Public Health Services, U.S. Department of Health and Human Services.

7. National Cancer Institute. 1992. *Strategies to Control Tobacco Use in the United States*. Public Health Services, U.S. Department of Health and Human Services.

8. Green, L.W., and M.W. Krueter. 1991. *Health Promotion Planning: An Educational and Environmental Approach*. Mountain View, CA: Mayfield Publishing.

9. Centers for Disease Control and Prevention. 1990. *Tuberculosis Among Foreign-Born Persons Entering the United States, Morbidity and Mortality Weekly Report*. Public Health Services, U.S. Department of Health and Human Services, Vol. 39, No. RR-18, December, 28.

10. Gallaher, M.M., D.W. Flemming, L.R. Berger, and C.M. Sewell. 1992. "Pedestrian and Hypothermia Deaths Among Native Americans in New Mexico," *Journal of the American Medical Association*, Vol. 267, No. 10, pp. 1345–1349, March 11.

11. Centers for Disease Control and Prevention. 1991. "Pedestrian Fatalities—New Mexico, 1958–1987, *Morbidity and Mortality Weekly Report*. Public Health Service, U.S. Department of Health and Human Services, Vol. 40, No. 19, May 17, pp. 312–314.

12. Centers for Disease Control and Prevention. 1991. "Fatal Carbon Monoxide Poisoning in a Camper-Truck—Georgia," *Morbidity and Mortality Weekly Report*. Public Health Service, U.S. Department of Health and Human Services, Vol. 40, No. 1, March 8, pp. 154–155.

13. Centers for Disease Control and Prevention. 1991. "Use of Smokeless Tobacco—Wisconsin," *Chronic Disease and Health Promotion Reprints from the MMWR, 1985–1989. Vol. 2. Tobacco Topics*. Public Health Service, U.S. Department of Health and Human Services, pp. 3–6.

14. Centers for Disease Control and Prevention. 1991. "Regional Variation in Smoking Prevalence and Cessation: Behavioral Risk Factor Surveillance, 1986," *Chronic Disease and Health Promotion Reprints from the MMWR, 1985–1989. Vol. 2. Tobacco Topics*. Public Health Service, U.S. Department of Health and Human Services, pp. 36–38.

15. Hakim, R.B., W. F. Stewart, J.K. Canner, and J.M. Tielsch. 1991. "Occupational Lead Exposure and Strabismus in Offspring: A Case-Control Study," *American Journal of Epidemiology*, Vol. 133, No. 4, pp. 351–356.

16. Infectious Disease Branch. 1992. "Preterm Births in California, 1989–1990: An Epidemiologic Profile," California Morbidity. Department of Health Services, California Health and Welfare Agency, #23/#24, June 12.

17. Lipscomb, W.R. 1971. "An Epidemiology of Drug Use-Abuse," *American Journal of Public Health*, Vol. 61, No. 9, pp. 1794–1800, September.

18. Centers for Disease Control and Prevention. 1992. "Death Rates of Malignant Melanoma Among White Men—United States, 1973–1988," *Morbidity and Mortality Weekly Report*. Public Health Service, U.S. Department of Health and Human Services, Vol. 41, No. 12, January 17, pp. 20–21 and 27.

19. Office of Vital and Health Statistics. 1992. "Office Visits for Diabetes Mellitus: United States, 1989," *Advanced Data*. Centers for Disease Control and Prevention, National Center for Health Statistics, Public Health Service, U.S. Department of Health and Human Services, No. 211, March 24.

20. Centers for Disease Control and Prevention. 1991. "Drinking and Driving and Binge Drinking in Selected States, 1982–1985—The Behavioral Risk Factor Surveys," *Chronic Disease and Health Promotion Reprints from the MMWR, 1985–1989. Vol. 3. Behavioral Risk Factor Surveillance System*. Public Health Service, U.S. Department of Health and Human Services, pp. 8–10.

21. Committee for the Study of the Future of Public Health Division of Health Care Services. 1988. *The Future of Public Health. Institute of Medicine*, National Academy of Sciences. Washington, D.C.: National Academy Press.

22. Mullen, P.D., J. Hersey, and D.C. Iverson. 1987. "Health Belief Models Compared," *Social Science and Medicine*, Vol. 24, pp. 973–981.

I

Case Studies

I

Snow on Cholera

"On the Mode of Communication of Cholera," by John Snow, MD. (Excerpted and adapted from the original 1855 Edition as found in *Snow on Cholera* by John Snow, Commonwealth Fund: New York, 1936.)

About Dr. John Snow: John Snow was born 1813 and died in 1858. Dr. Snow was alive at the beginning of the golden era of bacteriology and infectious disease discovery and was actively involved in his professional pursuits at the time of Ignas Semmelweis, MD, Louis Pasteur (1822–1895) of France, and John Koch, MD (1843–1910) of Germany. At the time these scientists led the world in the discovery of microbes, vaccines and advanced scientific and biomedical knowledge about communicable diseases. Dr. Snow was a distinguished anesthesiologist in England, who, among other accomplishments, administered chloroform to Queen Victoria at the birth of two of her children. Dr. Snow is most famous for his cholera investigations, including the epidemic in the Soho District of London, where he removed the handle from the Broad Street pump as a move to halt the cholera epidemic.

(A) CHOLERA—EXAMPLES, CASES, AND OBSERVATIONS

Communication (Transmission) of Cholera

"There are certain circumstances, connected with the progress of cholera, which may be stated in a general way. Cholera travels along the great tracks more slowly. In extending to fresh inland or continent, it always appears first at a sea-port. It never attacks the crews of ships going from a country free from cholera, to one where the disease is prevailing, till they have entered a port or had intercourse with the shore. Its exact progress from town to town cannot always be traced; but it has never appeared except where there has been ample opportunity for it to be conveyed by human intercourse."

"There are also innumerable instances which prove the communication of cholera, by individual cases of the disease, in the most convincing manner. Instances such as the following seem free from every source of fallacy . . . I called lately to inquire respecting the death of Mrs. Gore, the wife of a labourer, from cholera, at New Leigham Road,

---

Presented in its original text form.

Streatham. I found that a son of the deceased had been living and working at Chelsea. He came home ill with a bowel complaint, of which he died in a day or two. His death took place on August 18th. His mother, who attended on him, was taken ill on the next day and died the day following (August 20th). There were no other deaths from cholera registered in any of the metropolitan districts, down to the 26th of August, within two or three miles of the above place; the nearest being at Brixton, Norwood, or Lower Tooting . . .”

"John Barnes, aged 39, an agricultural labourer, became severely indisposed on the 28th of December, 1832; he had been suffering from diarrhoea and cramps for two days previously. He was visited by Mr. George Hopps, a respectable surgeon at Redhouse, who, finding him sinking into collapse, requested an interview with his brother, Mr. J. Hopps, of York. This experienced practitioner at once recognized the case as one of Asiatic cholera; immediately enquired for some probable source of contagion, but in vain: no such source could be discovered. When he repeated his visit on the day following, the patient was dead; but Mrs. Barnes (the wife), Matthew Metcalfe, and Benjamin Muscroft, two persons who had visited Barnes on the preceding day, were all labouring under the disease, but recovered. John Foster, Ann Dunn, and widow Creyke, all of whom had communicated with the patients above named, were attacked by premonitory indisposition, which was however arrested. Whilst the surgeons were vainly endeavouring to discover whence the disease could possibly have arisen, the mystery was all at once, and most unexpectedly, unravelled by the arrival in the village of the son of the deceased John Barnes. This young man was apprentice to his uncle, a shoemaker, living in Leeds. He informed the surgeons that his uncle's wife (his father's sister) had died of cholera a fortnight (2 weeks/14 days) before that time, and that, as she had no children, her wearing apparel had been sent to Monkton by a common carrier. The clothes had not been washed; Barnes had opened the box in the evening; on the next day he had fallen sick of the disease."

"During the illness of Mrs. Barnes, her mother, who was living in Tockwith, a healthy village five miles distant from Moor Monkton, was requested to attend her. She went to Monkton accordingly, remained with her daughter for two days, washed her daughter's linen, and sent out on her return home, apparently in good health. Whilst in the act of walking home she was seized with the malady, and fell down in collapse on the road. She was conveyed home to her cottage, and placed by the side of her bedridden husband. He, and also the daughter who resided with them, took the malady. All the three died within two days. Only one other case occurred in the village of Tockwith, and it was not a fatal case."

"A man came from Hull (where cholera was prevailing), by trade a painter; his name and age are unknown. He lodged at the house of Samuel Wride, at Pocklington; was attacked on his arrival on the 8th of September, and died on the 9th. Samuel Wride himself was attacked on the 11th September, and died shortly afterwards . . ."

"Liverpool. (Mr. Henry Taylor, reporter.) A nurse attended a patient in Great Howard Street (at the lower part of the town), and on her return home, near Everton (the higher part of the town), was seized and died. The nurse who attended her was also seized, and died. No other case had occurred previously in that neighborhood, and none followed for about a fortnight . . ."

"It would be easy, by going through the medical journal and works which have been published on cholera, to quote as many cases similar to the above as would fill a large volume. But the above instances are quite sufficient to show that cholera can be communicated from the sick to the healthy; for it is quite impossible that even a tenth part of these cases of consecutive illness could have followed each other by coincidence, without being connected as cause and effect."

"Besides the facts above mentioned, which prove that cholera is communicated from person to person, there are others which show, first, that being present in the same room with a patient, and attending on him, do not necessarily expose a person to the morbid poison; and, secondly, that it is not always requisite that a person should be very near to a cholera patient in order to take the disease, as the morbid matter producing it may be transmitted to a distance. It used to be generally assumed, that if cholera were a catching or communicable disease it must spread by effluvia given off from the patient into the surrounding air, and inhaled by others into the lungs. This assumption led to very conflicting opinions respecting the disease. A little reflection shows, however, that we have no right thus to limit the way in which a disease may be propagated, for the communicable diseases of which we have a correct knowledge may spread in very different manners. The itch, and certain other diseases of the skin, are propagated in one way; syphilis, in another way; and intestinal worms in a third way, quite distinct from either of the others . . ."

Cholera Propagated by Morbid Material Entering the Alimentary Canal

"Diseases which are communicated from person to person are caused by some material which passes from the sick to the healthy, and which has the property of increasing and multiplying in the systems of the persons it attacks. In syphilis, smallpox, and vaccinia, we have physical proof of the increase of the morbid material, and in other communicable diseases the evidence of this increase, derived from the fact of their extension, is equally conclusive. As cholera commences with an affection of the alimentary canal, and as we have seen that the blood is not under the influence of any poison in the early stages of this disease, it follows that the morbid material producing cholera must be introduced into the alimentary canal—must, in fact be swallowed accidentally, for persons would not take it intentionally; and the increase of the morbid material or cholera poison, must take place in the interior of the stomach and bowels. It would seem that the cholera poison, when reproduced in sufficient quantity, acts as an irritant on the surface of the stomach and intestines, or what is still more probable, it withdraws fluid from the blood circulating in the capillaries, by a power analogous to that by which the epithelial cells of the various organs abstract the different secretions in the healthy body. For the morbid matter of cholera having the property of reproducing its own kind, must necessarily have some sort of structure, most likely that of a cell. It is no objection to this view that the structure of the cholera poison cannot be recognized by the microscope, for the matter of smallpox and chancre can only be recognized by their effects, and not by their physical properties."

"The period which intervenes between the time when a morbid poison enters the system, and the commencement of the illness which follows, is called the period of incubation. It is, in reality, a period of reproduction, with regards to the morbid matter; and the disease is due to the crop of progeny resulting from the small quantity of poison first introduced. In cholera, this period of incubation or reproduction is much shorter than in most other epidemic or communicable diseases. From the cases previously detailed, it is shown to be in general from 24 to 48 hours. It is owing to this shortness of the period of the period of incubation, and to the quantity of the morbid poison thrown off in the evacuations, that cholera sometimes spreads with a rapidity unknown in other diseases . . ."

"The instances in which minute quantities of the ejections and dejections of cholera patients must be swallowed are sufficiently numerous to account for the spread of the disease. Nothing has been found to favour the extension of cholera more than want of personal cleanliness whether arising from habit or scarcity of water. The bed linen nearly always becomes wetted by the cholera evacuations, and as these are devoid of the usual colour and odour, the hands of persons waiting on the patient become soiled without their knowing it; and unless these person are scrupulously clean in their habits and wash their hands before taking food, they must accidentally swallow some of the excretion, and leave some on the food they handle or prepare, which has to be eaten by the rest of the family. The post mortem inspection of bodies of cholera patients has hardly ever been followed by the disease that I am aware, this being a duty that is necessarily followed by careful washing of the hands; and it is not the habit of medical men to be taking food on such occasion. On the other hand, the duties performed about the body, such an as laying it out, when done by women of the working class, who make the occasion one of eating and drinking, are often followed by an attack of cholera; and persons who merely attend the funeral, and have no connexion with body frequently contract the disease, in consequence, apparently of partaking of food which has been prepared or handled by those having duties about the cholera patient, or his linen and bedding."

"The involuntary passage of the evacuations in most bad cases of cholera, must also aid in spreading the disease. Mr. Baker, of Staines, who attended 260 cases of cholera and diarrhoea in 1849, chiefly among the poor, informed me in a letter with which he favoured me in December of that year, that 'when the patients passed their stools involuntarily the disease evidently spread.' It is amongst the poor, where a whole family live, sleep, cook, eat and wash in a single room, that cholera has been found to spread once introduced, and still more in those places termed common lodging amongst the vagrant class, who lived in a crowded state, that cholera was most fatal in 1832; but the Act of Parliament for the regulation of common lodging houses, has caused the disease to be much less fatal amongst these people in the late epidemics. When, on the other hand, cholera is introduced into the better kind of houses, as it often is by means that will be afterwards pointed out, it hardly ever spreads from one member of the family to another. The constant use of the hand-basin and towel, and the fact of the apartments for cooking and eating being distinct from the sick room, are the cause for this."

"If the cholera had no other means of communication than those we have been considering, it would be constrained to confine itself chiefly to the crowded dwellings of the poor, and would be continually liable to die out accidentally in a place, for want of the opportunity to reach fresh victims; but there is often a way open for it to extend itself more widely and reach well-to-do classes of the community; I allude to the mixture of the cholera evacuations with the water used for drinking and culinary purposes, either by permeating the ground, and getting into the wells, or by running along channels and sewers into the rivers from which entire towns are sometimes supplied with water."

"In 1849 there were in Thomas Street, Horsleydown, two courts close together, consisting of a number of small houses or cottages, inhabited by poor people. The houses occupied one side of each court or alley—the south side of Trusscott's Court, and the north side of the other, which was called Surrey Buildings, . . . divided into small back areas in which situated the privies of both courts, communicating with the same drain, and there was an open sewer which passed the further end of both courts. In Surrey Buildings the cholera committed fearful devastation, whilst in the adjoining court there was but one fatal case, and another case that ended in recovery. In the former court, the slops of dirty water, poured down by the inhabitants into a channel in front of the houses, got into the well from which they obtained their water; this being the only difference that Mr. Grant, the Assistant Surveyor for the Commissioners of Sewers, could find between the circumstances of the two courts."

"In Manchester, a sudden and violent outbreak of cholera occurred in Hope Street, Salford. The inhabitants used water from a particular pump/well. This well had been repaired, and a sewer which passes within nine inches of the edge of it became accidentally stopped up, and leaked into the well. The inhabitants of 30 houses used the water from this well; among these there occurred 19 cases of diarrhoea, 26 cases of cholera, and 25 deaths. The inhabitants of 60 houses in the same immediate neighbourhood used other water; among these there occurred eleven cases of diarrhoea, but not a single case of cholera, nor one death. It is remarkable, that, in this instance, out of the 26 persons attacked with cholera, the whole perished except one."

"Dr. Thomas King Chambers informed me, that at Ilford, in Essex, in the summer of 1849, the cholera prevailed very severely in a row of houses a little way from the main part of town. It had visited every house in the row but one. The refuse which overflowed from the privies and a pigsty could be seen running into the well over the surface of the ground, and the water was very fetid: yet it was used by the people in all the houses except that which had escaped cholera. That house was inhabited by a woman who took linen to wash, and she, finding that the water gave the linen an offensive smell, paid a person to fetch water for her from the pump in the town, and this water she used for culinary purposes as well as for washing."

"The following circumstance was related to me, at the time it occurred, by a gentleman well acquainted with all the particulars. The drainage from the cesspools found its way into the well attached to some houses at Locksbrook, near Bath, and the cholera making its appearance there in the autumn of 1849, became very fatal. The people complained of the water to the gentleman belonging to the property, who lived at Weston, in Bath, and he sent a surveyor, who reported that nothing was the matter. The tenants still complaining, the owner went himself, and in looking at the water and smelling it, he said that he could perceive nothing the matter with it. He was asked if he would taste it, and drank a glass of it. This occurred on a Wednesday; he went home, was taken ill with the cholera, and died on the Saturday following, there being no cholera in his own neighbourhood at the time."

Case Study Questions

A.1   Concerning John Barnes, how was the cholera being communicated? What were the modes of disease transmission presented in the Barnes case? What is the correct epidemiological term for the modes of transmission that were identified?

A.2   How long is a fortnight?

A.3   In the examples or circumstances presented, what were the various modes of transmission stated or at least alluded to? Which were correct? Which were incorrect and why? What role did personal hygiene and sanitation (including food preparation and hand washing) play in the transmission of the disease and continuation of an outbreak?

A.4   Several instances of *association* (cause-effect relations) were presented or alluded to in the examples presented in the case. List the various instances of *association* you can identify from the examples or situations presented in the case. What role did social class, poverty and housing arrangements play in *association*? What role did water play in *association*?

A.5   Describe the disease cholera as presented in the Snow case. Describe in detail cholera as it is known today. (Assistance of a *Merck Manual* or *Control of Communicable Diseases in Man* by A.S. Benenson, published by the American Public Health Association or other disease book is suggested.)

A.6   What hypotheses were developed by Dr. Snow about the cause (etiology), signs and symptoms, spread and course of the cholera disease? How do the observations and hypotheses of Dr. Snow conform with modern understanding and knowledge of cholera? Give several examples that support it and several examples that do not support it.

A.7   What is different about those who do not get ill from the disease compared to those who got ill?

A.8   What epidemiological phenomenon can be observed in the Locksbrook, near Bath, example?

(B) CHOLERA AND THE BROAD STREET PUMP OUTBREAK

"The most terrible outbreak of cholera which ever occurred in this kingdom, is probably that which took place in Broad Street, Golden Square, and the adjoining streets, a few weeks ago. Within 250 yards of the spot where Cambridge Street joins Broad Street, there were upwards of 500 fatal attacks of cholera in 10 days. The mortality in this limited area probably equals any that was ever caused in this country, even by the plague; and it was much more sudden, as the greater number of cases terminated in a few hours. The mortality would undoubtedly have been much greater had it not been for the flight of the population. Persons in furnished lodgings left first, then other lodgers went away, leaving their furniture to be sent for when they could meet with a place to put it in. Many houses were closed altogether, owing to the death of the proprietors; and in a great number of instances, the tradesmen who remained had sent away their families: so that in less than six days from the commencement of the outbreak, the most afflicted streets were deserted by more than three-quarters of their inhabitants."

"There were a few cases of cholera in the neighbourhood of Broad Street, Golden Square, in the latter part of August and the so-called outbreak, which commenced in the night between the 31st August and the 1st of September, was, as in similar instances, only a violent increase of the malady. As soon as I became acquainted with the situation and extent of this irruption of cholera, I suspected some contamination of the water of the much frequented street-pump in Broad Street, near the end of Cambridge Street; but on examining the water, on the evening of the 3rd of September, I found so little impurity in it of an organic nature, that I hesitated to come to a conclusion. Further inquiry, however, showed me that there was no other circumstance or agent common to the circumscribed locality in which this sudden increase of cholera occurred, and not extending beyond it, except the water of the above mentioned pump. I found, moreover, that the water varied, during the next two days, in the amount of organic impurity, visible to the naked eye, on close inspection, in the form of small white flocculent particles; and I concluded that, at the commencement of the outbreak, it might possibly have been still more impure. I requested permission, therefore, to take a list, at the General Register Office, of the deaths from cholera, registered during the week ending 2nd September, in the subdistricts of Golden Square, Berwick Street, and St. Ann's Soho, which was kindly granted. Eighty-nine deaths from cholera, were registered, during the week, in the three subdistricts. (See Figure I.1) Of these, only 6 occurred in the 4 first days of the week. Four (4) occurred on Thursday, the 31st of August; and the remaining 79 on Friday and Saturday. I considered therefore, that the outbreak commenced on the Thursday; and I made inquiry, in detail, respecting the 83 deaths registered as having taken place during the last 3 days of the week."

"On proceeding to the spot, I found that nearly all the deaths had taken place within a short distance of the pump. There were only 10 deaths in houses situated decidedly nearer to another street pump. In 5 of these cases the families of the deceased persons informed me that they always sent to the pump in Broad Street, as they preferred the water to that of the pump which was nearer. In three other cases, the deceased were children who went to school near the pump in Broad Street. Two of them were known to drink the water; and the parents of the third think it probable that it did so. The other two deaths, beyond the district which this pump supplies, represent only the amount of mortality from cholera that was occurring before the irruption took place. (See Figure I.1, map of the Broad Street and Golden Square area of London.)"

"With regard to the deaths occurring in the locality belonging to the pump, there were 61 instances in which I was informed that the deceased persons used to drink the pump-water from Broad Street, either constantly or occasionally. In six instances I could get no information, owing to the death or departure of everyone connected with the deceased individuals; and in 6 cases I was informed that the deceased persons did not drink the pump-water before their illness. (See Figure I.1, map of the Broad Street and Golden Square area of London.)"

"The result of the inquiry then was that there had been no particular outbreak or increase of cholera, in this part of London, except among the persons who were in the habit of drinking water of the above mentioned pump-well."

"I had an interview with the Board of Guardians of St. James's parish, on the evening of Thursday, 7th September, and represented the above circumstances to them. In consequence of what I said, the handle of the pump was removed on the following day."

"The additional facts that I have been able to ascertain are in accordance with those above related; and as regards the small number of those attacked, who were believed not to have drank the water from the Broad Street pump, it must be obvious that there are various ways in which the deceased persons may have taken it without the knowledge of their friends. The water was used for mixing with spirits in all the public houses around. It was used likewise at dining rooms and coffee shops. The keeper of a coffee shop in the neighbourhood which was frequented by mechanics, and where the pump water was supplied at dinner time, informed me (on 6th September) that she was already aware of 9 of her customers who were dead. The pump-water was also sold in various little shops, with a tea-spoonful of effervescing powder in it, under the name of sherbet; and it may have been distributed in various other ways with which I am unacquainted. The pump was frequented much more than is usual, even for a London pump in a populous neighbourhood."

"There are certain circumstances bearing on the subject of this outbreak of cholera which required to be mentioned. The workhouse in Poland Street is more than three-fourths surrounded by houses in which deaths from cholera occurred, yet out of 535 inmates only 5 died of cholera, the other deaths which took place being those of persons admitted after they were attacked. The workhouse has a pump-well on the premises, in addition to the supply from the Grand Junction Water Works, and the inmates never sent to the Broad Street pump for water. If the mortality in the workhouse had been equal to that in the streets immediately surrounding it on three sides, upwards of 100 persons would have died."

"There is a brewery in Broad Street, near to the pump, and on perceiving that no brewer's men were registered as having died of cholera, I called on Mr. Huggins, the proprietor. He informed me that there were above 70 workmen employed in the brewery, and that none of them had suffered from cholera, at least in a severe form, only two having been -

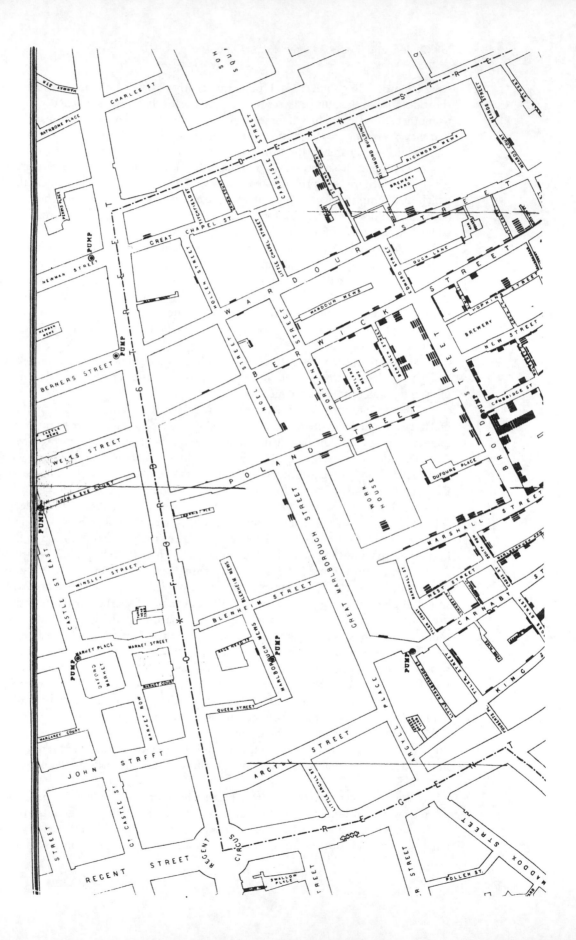

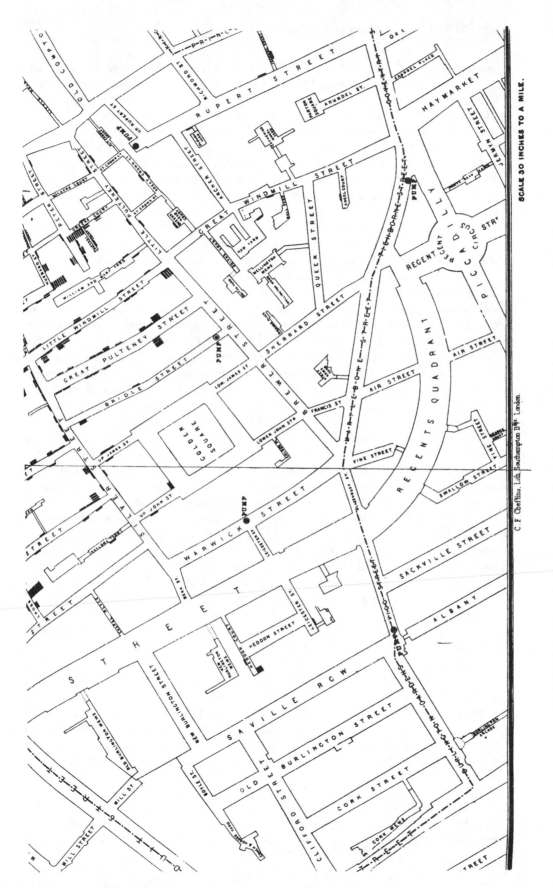

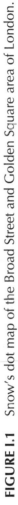

SCALE 30 INCHES TO A MILE.

C. F. Cheffins, Lith, Southampton B⁹⁹. London.

FIGURE I.1 Snow's dot map of the Broad Street and Golden Square area of London.

indisposed, and not that seriously, at the time the disease prevailed. The men are allowed a certain quantity of malt liquor, and Mr. Huggins believes they do not drink water at all; and he is quite certain that the workmen never obtained water from the pump in the street. There is a deep well in the brewery, in addition to the New River water."

"A 28 year old mother in the eighth month of pregnancy, went herself (although they were not usually water drinkers), on Sunday, 3rd September, to Broad Street pump for water. The family removed to Gravesend on the following day; and she was attacked with cholera on Tuesday morning at seven o'clock, and died of consecutive fever on 15th September, having been delivered. Two of her children drank also of the water, and were attacked on the same day as the mother, but recovered."

"In the 'Weekly Return of Births and Deaths' of September 9th, the following death is recorded as occurring in Hampstead district: At West End, on 2nd September, the widow of a percussion-cap maker, aged 59 years, diarrhoea two hours, cholera epidemic, 16 hours."

"I was informed by this lady's son that she had not been in the neighbourhood of Broad Street for many months. A cart went from Broad Street to West End every day, and it was the custom to take out a large bottle of the water from the pump in Broad Street, as she preferred it. The water was taken on Thursday, 31st August, and she drank of it in the evening, and also on Friday. She was seized with cholera on the evening of the latter day, and died on Saturday, as the above quotation from the register shows. A niece, who was on a visit to this lady, also drank of the water; she returned to her residence, in a high and healthy part of Islington, was attacked with cholera, and died also. There was no cholera at the time, either at West End or in the neighborhood where the niece died. Besides these two persons, only one servant partook of the water at Hampstead West End, and she did not suffer, or at least not severely. There were many persons who drank the water from the Broad Street pump about the time of the outbreak, without being attacked with cholera; but this does not diminish the evidence respecting the influence of the water, for reasons that will be fully stated in another part of this work. These activities are shown in Figure I.2, which presents the dates/chronological events of the Broad Street pump cholera epidemic."

"It is pretty certain that very few of the 56 attacks placed in the table to 31st August occurred till late in the evening of that day. The irruption was extremely sudden, as I learned from the medical men living in the midst of the district, and commenced in the night between the 31st August and 1st September. (See Figure I.2.) There was hardly any premonitory diarrhoea in the cases which occurred during the first three days of the outbreak; and I have been informed by several medical men, that very few of the cases which they attended on those days ended in recovery."

"The greatest number of attacks in any one day occurred on the 1st day of September, immediately after the outbreak commenced. The following day the attacks fell from 143 to 116 and the day afterwards to 54. A glance at Figure I.2 and Figure I.3 shows that the fresh attacks and deaths continued to become less numerous every day after 1st and 2nd of September. On September 8th—the day when the handle of the pump was removed—there were 12 attacks; on the 9th, 11 attacks; on the 10th and 11th 5 attacks and on the 12th only 1; after this time, there were never more than 4 attacks on one day. During the decline of the epidemic the deaths were more numerous than the attacks (compare Figure I.2 with Figure I.3.), owing to the decease of many persons who had lingered for several days in consecutive fever."

"There is no doubt the mortality was much diminished, by the flight of the population, which commenced soon after the outbreak; but the attacks had so far diminished before the use of the water was stopped, that it is impossible to decide whether the well still contained the cholera poison in an active state or whether, from some cause, the water had

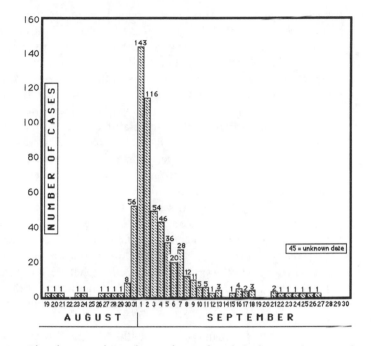

FIGURE I.2 The dates and numbers of **Attacks** of cholera in the Broad Street pump cholera epidemic, London.

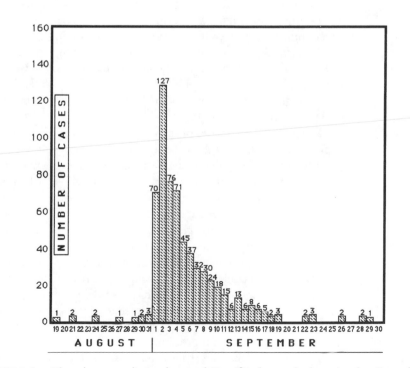

FIGURE I.3 The dates and numbers of **Deaths** from cholera in the Broad Street pump cholera epidemic, London.

become free from it. The pump-well has been opened, and I was informed by Mr. Farrell, the superintendent of the works, that there was no hole or crevice in the brickwork of the well, by which any impurity might enter; consequently in this respect the contamination of the water is not made out of the kind of physical evidence detailed in some of the instances previously related. I understand that the well is from 28 to 30 feet in depth, and goes through the gravel to the surface of the clay beneath. The sewer, which passes within a few yards of the well, is 22 feet below the surface. The water at the time of the cholera contained impurities of an organic nature, in the form of minute whitish flocculi visible on close inspection to the naked eye. Dr. Hassall, who was good enough to examine some of this water with a microscope, informed me that these particles had no organised structure, and he thought they probably resulted from decomposition of other matter. He found a great number of very minute oval animalcules in the water, which are of no importance except as an additional proof that the water contained organic matter on which they lived. The water also contained a large quantity of chlorides, indicating no doubt, the impure sources from which the spring is supplied. Mr. Eley, the percussion-cap manufacturer of 37 Broad street, informed me that he had long noticed that the water became offensive, both to the smell and taste, after it had been kept about two days. This, as I noticed before, is the character of water contaminated with sewage. Another person had noticed for months that a film formed on the surface of the water when it had been kept a few hours."

"I inquired of many persons whether they had observed any change in the character of the water, about the time of the outbreak of cholera, and was answered in the negative. I afterwards, however, met with the following important information on this point. Mr. Gould, the eminent ornithologist, lives near the pump in Broad Street, and was in the habit of drinking the water. He was out of town at the commencement of the outbreak of cholera, but came home on Saturday morning, 2nd September, and sent for some of the water almost immediately, when he was much surprised to find that it had an offensive smell, although perfectly transparent and fresh from the pump. He did not drink any of it. Mr. Gould's assistant, Mr. Prince, had his attention drawn to the water and perceived its offensive smell. A servant of Mr. Gould who drank the pump water daily, and drank a good deal of it on August 31st, was seized with cholera at an early hour on September 1st. She ultimately recovered."

"Whether the impurities of the water were derived from the sewers, the drains, or the cesspools, of which latter there are a number in the neighbourhood, I cannot tell. I have been informed by an eminent engineer, that whilst a cesspool in a clay soil requires to be emptied every six or eight months, one sunk in the gravel will often go for 20 years without being emptied, owing to the soluble matters passing away into the land-springs by percolation. As there had been deaths from cholera just before the great outbreak not far from this pump-well, and in a situation elevated a few feet above it, the evacuations from the patients might as a matter of course be amongst the impurities finding their way into the water, and judging the matter by the light derived from other facts and considerations previously detailed, we must conclude that such was the case. A very important point in respect to this pump-well is that the water passed with almost everybody as being perfectly pure, and it did in fact contain a less quantity of impurity than the water of some other pumps in the same parish, which had no share in the propagation of cholera. We must conclude from this outbreak that the quantity of morbid matter which is sufficient to produce cholera is inconceivably small, and that the shallow pump-wells in a town cannot be looked on with too much suspicion, whatever their local reputation may be."

"Whilst the presumed contamination of the water of the Broad Street pump with evacuations of cholera patients affords an exact explanation of the fearful outbreak of cholera in St. James's parish, there is no other circumstance which offers any explanation at all, whatever hypothesis of the nature and cause of the malady be adopted."

Case Study Questions

B.1   What are the **time** factors and implications for this case? Explain the time lag from Attacks in Figure I.2 to Deaths in Figure I.3.

B.2   What are the **place** factors and implications for this case? Compare the workhouse to the brewery to the pub. Discuss migration and its effect on the epidemic. What are **place** issues are important to this case?

B.3   What did the well persons do differently than the ill—those who got the disease (for example the inmates in the workhouse)?

B.4   From Figure I.2, what is the index case? What date is the beginning of the epidemic? What other **time** factors are discerned from this chart? How did Dr. Snow establish the time of onset?

B.5   What accurate observations were made about wells, cesspools and ground water, the purity of the water and its contamination? What inaccurate and misunderstood observations were made about the water, its flow and its contamination?

B.6   What evidence did Dr. Snow use to establish the fact that a cholera epidemic was occurring? Did Dr. Snow clearly demonstrate the cause and source of the outbreak of cholera in the Golden Square area? Explain.

B.7   What were Dr. Snow's initial and basic hypotheses concerning the epidemic? What processes and procedures did Dr. Snow use to establish his hypotheses (prove or disprove them) about the outbreak?

B.8   The obvious control measure applied was the removal of the handle from the Broad Street pump. What role did the removal of the pump handle play in the decline of the epidemic? Did the removal of the pump handle have an effect on the control epidemic? What other social and political roles did removing the handle from the pump play?

(C) CHOLERA EPIDEMIC OF 1853 AND TWO LONDON WATER COMPANIES

"London was without cholera from the latter part of 1849 to August 1853. During this interval an important change had taken place in the water supply of several of the south districts of London. The Lambeth Company removed their water works, in 1852, from opposite of Hungerford Market to Thames Ditton: thus obtaining a supply of water quite free from the sewage of London. The districts supplied by the Lambeth Company are, however, also supplied, to a certain extent by the Southwark and Vauxhall Co., the pipes of both companies going down every street, in the places where the supply is mixed (different houses getting water from one or the other water companies). Due to this intermixing of the sources of water, the effect of the alteration made by the Lambeth Co. on the progress of

TABLE I.1

Water Companies	Sources of Supply	Population	Deaths by Cholera in 13 Weeks Ending Nov. 19	Deaths in 100,000 Inhabitants
(1) Lambeth and (2) Southwark & Vauxhall	Thames, at Thames Ditton and at Battersea	346,363	211	61
Southwark & Vauxhall	Thames, at Battersea	118,267	111	94
(1) Southwark & Vauxhall (2) Kent	Thames, at Battersea; the Ravensbourne, in Kent, & ditches and wells	17,805	19	107

cholera was not so evident, to a cursory observer, as it would otherwise have been. It attracted the attention, however, of the Registrar-General, who published a table in the "Weekly Return of Births and Deaths," for 26th November 1853, of which the following is an abstract, containing as much as applies to the south districts of London."

"It thus appears that the districts partially supplied with the improved water suffered much less than the others, although, in 1849, when the Lambeth Company obtained their new supply, these same districts suffered quite as much as those supplied entirely by the Southwark and Vauxhall Co. The Lambeth water extends to only a small portion of some of the districts necessarily included in the groups supplied by the companies and when the division is made in a little more detail, by taking subdistricts, the effect of the new water supply is shown to be greater than appears in the Table I.1."

"As the Registrar-General published a list of all the deaths from cholera which occurred in London in 1853, from the commencement of the epidemic in August to its conclusion in January, 1854, I have been able to add up the numbers which occurred in the various subdistricts on the south side of the Thames, to which the water supply of the Southwark and Vauxhall Co. and the Lambeth Companies, extends."

"Although the facts shown in the Table I.2 afford very strong evidence of the powerful influence which the drinking of water containing the sewage of the town exerts over the

TABLE I.2

Subdistricts	Population in 1851	Deaths from Cholera—1853	Deaths by Cholera in Each 100,000 Living	Water Supply
First 12 subdistricts	167,654	192	114	South & Vauxhall
Next 16 subdistricts	301,149	182	60	Both
Last 3 subdistricts	14,632	0	0	Lambeth Company

spread of cholera, when that disease is present, yet the question does not end here; for the intermixing of the water supply of the Southwark and Vauxhall Company with that of the Lambeth Company, over an extensive part of London, admitted of the subject being sifted in such a way as to yield the most incontrovertible proof on one side or the other. In the subdistricts enumerated in the above table as being supplied by both companies, the mixing of the supply is of the most intimate kind. The pipes of each company go down all the streets, and into nearly all the courts and alleys. A few houses are supplied by one company and a few by the other, according to the decision of the owner or occupier at that time when the water companies were in active competition. In many cases a single house has a supply different from that on either side. Each company supplies both rich and poor, both large houses and small; there is no difference either in the condition or occupation of the persons receiving the waters of the different companies. Now it must be evident that, if the diminution of cholera, in the districts partly supplied with improved water, depended on this supply, the houses receiving it would be the houses enjoying the whole benefit of the diminution of the malady, whilst the houses supplied with the water from Battersea Fields would suffer the same mortality as they would if the improved supply did not exist at all. As there is no difference whatever, either in the houses or the people receiving the supply of the two water companies, or in any of the physical conditions with which they are surrounded. It is obvious that no experiment could have been devised which would more thoroughly test the effect of water supply on the progress of cholera than this, which circumstances placed ready made before the observer."

"The experiment, too, was on the grandest scale. No fewer than 300,000 people of both sexes, of every age and occupation, and of every rank and station, from gentlefolks down to the very poor, were divided into two groups without their choice, and in most cases, without their knowledge, one group being supplied with water containing the sewage of London, and amongst it, whatever might have come from the cholera patients, the other group having water quite free from such impurity."

"To turn this grand experiment to account, all that was required was to learn the supply of water to each individual house where a fatal attack of cholera might occur. I regret that, in the short days at the latter part of last year, I could not spare the time to make the inquiry; and indeed, I was not fully aware at that time, of the intimate mixture of the supply of the two water companies, and the consequently important nature of the desired inquiry."

CHOLERA EPIDEMIC OF 1854

"When the cholera returned to London in July of the present year, however, I resolved to spare no exertion which might be necessary to ascertain the exact effect of the water supply on the progress of the epidemic, in the places where all the circumstances were so happily adapted for the inquiry. I was desirous of making the investigation myself, in order that I might have the most satisfactory proof of the truth or fallacy of the doctrine which I had been advocating for five years. I had no reason to doubt the correctness of the conclusions I had drawn from the great number of facts already in my possession, but I felt that the circumstance of the cholera poison passing down the sewers into a great river, and being distributed through miles of pipes, and yet producing its specific effects, was a fact of so startling a nature, and so vast importance to the community, that it could not be too rigidly examined, or established on too firm a basis."

"I accordingly asked permission at the General Register Office to be supplied with the addresses of persons dying of cholera, in those districts where the supply of the two companies is intermingled in the manner I have stated above. Some of these addresses were published in the "Weekly Returns," and I was kindly permitted to take a copy of others. I commenced my inquiry about the middle of August with two subdistricts of Lambeth, called Kennington, first part and Kennington, second part. There were 44 deaths in these subdistricts down to 12th August, and I found that 38 of the houses in which these deaths occurred were supplied by the Southwark and Vauxhall Company, four houses were supplied by the Lambeth Company, and two had pump-wells on the premises and no supply from either of the companies."

"As soon as I had ascertained these particulars, I communicated them to Dr. Farr, who was much struck with the result, and at his suggestion the Registrars of all the South districts of London were requested to make a return of the water supply of the house in which the attack took place, in all cases of death from cholera. This order was to take place after the 26th August, and I resolved to carry my inquiry down to that date, so that the facts might be ascertained for the whole course of the epidemic."

"The inquiry was necessarily attended with a good deal of trouble. There were very few instances in which I could at once get information I required. Even when the water-rates are paid by the residents, they can seldom remember the name of the water company till they have looked for the receipt. In the case of working people who pay weekly rents, the rates are invariably paid by the landlord or his agent, who often live at a distance, and the residents know nothing of the matter. It would, indeed, have been almost impossible for me to complete the inquiry, if I had not found that I could distinguish the water of the two companies with perfect certainty by a chemical test. The test I employed was founded on the great difference in the quantity of chloride of sodium (salt) contained in the two kinds of water, at the time I made the inquiry. On adding solution of nitrate of silver to a gallon of the water of the Lambeth company, obtained at Thames Ditton, beyond the reach of the sewage of London, only 2.28 grains of chloride of silver were obtained, indicating the presence of .95 grains of chloride of sodium in the water. On treating the water of the Southwark and Vauxhall Company in the same manner, 91 grains of chloride silver were obtained, showing the presence of 37.9 grains of common salt per gallon. Indeed, the difference in appearance on adding nitrate of silver to the two kinds of water was so great, that they could be at once distinguished without any further trouble. Therefore when the resident could not find clear and conclusive evidence about the water company, I obtained some of the water in a small phial, wrote the address on the cover, when I could examine it after coming home. The mere appearance of the water generally afforded a very good indication of its source, especially if it was observed as it came in before it had entered the water-butt or cistern; and the time of its coming in also afforded some evidence of the kind of water, after I had ascertained the hours when the turncocks of both companies visited any street. These points were, however, not relied on, except as corroborating more decisive proof, such as the chemical test, or the company's receipt for the rates."

"According to a return which was made to Parliament, the Southwark and Vauxhall Company supplied 40,046 houses from January 1st to December 31st 1853, and the Lambeth Company supplied 26,107 houses during the same period; consequently, as 286 fatal attacks of cholera took place, in the first 4 weeks of the epidemic, in houses supplied by the former company, and only 14 in houses supplied by the latter, the proportion of fatal

TABLE I.3

	Number of Houses	Deaths from Cholera	Deaths in Each 10,000 Houses
Southwark and Vauxhall Company	40,046	1,263	315
Lambeth Company	26,107	98	37
Rest of London	256,423	1,422	59

attacks to each 10,000 houses was as follows. Southwark and Vauxhall 71. Lambeth 5. The cholera was therefore 14 times as fatal at this period, amongst persons having the impure water of the Southwark and Vauxhall Company, as amongst those having the purer water from Thames Ditton.”

“As the epidemic advanced, the disproportion between the number of cases in houses supplied by the Southwark and Vauxhall Company and those supplied by the Lambeth Company, became not quite so great, although it continued very striking.”

“Table I.3 is the proportion of deaths to 10,000 houses, during the first seven weeks of the epidemic, in the population supplied by the Southwark and Vauxhall Company, in that supplied by the Lambeth Company and in the rest of London. (See Figure I.4 map of River Thames area.)”

“The mortality in the houses supplied by the Southwark and Vauxhall Company was therefore between 8 and 9 times as great as in the houses supplied by the Lambeth Company. (See Figure I.4 map of River Thames area.)”

Case Study Questions

C.1 What are the various aspects of the *person* presented in the above water company case concerning the epidemic of cholera, especially as the person concept relates to the households which were recipients of the supplies of the water as compared to those who used different water supplies?

C.2 Concerning the water supply system and structure from the two different water companies, explain the soundness of the research approaches and short-comings encountered. Discuss and explain what type of research design this water supply structure would be if it were designed and planned by a epidemiologist today.

C.3 What were some of the practical problems and barriers that Dr. Snow faced which slowed his inquiry of the cholera epidemic of 1854? How would this relate to modern day epidemiological investigations?

C.4 “As the epidemic advanced, the disproportion between the number of cases in houses supplied by the Southwark and Vauxhall Company and those supplied by the Lambeth Company, became not quite so great. . . .” From an epidemiological point of view why was this so? Give detailed epidemiological reasoning and discussion addressing *time, place*, and *person* issues.

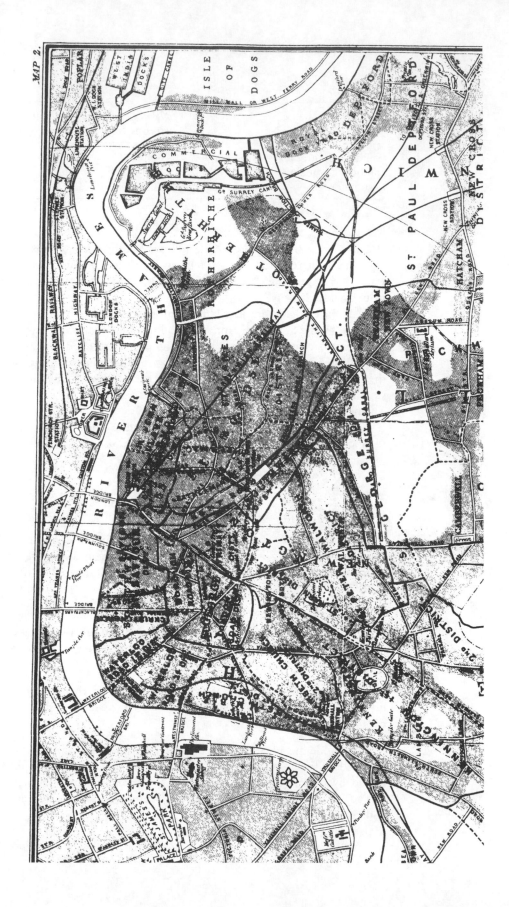

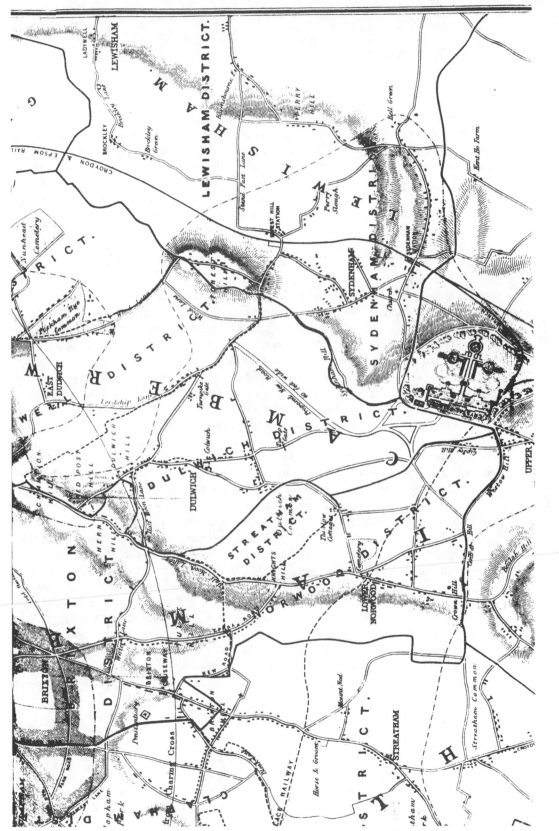

FIGURE I.4 River Thames area of London (shaded parts are the areas served by the two different water companies).

(D) EPIDEMIOLOGICAL ISSUES

Dr. Snow's Answers to Objections

"All the evidence proving the communication of cholera through the medium of water, confirms that with which I set out, of its communication in the crowded habitations of the poor, in coal-mines and other places, by the hands getting soiled with evacuations of the patients, and by small quantities of these evacuations being swallowed with the food, as paint is swallowed by house painters of uncleanly habits, who contact lead-colic in this way."

"There are one or two objections to the mode of communications of cholera which I am endeavouring to establish, that deserve to be noticed. Messrs. Pearse and Marston state, in their account of the cases of cholera treated at the Newcastle Dispensary in 1853, that one of the dispensers drank by mistake some rice-water evacuation without any effect whatever. In rejoinder to this negative incident, it may be remarked, that several conditions may be requisite to the communication of cholera with which we are as yet unacquainted. Certain conditions we know to be requisite to the communication of other diseases. Syphilis we know is only communicable in its primary state, and vaccine lymph must be removed at a particular time to produce its proper effects. In the incident above mentioned, the large quantity of the evacuation taken might even prevent its action. It must be remembered that the effects of a morbid poison are never due to what first enters the system, but to the crop of progeny produced from this during a period of reproduction, termed the period of incubation; and if a whole sack of grain, or seed of any kind, were put into a hole in the ground, it is very doubtful whether any crop whatever would be produced."

"An objection that has repeatedly been made to the propagation of cholera through the medium of water, is, that every one who drinks of the water ought to have the disease at once. This objection arises from mistaking the department of science to which the communication of cholera belongs, and looking on it as a question of chemistry, instead of one of natural history, as it undoubtedly is. It cannot be supposed that a morbid poison, which has the property, under suitable circumstances, of reproducing its kind, should be capable of being diluted indefinitely in water, like a chemical salt; and therefore it is not to be presumed that the cholera-poison would be equally diffused through every particle of water. The eggs of the tape-worm must undoubtedly pass down the sewers into the Thames, but it by no means follows that everybody who drinks a glass of water should swallow one of the eggs. As regards the morbid matter of cholera, many other circumstances, besides the quantity of it which is present in a river at different periods of the epidemic must influence the chances of it being swallowed, such as its remaining in a butt or other vessel till it is decomposed or devoured by animalcules, or its merely settling to the bottom and remaining there. In the case of the pump-well in Broad Street, Golden Square, if the cholera-poison was contained in the minute whitish flocculi visible on close inspection to the naked eye, some persons might drink of the water without taking any, as they soon settled to the bottom of the vessel."

Duration of Epidemic and Size of Population

"There are certain circumstances connected with the history of cholera which admit of a satisfactory explanation according to the principles explained above, and consequently tend to confirm those principles. The first point I shall notice, viz., the period of duration of the epidemic in different places, refers merely to the communicability of the disease, without regard to the mode of communication. The duration of cholera in a place, is usually in direct proportion to the number of the population. The disease remains but two or three weeks in a village, two or three months in a good-sized town, whilst in a great metropolis it often remains a whole year or longer. I find from an analysis which I made in 1849 of the valuable table of Dr. Wm. Merriman, of the cholera in England in 1832, that fifty-two places are enumerated in which the disease continued less than 50 days, and that the average population of these places is 6,624. Forty-three places are likewise down in which the cholera lasted 50 days, but less than 100; the average population of these is 12,624. And there are, without including London, 33 places in which the epidemic continued 100 days and upwards, the average population of which is 38,123; if London be included, 34 places, with an average of 78,832."

"There was a similar relation in 1849 between the duration of the cholera and the population of the places which it visited; a relation which points clearly to the propagation of the disease from patient to patient; for if each case were not connected with a previous one, but depended on some unknown atmospheric or telluric condition, there is no reason why the 20 cases which occur in a village should not be distributed over as long a period as twenty hundred cases which occur in a large town."

Effect of Season

"Each time when cholera has been introduced into England in the autumn, it has made but little progress, and has lingered rather than flourished during the winter and spring, to increase gradually during the following summer, reach its climax at the latter part of the summer, and decline some what rapidly as the cool days of autumn set in. In most parts of Scotland, on the contrary, cholera has each time run through its course in the winter immediately following its introduction. I have now to offer what I consider an explanation, to a great extent, of the peculiarities in the progress of cholera. The English people, as a general rule, do not drink much unboiled water, except in warm weather. They generally take tea, coffee, malt liquor, or some other artificial beverage at the meals, and do not require to drink between meals except when the weather is warm. In summer, however, a much greater quantity of drink is required, and it is more usual to drink water at that season than in cold weather. Consequently, whilst the cholera is chiefly confined in winter to the crowded families of the poor, and to the mining population, who, . . . eat each others excrement at all times, it gains access as summer advances to the population of the towns, where there is a river which receives the sewers and supplies the drinking water at the same time; and, where pump-wells and other limited supplies of water happen to be contaminated with the contents of the drains and cesspools, there is a greater opportunity for the disease to spread at a time when unboiled water is more freely used."

"In Scotland, on the other hand, unboiled water is somewhat freely used at all times to mix with spirits; I am told that when two or three people enter a tavern in Scotland and ask for a gill of whiskey, a jug of water and tumbler-glasses are brought with it. Malt liquors are only consumed to a limited extent in Scotland, and when persons drink spirits without water as they often do, it occasions thirst and obliges them to drink water afterwards."

"There may be other causes besides the above which tend to assist the propagation of cholera in warm, more than in cold weather. It is not unlikely that insects, especially the common house-flies, aid in spreading the disease. An ingenious friend of mine has informed me that, when infusion of quassia has been placed in the room for the purpose of poisoning flies, he has more than once perceived the taste of it on his bread and butter."

Alternative Theories

"Dr. Farr discovered a remarkable coincidence between the mortality from cholera in the different districts of London in 1849, and the elevation of the ground; the connection being of an inverse kind, the higher districts suffering least, and the lowest suffering most from this malady. Dr. Farr was inclined to think that the level of the soil had some direct influence over the prevalence of cholera, but the fact of the most elevated towns in this kingdom, as Wolverhampton, Dowlais, Merthyr Tydvil, and Newcastle-upon-Tyne, having suffered excessively from this disease on several occasions, is opposed to this view, as is also the circumstance of Bethlehem Hospital, the Queen's Prison, Horsemonger Lane Gaol, and several other large buildings, which are supplied with water from deep wells on the premises, having nearly or altogether escaped cholera, though situated on a very low level, and surrounded by the disease. The fact of Brixton, at an elevation of 56 feet above Trinity high-water mark, having suffered a mortality of 55 in 10,000 whilst many districts on the north of the Thames, at less than half the elevation, did not suffer one-third as much, also points to the same conclusion."

"I expressed the opinion in 1849, that the increased prevalence of cholera in the low-lying districts of London depended entirely on the greater contamination of the water in these districts, and the comparative immunity from this disease of the population receiving the improved water from Thames Ditton, during the epidemics of last year and the present, as shown in the previous pages, entirely confirms this view of the subject; for the great bulk of this population live in the lowest districts of the metropolis."

"It is not necessary to oppose any other theories in order to establish the principles I am endeavouring to explain, for the field I have entered on was almost unoccupied. The best attempt at explaining the phenomena of cholera, which previously existed, was probably that which supposed that the disease was communicated by effluvia given off from the patient into the surrounding air, and inhaled by others into the lungs; but this view required its advocates to draw very largely on what is called predisposition, in order to account for the numbers who approach near to the patient without being affected, whilst others acquire the disease without any near approach. It also failed entirely to account for the sudden and violent outbreaks of the disease, such as that which occurred in the neighbourhood of Golden Square."

"Another view having a certain number of advocates is, that cholera depends on an unknown something in the atmosphere which becomes localized, and has its effects increased by the gases given off from decomposing animal and vegetable matters. This hypothesis is, however, rendered impossible by the motion of the atmosphere, and, even in the absence of wind, by the laws which govern the diffusion of aeriform bodies; moreover, the connection between cholera and offensive effluvia is by no means such as to indicate cause and effect; even in London, as was before mentioned, many places where offensive effluvia are very abundant have been visited very lightly by cholera, whilst the comparatively open and clean districts of Kennington and Clapham have suffered severely. If inquiry were made, a far closer connection would be found to exist between offensive effluvia and the itch, than between these effluvia and cholera; yet as the cause of itch is well known, we are quite aware that this connection is not one of cause and effect."

"Mr. John Lea, of Cincinnati, has advanced what he calls a geological theory of cholera. He supposes that the cholera-poison, which he believes to exist in the air about the sick, requires the existence of calcareous or magnesian salts in the drinking water to give it effect. This view is not consistent with what we know of cholera, but there are certain circumstances related by Mr. Lea which deserve attention. He says that, in the western districts of the United States, the cholera passed round the arenacious, and spent its fury on the calcareous regions; and that it attacked with deadly effect those who used the calcareous water, while it passed by those who used sandstone or soft water. He gives many instances of towns suffering severely when river water was used, whilst others, having only soft spring water or rain water, escaped almost entirely; and he states that there has been scarcely a case of cholera in families who used only rain water. The rivers, it is evident, might be contaminated with the evacuations, whilst it is equally evident that the rain water could not be so polluted. As regards sand and all sandstone formations, they are well known to have the effects of oxidizing and thus destroying organic matters; whilst the limestone might not have that effect, although I have no experience on that point. The connection which Mr. Lea has observed between cholera and the water is highly interesting, although it probably admits of a very different explanation from the one he has given."

Case Study Questions

D.1   What are the epidemiological implications of Dr. Snow's observations about sizes of cities and length of epidemics?

D.2   Dr. Snow suggested several reasons for the failure of contaminated water to produce disease in all who consume it. Why is it that not everyone gets ill or dies, who consumes cholera pathogens? What was correct about his explanations and what was incorrect? Why?

D.3   What principles were correct and what were incorrect in Snow's observations about time and seasons and the effects on epidemics? Why?

D.4   Several different theories and hypotheses have been presented. Which of these are consistent with known scientific and biomedical knowledge and common sense? Which of these were not consistent nor supported by scientific and biomedical knowledge and common sense? Why? Explain.

II

Working through a Foodborne Illness Epidemic Investigation— Typhoid Fever in Schenectady

Excerpted and adapted from "Typhoid in Schenectady: A Foodborne Outbreak," *Case Studies in Epidemiology*, by El-Ahraf, A., and Brin, B.N., Course Syllabus for Principles of Epidemiology, California State University, San Bernardino.

Typhoid fever, cholera, and salmonellosis, also referred to as alvine discharge diseases, are infections of the digestive system. Such diseases are often spread because of lack of such sanitary measures as hand washing before handling food. The lack of food protection and good sanitary measures in food preparation are major contributing causes of food poisoning from these and other diseases.

Typhoid fever was made famous by Typhoid Mary. Mary Mallon, a food service worker, caused many deaths and several typhoid outbreaks in New York in the early 1900's. When finally identified as the source of the typhoid epidemics, bacteriological examination of her feces showed that she was a chronic typhoid carrier. Having made her mark in the pages of history, Mary Mallon, better known by her alias as Typhoid Mary, has been taught in history and social studies related classes in schools and colleges ever since.

Typhoid fever is one of the multitude of salmonella infections and becomes pathogenic due to the endotoxins it produces. The source of infection is usually the feces of asymptomatic carriers. About 2 to 5% of patients become chronic carriers. Persistent carriers by law must be reported to public health departments and are prohibited from handling food. The stool or urine of ill patients who have an active case of the disease is also a source. The organism enters the GI tract and invades the blood stream and lymph system. Incubation period relates to the numbers of organisms taken in (3 to 25 days). Symptoms include: slow onset, chills, malaise, headache, anorexia, muscle aches, fever/elevated temperature, and constipation. As the disease progresses, bradycardia, discrete rounded rose-colored spots in crops emerge on abdomen and chest and splenomegaly occurs. Prevention is by purification of drinking water, pasteurization of milk, sanitation and food protection and control of carriers. Tests include blood and stool cultures, as well as bone marrow, rose spots and liver tests. Food, water, milk and seafood are common sources of the typhoid salmonella pathogen. (Source: Berkow, R. (Editor-in-Chief), *The Merck Manual*, 14th Edition, Merck and Co. Inc.: Rahway, N.J. 1982.)

CASE OF TYPHOID FEVER IN SCHENECTADY, NEW YORK

In 1939, Schenectady was a city of approximately 90,000 people. On June 20th of this same year, the Public Health Department's Health Officer received reports of 5 cases of typhoid fever within the city. The Health Officer also received a report of one case of typhoid fever in a person who lived about 100 miles away in Massachusetts. The person had visited Schenectady in recent weeks preceding. No cases of typhoid had been reported for the past year up to that date in the city. In the preceding 5 years the average annual prevalence of typhoid had been 2 cases per year.

Schenectady's water supply was obtained from surface water. A stream with drainage from relatively uninhabited areas was the main water source. About eight years prior to the typhoid outbreak, a modern rapid sand filtration water treatment plant was installed and competently operated by a sanitary engineer. The water supply for the city was chlorinated. Daily bacteriological analyses of water from 6 points in the water distribution system were conducted and reported to the Health Officer. Schenectady had a modern sewer system. Within the city, 95% to 98% of the houses were connected to the sewer system, which was a good record for 1939.

City ordinances prohibited sale of unpasteurized milk or sale of milk other than by certified dairies. Approximately 75% of the city's milk was supplied by two large dairies. One other dairy distributed about 300 quarts of pasteurized milk daily. Consumers, using their own containers, purchased a small but unknown amount of unpasteurized milk from nearby farmers. About 95% of all ice cream was supplied by two large manufacturers. They also supplied ice cream to nearby cities. All shellfish dealers were required to be licensed by the local health department. Shellfish dealers were also required to keep records of the receipt and distribution of all shellfish stock handled.

Typhoid carriers were required to be registered with the public health department. Twenty one carriers were known and tracked by the health department. A survey of the city's hospitals and all physicians showed a total of 13 known or suspected cases of typhoid, which included the one reported from Massachusetts. From interviewing each case in their homes epidemiological data were collected. With the use of a dot map, it was observed that there was no geographical clustering of cases.

From the interviews and epidemiological investigations with the 13 cases, a table of the information was compiled and tabulated and is presented in Table II.1. The epidemiological interview gathered usual information from each case as found in most any survey; name, age, sex, occupation. For this particular epidemic as in most foodborne outbreaks, certain specific data must be gathered, and in this outbreak included: date of onset, sewerage, water supply, dairy products eaten, uncooked foods eaten, trips, and foods taken away from home. After studying Table II.1, answer the following questions. See Table II.1 Summary of Dates Relevant to Cases of Typhoid Fever in Schenectady Outbreak.

Case Study Questions

1. What key activities, and important facts tie each of the individual cases together?

2. Prepare a line graph chart showing the dates and numbers of cases per day of the outbreak by date of onset for each typhoid case. Is this an epidemic curve? Why? Defend your answer.

3. From the case and epidemiological data can you estimate possible date of common exposure? (Present evidence and facts other than just the date.)

TABLE II.1 Summary of dates relevant to cases of typhoid fever in Schenectady outbreak

Name	Age	Sex	Occupation	Onset Date	Home Sanitation		Dairy Products	Use of Uncooked Foods	Trips	Meals Away from Home
					Sewerage	Water				
Christiansen, Estelle	15	F	Student	6/7	City	City	Dairylea, Blair's	Clams 6/2	None	Daily at school; Blair's 6/2; M.E. picnic 5/30
Blair, Florence	55	F	Housewife	6/9	Septic tank	Own well	Own cows, Dairylea	Own garden vegetables	Schenectady	M.E. picnic 5/30; Potters 6/4
Dencher, Mary	65	F	Housewife	6/5	City	City	Borden's, Blair's	Market vegetables	Lebanon 5/1–14	M.E. picnic 5/30
Howard, Flora	64	F	Housewife	6/7	Septic tank	Own well	Own cows	Oysters 5/1; fresh tomatoes	None	M.E. picnic 5/30
Jones, Theda	21	F	Teacher	6/7	City	City	Borden's, Dairylea	Clams 5/21; Garden vegetables	Altaville 5/20–21	Altaville 5/20–21; M.E. picnic 5/30
Ostrander, Edith	49	F	Housewife	6/11	City	City	Kingning, Dairylea	Garden vegetables	None	M.E. picnic 5/30
Thurber, Walter	25	M	Mechanic	6/25	City	City	Borden's Good Humor	Garden vegetables	None	Shares lunch daily with fellow workers
Kmiecziak, Robert	14	M	Student	6/18	City	City	Canned	None	None	M.E. picnic 5/30
Wagoner, Dorothy	16	F	Housework	6/16	City	City	Borden's Good Humor	None	None	M.E. picnic 5/30; Pep club 5/3
Wagoner, Grace	44	F	Housewife	6/9	City	City	Borden's	None	None	M.E. picnic 5/30
Wagoner, Robert	40	M	Grocer	6/28	City	City	Borden's	None	None	M.E. picnic 5/30
Woods, Alice	53	F	Housewife	6/7	Septic tank	Own well	Own cows	Garden vegetables	None	M.E. picnic 5/30
Vogel, Ethel	41	F	Mill worker	6/7	Pit privy	Chicopee Falls, Mass.	Canned	None	Schenectady 5/29–6/12	Sister's home—Schenectady; M.E. picnic 5/30

4. Several unrelated cases appeared in the investigation. Explain the exposure to typhoid and implications of the unrelated cases of typhoid and give several examples or possibilities.

5. Briefly outline additional steps that are needed in order to complete this particular investigation.

The Schenectady Methodist Episcopal Church held a Memorial Day celebration at the church which included a buffet picnic supper. On the afternoon of May 30th, the annual Memorial Service was held at the Methodist cemetery in Schenectady and was followed by a late afternoon picnic supper. A potluck approach was used to furnish the food and was provided by a number of the participants. Supper was served to 33 of the persons who attended the service.

An epidemiological investigation was held at the Schenectady Methodist Episcopal church. In the investigation, inquiries were made of persons attending the picnic. All persons who attended the supper were interviewed. Interviewers recorded as accurately as possible all the foods consumed by each individual. Information about any previous history of typhoid, or any possible symptoms was recorded, as well as information concerning the preparation and serving of foods. Food samples were not available as all food had either been eaten or discarded. An attempt was made to obtain fecal specimens from all individuals who were at the picnic. A series of three specimens was acquired from all persons who prepared and provided food for the picnic.

No previous history of any typhoid illness was confirmed in any case. Laboratory studies, mostly consisting of stool cultures that came out positive, confirmed the clinical diagnosis of typhoid fever in all 13 cases. Additionally the following laboratory data were obtained for persons who attended the picnic but showed no evidence of the typhoid disease.

- Irene Picket = positive stools on July 4, July 5 and July 6, and negative stools on July 23 and Aug 2.

- Margaret Bennett = 11 consecutive positive stools, July 2, through Oct. 4.

- Kenneth Rineheardt = positive stools July 4 and 3, negative stools at a later date.

6. Of the three persons, Pickett, Bennett and Rineheardt, who was most likely to have been infected during the church picnic outbreak? Who was most likely to have been infected previously, before the picnic?

7. Which laboratory tests might be administered nowadays which were not generally available in 1939? (Some outside research in medical diagnostic books might be needed to answer this question.) How would these tests help the church picnic investigation?

See Table II.2, which is a checklist of the foods eaten at the Methodist church picnic. Included in the table are the names of the 35 persons/cases involved in the outbreak. The table provides information on whether a person was a case or not a case, and the different foods each consumed, with a key at the bottom about each person's eating of different foodstuffs and the ability to recall the foods each had eaten. See Table II.2 and use the "Worksheet for food-specific attack rates," Table II.3.

TABLE II.2 Checklist of foods eaten at the Memorial Day church supper

Name	Case	Potato Salad	Macaroni Salad	Cabbage Salad	Summer Sausage	Spiced Ham	Baked Beans	Rolls	Cakes	Coffee	Pickles
S. Christian	Yes	1	1	2	2	2	2	1	2	1	1
S. Blair	Yes	3	3	2	2	2	2	1	2	1	1
M. Dencher	Yes	1	2	2	2	1	2,4	1,4	1	2	2
F. Howard	Yes	1	1	2	2	2	2	2,4	1,4	2	2
T. Jones	Yes	1	3	2	1	2	1	1	1	2	2,4
E. Ostrander	Yes	2	1	2	2	2	2	1	2	1	2
W. Thurber[5]	Yes	1	2	2	1	2	2	2	2	2	2
R. Kmiecziak	Yes	1	1	2	1	2	1				1
D. Wagner	Yes	1	1	1	2	1	2	1	1	1	2
G. Wagoner	Yes	3	1	3	1	1	2	1	1,4	1	2
R. Wagoner	Yes	1	1	1	1	1	1	1	1	1	1
A. Woods	Yes	1	1	2	1,6	2,6	2,6	1,4	1	1	3
E. Vogel	Yes	1	1	3	2	2	1	1	1	1	2
G. Harmon	No	1	2	2	2	2	1	1	2	1	2
J. Stoddard	No	1	1	1	2	8	8	8	8		1
I. Pickett	No	1	1	1	2	2	1	1	1	1	1
J. Bennett	No	1	1	1	1	2	1	1	1	1	1
C. Carrol	No	1	2	1	1	2	1		2		1
G. Anderson[5]	No	1	2	2	2	2	2	2	2	2	2
N. Brothers	No	1	2	2	2	1	2	2			2
E. Conrad	No	1	2	1	2	2	1	1			2
E. Gray	No	1	2	2	2	2	1	1	2		2
G. Harrington	No	2	2	2	2	2	1	1		1	2
S. McAuliffe	No	1	2	2	2	2	2	2	1	1	2
E. Pickett	No	1,4	2	2	1	2	2	1	1,4	1	1
J. Sailsburgh	No	2	2	2	2	2	2	1	1	1	2
L. Smith	No	1	3	3,4	2	2	1	1	2	1	1
M. Bennett	No	1,4	2,4	2	2	2	2	2	1	2	2
E. Thurber	No	2,4	2	2	2	2	2	1	2	2	2
K. Rhinehardt	No	1	1	1	2	2	1	1	2	1	2
A. Wagoner	No	1	1	1	1	2	1	1	1	2	2
H. Wagoner	No	1	1	2	1	2	1	1	1	1	2
B. Alexander[7]	No	Unavailable for interview									
C. Scofield[7]	No	Unavailable for interview									
M. Harrison	No	1	3	2	2	2	1	1		1	2

[1] Recalled having eaten the food
[2] Recalled having not eaten the food
[3] Could not remember
[4] Brought or prepared food indicated

[5] Ate food brought home by Mrs. Thurber
[6] Foods store bought
[7] Not located
[8] Gave contradictory responses regarding the food

TABLE II.3   Worksheet for food-specific attack rates

Food	Persons Contracting Typhoid	Persons Not Contracting Typhoid	Total Persons	Attack Rate %	Relative Risk
Potato salad:	Eating Not eating Unknown				
Macaroni salad:	Eating Not eating Unknown				
Cabbage salad:	Eating Not eating Unknown				
Summer sausage:	Eating Not eating Unknown				
Spiced ham:	Eating Not eating Unknown				
Baked beans:	Eating Not eating Unknown				
Rolls:	Eating Not eating Unknown				
Cakes:	Eating Not eating Unknown				
Coffee:	Eating Not eating Unknown				
Pickles:	Eating Not eating Unknown				

8. Compute the attack rates for those **eating** and for those **not eating** each food and the unknowns. Calculate a relative risk for **each** food. Include data for all 35 individuals. (Include the use of food specific attack rate.)

9. From the array of foods provided, list those which you think would be most susceptible to mass contamination. Identify those foods and conditions that provide a good growth medium for bacteria. Which foods are at high risks for contamination during preparation, serving and storage, thus making them high possibilities as sources for typhoid transmission? Based on the foodstuff type, and conditions that provide a poor growth medium for bacteria, list those foods that would be least susceptible in typhoid transmission.

10. As a result of the worksheet that included food-specific attack rates that you prepared, determine the food or foods most likely to be involved in the typhoid outbreak. Base your determination on the following epidemiological concepts:

    - A majority of cases should have eaten the food.
    - The relative risk.
    - The ease of mass contamination of the food.
    - List of foods that appear to be of high risk in the transmission of disease but have minimum likelihood due to the scientific basis for not being probable of transmitting the disease. Explain why they are not likely to be suspect.

11. How should an epidemiologist deal with circumstances in which an individual cannot recall a food eaten or who gave contradictory responses about whether or not the food items were eaten?

12. Why is an epidemiologist concerned about attack rates and relative risk among persons not eating particular foods?

13. To incriminate a particular food as a source of disease transmission, what epidemiological and scientific/biomedical findings are necessary?

14. Are pieces of information missing that leave the investigation incomplete? What are the missing pieces of information or gaps in the investigation? For 1939? For this year; this modern day?

15. Considering all the data, information, and evidence, what is the most likely and probable explanation for this epidemic? Be specific about the individual persons and the foodstuffs and other supporting factors include *time*, *place*, and *person*.

16. As an epidemiologist, how would you prevent and control future typhoid fever epidemics such as this one?

III

Common-Source Outbreak of Waterborne Shigellosis at a Public School

Adapted from Bain, W.B., Herron, C.A., Keith, Bridson, et al. "Waterborne Shigellosis at a Public School," *American Journal of Epidemiology*, Vol. 101, No. 4, 1975.

Shigellosis is a intestinal tract infection caused by shigella organisms, and has 4 major subgroups of pathogens. The source of infection is excreta of infected individuals or carriers. Shigellosis is usually spread by ingesting food or water contaminated by fecal matter. Flies are also a vehicle/vector of contamination. Fomites have also been implicated in the spread of the disease. Epidemics are often found in crowded populations living with poor sanitation and are a source of bacillary dysentery found in children living in endemic areas.

The incubation period is 1 to 4 days. In younger children onset can be sudden. Symptoms include fever, irritability, drowsiness, anorexia, nausea or vomiting, diarrhea, abdominal cramps. Within three days, blood, pus and mucus appear in the stools. Number of stools increase rapidly to about 20 or more a day; severe diarrhea. In the laboratory findings of sample specimens, the shigella bacteria is found in the stools. The white blood count is often reduced at onset and goes up to 13,000. Plasma CO_2 is usually low, showing a response from the diarrhea-induced metabolic acidosis. Prevention and control is by preventing the spread through contaminated food, water and flies by having good sanitation, including thorough hand washing before food handling, soaking contaminated clothes in soap and water until boiled; isolation of patients and carriers, and stool isolation. (Source: Berkow, R. (Editor-in-Chief), *The Merck Manual*, 14th Edition, Merck and Co. Inc.: Rahway, N.J. 1982)

CASE OF COMMON-SOURCE OUTBREAK OF WATERBORNE SHIGELLOSIS AT A PUBLIC SCHOOL

In November, 1972 a public school in Stockport, Iowa (population 334) experienced an outbreak of gastro-intestinal illness. Of the 269 pupils who attended the public school, 194 (72%) were affected and 14 out of the 23 (61%) faculty and staff were also affected. Laboratory and clinical exams showed that the etiological agent was *Shigella sonnei*. When assessing secondary infections, of the 698 student contacts with members of households, 97 (14%) also developed diarrhea. Secondary cases also occurred in 3 out of 32 members of households of the school's staff.

Shigellosis is most often spread from person-to-person; common-source outbreaks also occur and must be considered in any epidemiological investigation. Water or food should both be considered as a mode of transmission.

In the second week of November of 1972, a physician in Fairfield, Iowa contacted the Iowa State Department of Health by telephone to report a case of shigellosis infection in a young woman who was from Stockport Iowa. The young woman/patient lived in an apartment across the street from a county middle school. The young woman shared a common water supply with the school. Several guests who attended a gathering at her apartment on November 4th, had experienced gastrointestinal illness.

It was discovered that there were high levels of absenteeism at the school due to gastrointestinal illnesses. Similar illnesses were also reported among members of the local high school's boys basketball team. A high school boys basketball team from the neighboring town also reported gastrointestinal illnesses. The two teams had played a scrimmage at the middle school's gym on November 15th.

Van Buren County, with a population of 8,643 according to the 1970 census, is a small county located in southeastern Iowa near the Missouri border. This is a rural county, with 37% of the mostly White residents living on farms. Almost 22% of the residents lived below the federal poverty level and 755 or 22% of the 3,399 households in the county lacked in some or all standard plumbing facilities. All 6th, 7th and 8th grade students in the Van Buren School District attend the middle school in Stockport. In November of 1972, the enrollment at the middle school was 289 and 25 teachers and staff.

The layout of the school is an important epidemiological consideration in this case of a common-source outbreak. The school included a main building; an annex housed the gym and several classrooms. The gym was used for physical education classes, and high school teams in the region used it for practice games. Included in the buildings of the school was an old garage, across the street from the school and east of the main building. The building was used as a shop for industrial arts classes. The easternmost third of the shop building was the private residence/apartment of the young woman mentioned above, who also developed shigellosis (see building map in Figure III.1).

The water supplies for the middle school, the gym, the shop and the private apartment all came from wells on the school grounds (see Figure III.1). Environmental studies were conducted to test the school's water supply. Microbiological testing of the wells was done. Assessment of the well's construction was studied. Water flow and cross connection tests were carried out on the water supply and the sewage system of the middle school and nearby buildings, with fluorescent dye studies.

The family and guests at the gathering in the young woman's apartment on Nov. 4th were questioned about gastrointestinal illness. The students and faculty and staff of Van Buren on Nov. 30th were interviewed and surveyed. Interviews included customary daily consumption of the water at the school, including the fountain in the Gym, illnesses, date of onset, symptoms, school absenteeism, physician visits or hospitalizations. The two basketball teams also were surveyed plus an estimated amount of water consumption at the scrimmage on Nov. 15. Most symptomatic and some asymptomatic cases submitted rectal swabs for bacteriological culture using standard laboratory procedures.

To investigate secondary transmission of the disease, questionnaires were distributed to families of students, faculty, staff and all of the basketball players in order to determine

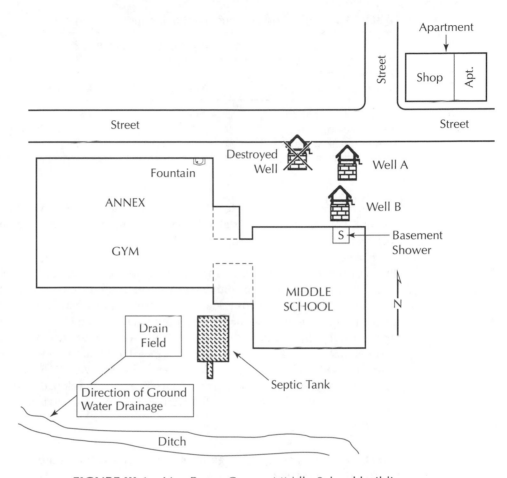

FIGURE III.1   Van Buren County Middle School building map.

incidence (see Table III.1). A secondary case was defined as diarrhea beginning between Nov. 10th and Dec. 4th, among household members (or contacts) of students, faculty and staff and ballplayers. Rectal swabs for culture were obtained from available family members of the groups. Those groups consisted of 10 families chosen at random from the first 40 families to report an apparent secondary infection, 3 families out of 5 of students in which there were apparent secondary cases without illness in the pupil and 3 families of faculty and staff with apparent secondary infection. Cultures were obtained from the index case, an 8th grader and two of the participants in the apartment gathering; all were positive. In the questionnaire, gastrointestinal illness was defined by symptoms: nausea; vomiting; bowel movements that were loose, frequent or bloody; cramps or tenesmus. Questionnaires were retrieved from 93% of the students and 92% of the faculty and staff; 194 students, 14 faculty and staff reported gastrointestinal illness in November.

Of the families of the middle school faculty and staff, three returned questionnaires on secondary attacks at 88% or 22 out of 25. Three (3) of 32 household contacts had diarrhea, for a secondary attack rate of 9%.

TABLE III.1   Shigellosis secondary attack rates

	General Secondary Attack Rates		
Questionnaires Returned by	Total Number	Number Returned	Attack Rate%
Families of students	245	169	—
Household contacts	698	97	—
Asymptomatic students	5	37	—

Rectal swabs were positive for *Shigella sonnei* for 96 out of 123 symptomatic staff members, and 3 out of 6 faculty and staff. Rectal swabs from 13 of 23 asymptomatic students were positive for *Shigella sonnei* as shown by cultures.

Eleven (11) out of 12 of those at the apartment gathering developed gastrointestinal illness within 4 days of the Nov. 4th date. Several students and faculty and staff reported illness in the first week of November (see Tables III.2 and III.3). The first peak in the epidemiology curve occurred on Friday, November 10th, with an average of 12 cases a day for the next 5 days. 45 cases occurred on Thursday, November 16th. The outbreak then tapered off rapidly. Male and female attack rates were about the same; grade level showed no difference in attack rates. No clear trends in water consumption and illness attack rates were seen (see Table III.4). From November 16th–19th, 7 of 18 high school ball players on the visiting team and 10 local high school ball players developed diarrhea. Four (4) out of 25 rectal swabs were positive, all 4 were symptomatic. Diarrhea attack rates among

TABLE III.2   Date of onset of gastrointestinal illness, Van Buren Middle School, Stockport, Iowa, 1972

Date of Onset of Illness	Number of Cases	Date of Onset of Illness	Number of Cases
November		November	
2	1	16	45
3	1	17	30
4	2	18	7
5	2	19	1
6	1	20	6
7	2	21	3
8	2	22	0
9	3	23	1
10	19	24	3
11	11	25	0
12	12	26	0
13	9	27	2
14	6	28	2
15	14	29	0
		30	1

TABLE III.3   Date of onset of secondary attack rates of gastrointestinal illness in faculty and staff, Van Buren Middle School, Stockport, Iowa, 1972

Date of Onset of Illness	Number of Cases	Date of Onset of Illness	Number of Cases
November		November	
7	1	22	8
8	0	23	2
9	0	24	3
10	1	25	13
11	3	26	4
12	1	27	4
13	4	28	2
14	0	29	9
15	0	30	8
16	5	December	
17	2	1	3
18	5	2	0
19	3	3	5
20	7	4	0
21	3	5	0

basketball players were directly correlated to water consumption at the school's fountain in the gym.

The main water sources for the school complex were from the water-wells in the school-yard north of the school house and when the shigellosis outbreak occurred, water-well A was in use. Well A supplied water to the shop and to the apartment. Even though shigellosis is rarely transmitted by water, at the time of the outbreak, the water supply for the school became suspected. The suspect well was not chlorinated at the time of the outbreak, and because it was suspected it was superchlorinated on Nov. 17th. The Stockport municipal water company had a water system under construction and special priority was given to connecting the school to the new water supply. The water was connected on Nov. 21st. One of the

TABLE III.4   Attack rates of gastrointestinal illness by usual amount of water consumed daily at the Middle School

Estimated Amount of Water Drunk	Students		Faculty & Staff	
	No. Ill/Total	Attack Rate (%)	No. Ill/Total	Attack Rate (%)
0 glasses	4/11		3/3	
1 glass	14/19		2/5	
2 glasses	24/36		1/2	
3 glasses	38/57		1/3	
4 glasses	43/56		2/2	
5 glasses	28/38		0/1	
6+ glasses	43/50		3/3	

three wells was destroyed in the process of hooking up the municipal water system. Investigation of the two remaining wells showed that they were shallow bored well cases with ceramic pipe segments, having joints that were not watertight. The outflow pipes of the submersible pump pierced the lining of the well below ground level. The hole allowed seepage of ground water into the well. Well B, which was closer to the school, was not in use at the time of the shigellosis epidemic, however when the pump in one well was turned on it lowered the water table in both wells. Well B was located in a slight depression on the surface of the earth and could be contaminated by surface water as well as ground water sources. Indeed, debris was found floating in well B. On the opposite side of the school from the wells was a septic tank that fed a drain field emptying into a ditch southeast of the school. Attempts with dye were made to show cross contamination. All efforts failed to reveal any cross contamination by the appearance of the dye in the school well-water supply. Other attempts to show cross contamination involved using fluorescent dye in the toilet in the apartment located in the shop building, across the street from the school as well as the school yard storm drains; all failed, with one exception, to show cross contamination of the well water.

Showers for the students were adjacent to the Gym but visiting teams used the shower located in the utility room on the basement floor of the school. The shower was installed only shortly before the shigellosis outbreak. The shower drained down into a bed of gravel under the basement floor, and was known to drain well. Hooking the shower up to the sewer system had been considered unnecessary as it drained well. Dye studies flushed down the drain of the shower, located only a few feet from the wells, showed up in the well water within 3 hours. This same shower was used by 3 faculty members during the time period of the outbreak. Two (2) of the 3 faculty members were among those documented with shigellosis on November 13th and the other was identified with the disease on November 15th and had febrile diarrhea. On Nov. 16th, water samples were taken from the tap in the boy's restroom which revealed a total coliform count of 125 per 100 ml. A second water sample was obtained from the school on Nov. 17th prior to the superchlorination of the supply. The second water sample revealed a coliform most probable number of 16+, and *Shigella sonnei* was recovered from a 1600 ml sample.

Case Study Questions

1. The common-source and first cases of the outbreak were from the wellwater. Explain how the secondary cases of shigellosis probably occurred; identify the probable mode(s) of transmission in the secondary cases.

2. Was the basketball team from the neighboring community primary transmission cases or secondary? Why? What role did the neighboring basketball team play in secondary cases?

3. In this case, a secondary case was defined as diarrhea beginning between Nov. 10th and Dec. 4th. Why are these dates chosen for this purpose and how do they help determine what a secondary case is in this investigation?

4. Much concern was given to whether or not a case was symptomatic or asymptomatic. What is the significance of these two states of illness and why is this important in this particular disease?

5. Calculate the secondary attack rates for Table III.1.

6. What problems or shortcomings did you see in this study? What would be necessary to overcome such shortcomings?

7. What type of sewage system in the school complex was used and how effective was it? What role did it play in disease transmission?

8. What was the attack rate for the students for November?

9. What caused the epidemic to taper off after November 16th?

10. What was the attack rate for the faculty and staff for November?

11. What is the sensitivity for the symptomatic students and faculty and staff using the rectal swab test?

12. What is the specificity for the asymptomatic students and faculty and staff using the rectal swab test?

13. Develop and construct a bar chart of the epidemiological curve for the shigellosis outbreak using the data in Table III.2. Identify the index case and date, and explain who the index case was. What date was the water chlorinated? What did chlorinating the water do to the epidemic curve?

14. Develop a bar graph of the secondary attack rate for the shigellosis epidemic using the data from Table III.3. Explain why the secondary epidemic curve is different than that of the primary epidemic curve.

15. Calculate the attack rates for the various amount of water consumption as it related to illness onset, found in Table III.4.

16. What are your observations as to the source of the contamination of the well water with *Shigella sonnei*, that caused the outbreak? Give two possible sources for the pathogen getting into the water supply, (1) direct and (2) indirect.

17. What are the control and prevention measures needed for this case and shigellosis general?

IV

Retrospective Analysis of Occupation and Alcohol-Related Mortality

Adapted from Brooks, S.D. and Harford, T.C., "Occupation and Alcohol-Related Causes of Death," Drug and Alcohol Dependence, Vol. 29, No. 3, pp. 245–251, 1992.

The liver is the organ most often seriously damaged by heavy drinking. Even moderate drinking damages body tissues, which are quickly mended. The more one drinks and the longer, the more lasting and serious the effects on the body. The connection between heavy drinking of alcohol and heart disease has been known for over 100 years. For years, malnutrition was pointed to as the cause of the physiological damage. Malnutrition is still a major factor, but now it known that the alcohol does the damage to the body tissues and organs directly. A direct causative association between heavy alcohol consumption and heart disease has been established. Areas of the heart affected are the mitochondria (energy-producing cells in the cardiac muscle), which results in alcoholic cardiomyopathy (heart muscle degeneration). Without energy the heart's pumping action fails over time. Arrhythmia of the heart is also seen in heavy drinkers, because, alcohol disrupts the natural heart rhythms. High blood pressure is also seen. Cancer is also caused by heavy drinking. Cancer of the liver, larynx, nasopharynx and esophagus are seen more frequently in heavy drinkers. Ulcerative lesions are seen in the small intestine. The pancreas is vulnerable to alcohol abuse, resulting in pancreatitis. Alcoholic myopathy or muscle weakness is also seen at serious clinical levels in heavy drinkers. (Source: Schlaadt, R.G. *Wellness: Alcohol Use and Abuse*, Dushkin Publishing Group: Guilford, CT 1992.)

CASE OF OCCUPATION AND ALCOHOL-RELATED CAUSES OF DEATH, CALIFORNIA

Are alcohol-related causes of death associated with similar occupational groups? Is heavy drinking associated with different occupations? Most studies have focused on cirrhosis of the liver deaths related to alcohol drinking. Several research studies found that cirrhosis mortality has been shown to be associated with the following occupations: bartenders, waiters, cooks, longshoremen, seamen, salesmen, wholesale and retail trades, entertainment and recreation workers, truck drivers, garage proprietors and personal service workers. The studies also found that cirrhosis is highest in lower status jobs; blue collar workers. Also, jobs with high exposure to alcohol use and/or consumption have high drinking levels. Only 8 to 12% of heavy drinkers die from cirrhosis.

Many other alcohol and occupation associated conditions occur but do not get as much focus as cirrhosis of the liver. The more common conditions in which alcohol is implicated as a cause of death include: digestive tract cancers, pancreatic disorders, certain cardiovascular diseases, and accidents and injuries.

Which alcohol-related causes of death are associated with which occupations?

The California Occupational Mortality Study (COMS) data set was employed to assess mortality data for the years 1979–1981. A 2% sample of employed persons from the 1980 census of California was used. The COMS contains the occupation of each decedent (person who died).

This study, as any occupation based study, is restricted to the work life span as far as age of subjects is concerned. This study used ages 16 through 64. Certain persons, due to their source of work were excluded as subjects; homemakers, retired persons, students, disabled, military personnel, etc. Only mainstream type employment was used in this study to establish occupations at risk for heavy alcohol drinking. Military/nonworkers/unknowns were also analyzed. Underlying causes of death were used from the ICD-9-CM (see Chapter 2) for cirrhosis, digestive organ cancers, injuries, suicide and homicide (see Table IV.1).

Thirteen occupational groups were identified, using the Census Bureau's 1980 Alphabetical Index of Industries and Occupations. Age adjusted mortality rates per 100,000 were calculated for each of the 13 occupational groups (see Table IV.2). The **numerator** used was the number of occupation-specific deaths in each category of underlying cause of death in California 1979–1981. The **denominator** for each occupational group was from the 20% sample of the 1980 Census of California used in the COMS which was 173,438 deaths in California 1979–1981.

Males and Caucasians had the highest percent for each of the causes of death. Older age groups had the large percent of deaths for cirrhosis and digestive organ cancers. Younger age groups had higher percents in injuries, suicide and homicide. Military/nonworkers/unknowns, had a pattern similar to that of workers, except for females, who had higher deaths rates related to alcohol than the female workers. The age-adjusted mortality rate for "all other causes of death per 100,000 for the State of California was 238.77.

Research findings show that individuals in certain occupations drink alcohol more heavily than persons in other occupations. Factors which contribute to heavy alcohol consumption include: opportunity to drink, time, location and availability of alcohol, work group or social group that has drinking as a custom, job stress, time pressures and work rotations. Additionally, heavy drinking may occur in jobs that have: low job visibility, high

TABLE IV.1   Alcohol deaths in California

Alcohol Related Deaths in California, 1979–1981	
Cirrhosis	5.5%
Digestive organ cancers	5.7%
Injuries	13.7%
Suicide and homicide	5.1%
All other causes	64.9%

TABLE IV.2   Age-adjusted mortality rates for occupational groups and cause of death

Age-Adjusted Mortality Rates for Occuaptional Groups and Cause of Death per 100,000

Occupational Group	Digestive Cirrhosis Mortality Rate	Cancer Mortality Rate	Injury Mortality Rate	Suicide Mortality Rate	Homicide Mortality Rate
Executive, administrative and managerial	13.60	25.10	32.47	13.72	10.02
Professional specialty	15.24	23.76	35.79	20.39	7.97
Technicians and related support areas	19.82	26.47	54.86	22.99	8.83
Sales	16.72	26.17	35.58	17.43	12.62
Administrative support, including clerical	13.50	20.07	23.97	12.15	7.58
Private household service	15.07	22.46	16.79	7.14	17.14
Protective service	36.17	40.46	61.02	33.95	38.13
Other service	29.66	26.46	47.97	18.28	25.60
Farming, forestry and fishing	41.23	28.56	158.87	23.75	56.68
Precision production, craft and repair	33.98	34.69	91.29	32.78	30.51
Machine operators and assemblers	25.67	27.76	55.66	19.23	26.49
Transportation and material moving	39.58	38.45	112.84	28.41	34.64
Handlers, equipment, cleaners, helpers and laborers	75.97	52.26	129.14	39.33	77.11
State of California	**20.07**	**21.01**	**50.44**	**18.71**	**18.64**

turnover, little supervision and minimal job qualifications. High stress on the job, low accountability, and easy access to alcohol are factors that may contribute to heavy and destructive use of alcohol. From an epidemiological research point of view, all of these factors may serve as confounding variables to occupation and alcohol abuse research.

Certain occupations may allow drinking on the job, as supervisors know little about it. Some people work in the field independently, away from the work site and other jobs may actually encourage drinking on the job or at lunch. Many studies fail to differentiate between drinking on the job, job-related alcohol consumption, and non-job related drinking. It is suspected that workplace drinking risks are low as compared to after-hours or lunchtime drinking. Other factors that may contribute to heavy drinking regardless of the work setting are the biological/physiological, psychological, familial, social class, religious influences, peer pressure, and other nonwork related factors and variables.

Case Study Questions

1. What occupations are most vulnerable to acquiring cirrhosis of the liver from heavy drinking? List several of the occupations identified by research studies which are more vulnerable to alcohol induced cirrhosis related deaths and that have the highest mortality rates.

2. Other than cirrhosis, what major diseases have heavy alcohol use implications as far as causation? List several.

3. Discuss why this study was restricted to ages 16–64. Discuss the research design implications of the age span restrictions in occupational studies.

4. In this study, which occupations had the highest digestive organ cancer mortality rate?

5. In this study, which occupations had the highest injury mortality rate?

6. In this study, which occupations had the highest suicide mortality rate?

7. In this study, which occupations had the highest homicide mortality rate?

8. Two occupational groups repeatedly exceeded the state average for alcohol-related deaths. Which two were they? Why? Provide an explanation.

9. What figures were used for the numerator of this study? What figures were used for the denominator of this study? Was the use of the numerator and denominator appropriate for age adjusted rates?

10. Develop and show the formula for the age-adjusted digestive cancer mortality rate for the top 4 at-risk occupations for this disease found in Table IV.2.

11. What are the possible confounding variables for research in occupations and heavy drinking that lead to fatal diseases? Identify and explain which factors are confounding variables and how they serve as confounding variables.

12. Develop and construct a *web of causation* along with appropriate decision trees for occupational group related alcohol deaths.

V

Retrospective Cohort Study of the Association of Congenital Malformations and Hazardous Waste

Adapted from Geschwind, S.A., Stolwijk, J.A.J., Bracken, M., et al., "Risk of Congenital Malformations Associated with Proximity to Hazardous Waste Sites," *American Journal of Epidemiology*, Vol. 135, No. 11, pp. 1197–1207, 1992.

Congenital anomalies or malformations are difficult to pinpoint as to cause. Some congenital malformation causes are understood, many are not. Causes may be single isolated cases where others are multiple and varied. Some malformations at birth are inherited, and some are sporadic in their manifestation. Congenital defects are sometimes apparent, others hidden, taking years to become obvious; others are gross and easily seen while others are subtle and not easily detected even by physicians at first. About 10% of neonatal deaths are caused by congenital malformations. A major malformation is apparent at birth in 3 to 4% of newborns. By the fifth year, up to 7.5% of all children manifest a congenital malformation. The incidence of certain congenital malformations varies with the defect (cleft lip occurs at the rate of 1 per 1,000 births in the U.S.) and the geographic area (spina bifida is about 4 per 1,000 births in Ireland and 2 per 1,000 in the U.S.). Interfamily marriage and culture practices can contribute to congenital malformations as can perinatal problems and environmental exposures. Genetic factors are responsible for many congenital anomalies and syndromes. On the other hand, multiple factors are often involved in causing congenital malformations. Drugs taken while pregnant, infectious agents and irradiation are known to cause birth defects. Chemicals in the environment as well as exposure to hazardous materials and waste in the environment and exposure to radiation in the worksite or environment have also been implicated. (Source: Berkow, R. (Editor-in-Chief), *The Merck Manual*, 14th Edition, Merck and Co. Inc.: Rahway, N.J. 1982).

CASE ON CONGENITAL MALFORMATIONS ASSOCIATED
WITH PROXIMITY TO HAZARDOUS WASTE SITES

Much concern has been expressed by the general public and public health scientists alike, over the effects of exposure to environmental pollutants and how they have increased in modern society. It remains unclear whether chronic exposure to toxic chemicals in the environment is present in sufficiently high doses to produce adverse medical effects in humans. Inadvertent exposure to hazardous waste such as Love Canal has increased concern about any adverse effects the exposure might have on reproductive health. It also remains unclear whether individuals who live near toxic chemical waste sites receive doses in sufficient amounts to pose a health hazard, especially to reproductive functions. One concern is that many toxic chemicals present in toxic waste landfills and hazardous waste sites are cytotoxic. That is, they affect cells, tissues and organs at specific stages of development and inhibit or interfere with normal growth, especially in embryo and fetus growth and developmental stages.

High rates of birth defects have been reported in children exposed to mercury, solvents and certain toxic chemicals. Community based studies have been conducted based on reports of clustering of disease around hazardous waste sites. Rarely have congenital defects in infants born to exposed parents been well documented.

This uses a 4-tiered hypothesis approach in order to evaluate the relationship between birth defects and the potential exposure to toxic waste sites. 1. Does residential proximity to a waste site when pregnant increase risk of bearing a child with a defect? 2. Do defects of specific organ systems correlate with proximity to a toxic waste site? 3. Were defects associated with off-site migration of chemicals? How does the epidemiologist clarify whether this increased potential health risks? 4. Have chemical types associated with certain organ system defects been evaluated?

Pesticides have been associated with oral cleft (lips or palate), or musculo-skeletal defects, heavy metals with nervous system defects, solvents have been associated with nervous system defects or digestive system defects, and plastics with chromosomal anomalies. Do the later phases corroborate the initial findings? Finally this study was to test the association of environmental and health data bases and geographic mapping methods for ascertaining environmental exposures.

The data bases of the New York State Department of Health were used; Congenital Malformation Registry (CMR) and the Hazardous Waste Site Inspection Program. The two programs were linked together for analysis of the 4 tiers of hypotheses. The Congenital Malformation Registry includes reports of all congenital malformations for the state's hospitals, medical facilities and private physicians diagnosed in children up to two years of age. In the state of New York, 917 waste sites in 62 counties were available. New York City sites as well as several other sites were eliminated due to inadequate information. For final study, 590 waste sites in 20 counties were used. Epidemiological map study approaches included each site being assigned a longitude and latitude using EPA and New York Department of Environmental Conservation records. (See Figure V.1, map of New York State with waste sites identified as small black triangles.)

A total of 34,411 cases of malformations were recorded in the CMR for the years 1983–85 and 1984–86 birth cohorts. Any cases that were unusual were eliminated: multiple births, redundant cases, CDC exclusions list to avoid misclassification of malformations, census mapping coordinates missing, addresses incomplete and locations without a census

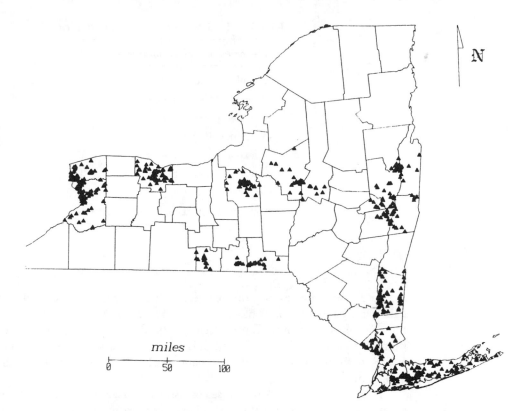

FIGURE V.I   Map of New York State with waste sites identified.

tract. The study was based on 12,442 congenital malformations and 9,313 cases. One case could have more than one defect.

Eight categories of malformations were used from ICD-9-CM (see Chapter 2) that have been reported by research studies in the literature as being associated with exposures to chemicals or toxic substances (see Table V.1). Each individual exposure was unknown and each probably could have had multiple exposures to a complex mix of chemicals. All cases were put under one general analysis. Each case was then placed in one of the 8 categories and analyzed. More than one defect was found present in each case.

Controls were selected from birth certificate records; 17,802 or 12% of the 506,183 live birth for 1983–1984 in the State of New York. Cross checks were made to assure no congenital malformations were included in the control. Confounding variables were excluded from both cases and controls and the information included:

- Maternal age
- Race
- Education
- Address and county of residence
- Any pregnancy complications

- Parity
- Birth weight of the child
- Length of gestation
- Sex of the child

TABLE V.1   Categories of malformations

8 Categories of Malformations ICD-9-CM

- Oral clefts defects
- Musculo-skeletal defects
- Nervous system defects
- Integument defects
- Digestive system defects
- Chromosomal anomalies
- Syndromes
- Remaining defects without category

Addresses for cases and controls were each assigned a latitude and longitude. Coordinates were based on census blocks based on Standard Metropolitan Statistical Areas, and Post Carrier Route centroids were used. (centroid is the center point of the Postal Carrier Route boundary) and Zip code centroids. A sample of 500 addresses was taken at random as a test of the mapping methods. The mapping procedure was accurate within 200 feet, 80% of the time.

Hazardous waste sites were assessed using the Hazardous Waste Site Inspection Program (HWSIP) which estimates the likelihood of human exposure. Possible exposure routes into humans include inhalation, ingestion and dermal contact which occurs by environmental exposure transmission from air, groundwater, surface, water, or soil. This study included all residents within a 1 mile radius of the waste site edge. Still, absolute risk of exposure was uncertain. Assessment was based on a set of scores of a variety of factors: Chemical exposure, a probability score chance of contaminant transport from the site, a target factor score which accounts for the population and distance from the waste site and a weighting factor score giving each exposure a level of relative importance. The assessment excluded the total population portion of the target factor score, to give greater weight to the residents surrounding the waste sites.

Four general categories of chemicals grouped by chemical properties were developed. The five categories were

1. pesticides
2. metals
3. solvents
4. plastics
5. unknown

An exposure risk index was completed for each case. The index accounted for distance and hazard ranking score within a 1 mile radius of the birth residence. Waste sites based on evidence of off-site migration of contaminants were separated from nonmigration sites.

All cases and controls coordinates were matched to hazardous waste sites by a matching program. Distance and direction from the hazardous waste site for the residence of each case or control living within a 1-mile radius of the edge of the site were considered potentially exposed. Risk was determined by association between mothers' (maternal) proximity to waste sites and presence of congenital anomalies (birth defects).

A 12% increased risk for birth defect associated with maternal proximity to toxic waste sites was found. Odds ratios were used to assess the association between proximity to toxic sites and maternal residence. An odds ratio score above 1.01 shows a positive association and the higher the score the stronger the association. Table V.2 presents the odds ratios for congenital malformation with residential proximity to selected hazardous waste sites. Table V.3 presents odds ratios and exposure risk index for all congenital malformations and for three specific body systems affected by documented chemical leaks at hazardous waste sites. Table V.4 presents odds ratios for congenital malformations for all infants with specific malformations and residential proximity to selected toxic waste sites and chemical groups.

TABLE V.2 Odds ratios for congenital malformations with residential proximity to selected hazardous waste sites

Odds ratios for all congenital malformations and for specific malformations in infants with residential proximity to selected hazardous waste sites, New York State, 1983–1984

No. of Cases[‡]	Congenital Malformation(s)	OR[†,§]
9,313	All malformations combined	1.12**
421	Nervous system	1.29*
2,730	Musculoskeletal system	1.16**
1,370	Integument system	1.32**
232	Oral clefts	1.15
429	Digestive system	0.89
245	Chromosomal anomalies	1.18
575	Syndromes[‖]	1.15
4,003	Other (data too limited to infer associations with chemical exposure)	1.01

*p < 0.05; **p < 0.01

[†]ICD-9, International Classification of Diseases, Ninth Revision; OR, odds ratio; CI, confidence interval.

[‡]The numbers of cases for the individual organ systems do not add up to the total number of cases for all defects combined because individuals may have had more than one defect.

[§]Adjusted for maternal age, race, education, complications during pregnancy, parity, population density for county of residence, and sex of the child, by logistic regression.

[‖]Syndromes include all defects coded as "syndrome" in the New York State Congenital Malformations Registry, or any child with four or more defects.

TABLE V.3   Odds ratios and exposure risk index for all congenital malformations and for three specific body systems affected by documented chemical leaks at hazardous waste sites

Exposure	*All Malformations Combined (740–759)*[‡]	*Nervous System (740–742)*	*Musculoskeletal System (754–756)*	*Integument System (757)*
	Exposure Risk Index			
No exposure risk	1.00	1.00	1.00	1.00
Low exposure risk	1.09** (1.04–1.15)[§]	1.27* (1.03–1.57)	1.09 (1.00–1.18)	1.22** (1.08–1.38)
High exposure risk	1.63** (1.34–1.99)	1.48 (0.69–3.16)	1.75** (1.31–2.34)	2.63** (1.90–3.67)
	Chemical Leaks			
Not exposed	1.00	1.00	1.00	1.00
Exposed, but no leaks found at site	1.08* (1.02–1.15)	1.35* (1.06–1.72)	1.08 (0.98–1.20)	1.22* (1.06–1.40)
Exposed, and leaks found at site	1.17** (1.08–1.27)	1.16 (0.87–1.55)	1.16* (1.03–1.31)	1.38** (1.17–1.62)

*$p < 0.05$; **$p < 0.01$.

[†]Adjusted for maternal age, race, education, complications during pregnancy, parity, population density for county of residence, and sex of the child, by logistic regression.

[‡]International Classification of Diseases, Ninth Revision, code(s).

[§]Numbers in parentheses, 95% confidence interval.

Case Study Questions

1.   What are controls in a research study and how are they used? How are controls used in this study?

2.   What are confounding variables? How do they affect a research study? What are the problems and limitations of confounding variables in this study?

3.   From Table V.2 which malformations had the highest odds ratio? Which malformations had the lowest odds ratio score? What is the significance of each?

4.   From Table V.3 which body systems were at the most risk of exposure to chemical leaks? What is the significance of such determination?

5.   From Table V.4 which three combinations of "chemicals associated with congenital malformation" were the highest? Which chemicals were linked to and associated with malformations according to the odds ratio score? Explain the assessment and the meaning of Table V.4?

TABLE V.4 Odds ratios for congenital malformations for specific malformations and residential proximity to selected toxic waste sites and chemical groups

*Odds ratios for congenital malformations for all infants with specific malformation codes†
and residential proximity to selected toxic waste sites containing associated chemical
groups: New York State, 1983–1984*

Chemical and Associated Malformation (Reference)	OR [†,§]	CI[‡]
Pesticides/oral clefts (13–15)	1.27	0.84–1.92
Pesticides/musculoskeletal system (16, 17)	1.20*	1.05–1.38
Metals/nervous system (18–20)	1.34*	1.07–1.67
Solvents/nervous system (21–23)	1.24*	1.01–1.54
Solvents/digestive system (24, 25)	0.91	0.73–1.13
Plastics/chromosomal anomalies (26–29)	1.46*	1.01–2.11

*$p < 0.05$.

†Previously related to chemical exposures in the literature.

‡ICD-9, International Classification of Diseases, Ninth Revision; OR, odds ratio; CI, confidence interval.

§Adjusted for maternal age, race, education, complications during pregnancy, parity, population density for county of residence, and sex of the child, by logistic regression.

6. From the three tables and the final assessments, what are the findings of this study with regards to exposure and proximity to hazardous waste sites and congenital malformation? Explain your answer.

7. Pick one form of congenital malformation, develop and construct a *web of causation* for the disorder, including appropriate *decision trees*.

8. What prevention and control programs can be implemented to reduce congenital malformations from environmental exposure?

VI

History and Epidemiology of Polio Epidemics

Instructions: Read the paragraphs preceding the questions then answer the questions that pertain to those paragraphs. Continue through the case until all questions are answered.

Infantile paralysis, as it was first known, was a most difficult disease to understand. For centuries, people became crippled and no one seemed to know why, for the paralysis was not associated with a disease. It was observed that mostly young people were paralyzed, and often the legs or back and also the arms were affected. Historically, this crippling disease was called infantile paralysis or anterior infantile and a variety of other names. The term *infantile paralysis* became popular because this disease was thought to be confined to children, although it had been observed in almost all ages.

Infantile paralysis was studied by physician/epidemiologists, and the disease was eventually called poliomyelitis. The real breakthrough came when the infection was finally discovered to be a biphasic disease (see page 475). The first phase of the disease has symptoms similar to those of the flu or a bad cold. It was the second phase in which the crippling occurs, as the virus moves from the blood into the central nervous system (CNS), where nerve cells in the spinal cord and/or brain are destroyed and replaced with fatty deposits. The devastating result is the irreversible loss of control of the lungs, limbs, or other musculoskeletal structures. Atrophy of muscles is caused by loss of neuromotor control of the affected muscles. The sensory nerves are mostly unaffected, and feelings remained. The part of the spinal cord affected by the virus is the anterior horn of the gray matter of the spinal cord.

When the two levels of the disease were finally discovered, the door was opened for more effective epidemiological investigations. The disease, when running its course, did not always progress into the second phase in all people; and those fortunate enough to experience only the first phase usually escaped paralysis.

The virus, when finally discovered, was thought to be harbored only in the upper respiratory tract, but was later found throughout the body, with its highest concentrations in the gastrointestinal tract.

The Salk killed virus vaccine, injected intramuscularly, has a moderate level of effectiveness. Sabin developed a more effective vaccine in the form of a weakened live vaccine taken orally in sugar cubes, thus targeting the higher concentration of the virus in the gastrointestinal tract with the Sabin vaccine being the more effective of the two. From the use of these vaccines, millions of people have escaped the crippling paralysis caused by the poliovirus.

(A) BRIEF REVIEW OF POLIOMYELITIS AS IT IS KNOWN TODAY

The virus responsible for polio is very small compared to many other viruses, such as the smallpox and chickenpox viruses. The poliovirus falls in the Enterovirus class of the Picornavirus group. It exists in three immunological virus types: Type I is the most likely to cause paralysis and lead to identifiable epidemics due to the observed paralysis. The infection is highly contagious and is spread via fecal-oral and pharyngeal-oropharyngeal (mouth-throat) routes.

The main source of spread is from the lesser types, labeled as inapparent infections, which occur widely in unimmunized populations. The risk of direct person-to-person transmission comes from the fact that inapparent cases are mistaken for colds or influenza. The apparent/overt (easily seen) outbreak is rare except during epidemics, and even then the ratio of inapparent infections to clinical cases exceeds 100:1. Epidemics are most likely to occur when basic public health measures such as hand washing are neglected, when food sanitation is poor, and through interpersonal transmission by those who think the infection is only the flu. Where sanitation and hygiene are poor, virus circulation can be extensive. When the infection and immunity are acquired in the first few years of life, cases are sporadic, confined largely to children under five years, and epidemics do not occur. Polio is a seasonal disease occurring in the summer and fall in temperate climates. Tropical climates and underdeveloped countries experience epidemics year round. Unvaccinated populations are at high risk of epidemics.[1]

The virus multiplies in the pharynx and intestinal tract and is present in the blood, throat, and feces during the incubation period. After onset it can be recovered from the throat for about 1 to 2 weeks and from the feces for 3 to 6 weeks or longer. CNS involvement lasts several days, disappearing as antibodies develop. Factors predisposing patients to serious neurologic involvement include increasing age, recent innoculations (recent DTP is commonly found connected to the onset of poliomyelitis), recent tonsillectomy, pregnancy, and physical exertion concurrent with onset of the CNS phase. In older cases, the first phase might not be accounted for, or the minor illness might go unobserved.[1]

Rotary International has been working toward a goal of eradicating poliomyelitis from the earth by eventually vaccinating each and every person in all countries, especially underdeveloped countries. There is also much effort being put forth to eliminate the polio vaccination activities in the U.S., much as was done with smallpox. The eventuality is that all people are to be protected by vaccination, and the source of the pathogen will be eliminated. Some segments of the public health community are warning that to halt polio immunizations is a bad move and have issued similar warnings about smallpox vaccinations' being stopped. In regard to smallpox, the world now has a massive population of susceptibles who could become infected with smallpox—all those born after 1978. Much media attention has been focused on the few rare cases of children acquiring polio from the immunization process. However, the media fails to point out the millions of persons who could be crippled today from paralytic polio, if it were not for the polio vaccine.

Case Study Questions

A.1   Identify the pathogenic agent and the group to which infantile paralysis belongs.

A.2   Identify the locations in the body where this pathogen is harbored.

A.3   Identify the current accepted mode of disease transmission and related epidemiological implications.

(B) FIRST POLIO EPIDEMICS STUDIED AND REPORTED: SWEDEN

Some early observations of Dr. Ivar Wickman in several cities in Sweden (Umea, Goteborg, Stockholm, and Tingsryd [population 3,000, 200 miles southwest of Stockholm] in the summer of 1905) follow.

A minor case of the illness, with its outward symptoms (as opposed to the inward progress of the disease as it occurs when it has moved into the CNS) is what Swedish epidemiologist Ivar Wickman observed in the early part of the twentieth century. These observations were crucial to detecting and understanding the total picture and scope of the disease and its two-phase process.[2]

Names of Polio

Wickman referred to this child-crippling disease as Heine-Medin Disease in 1907. Jacob Von Heine (1799–1878) was a German orthopedist and Wickman's teacher. Oskar Medin (1847–1927) was a Swedish pediatrician. Wickman named polio after Heine and Medin because they had both conducted the earliest adequate study of the disease.[2]

Other names of polio included "debility of the lower extremities," a term used in the late 1700s; "morning paralysis," used in the mid-1800s, and "Heine-Medin Disease," used in the late 1800s and early 1900s. Most commonly in the early 1900s it was called "infantile paralysis." "Anterior *poliomyelites*," is a term later derived from the work of Dr. John Shaw. With the discovery of the virus it was called "*poliomyelites*" and shortened to "polio."[2,3,4,5]

The mid-1800s through the early 1900s was an amazing era for advances in microbiology, epidemiology, medicine, and science, all of which in some way contributed to the understanding of polio and the discovery of the poliovirus.[2] Wickman and Medin believed that Bergenholtz deserved credit for observing the first polio epidemic, a minor outbreak of 13 cases in the small village of Umea in northern Sweden in 1881.[2,3,4,5]

Age Issues—Not Just a Child's Disease

As early as 1858, Q. Vogt described the first case of poliomyelitis in an adult (Switzerland). Polio was previously thought to occur only in children. In the 1905 epidemic, it was reported by Wickman that 45% of those stricken with the disease were over the age of 10, and 21% were over the age of 15. Wickman observed that poliomyelitis was not limited to children and that, as epidemics recurred, they included older age groups. The concept of the disease as "infantile paralysis" became obscured.[2]

In 1884, the first accurate account of the encephalitic form or cerebral type of polio was documented by Adolf von Strümpell in Vienna. He suggested that the causative agent could be localized in the brain and the spinal cord.[2]

Epidemiologists struggled for the longest time trying to understand the disease and identify true outbreaks, as the disease goes through a two-phase process before getting to the paralytic phase. At first, only the paralytic phase was clearly recognized and identified as infantile paralysis, because the first phase was so easily confused with other diseases such as the flu, common colds, and related conditions. This was the case with an outbreak of polio in Oslo, Norway, which was thought to be spinal meningitis. Epidemics of influenza have also been confused with the first phase of poliomyelitis because the symptoms are quite similar. Such a mistaken occurrence took place in Los Angeles in the mid-1930s, causing a panic among health care professionals. Mild cases of the disease that did not reach the paralytic stage were thought to constitute 5 to 25% of all cases.[2]

Disease investigators of the day were a frustrated lot due to the lack of clear understanding and diagnosis of the disease. Numerous field workers, such as nurses, who were hired to trudge through communities during polio outbreaks in an attempt to trace relationships between multiple paralytic cases, often found only dead ends. Countless case questionnaires and forms were completed with the assistance of families in an effort to trace the disease and its transmission. The data from these questionnaires were analyzed in order to trace the spread of the disease.[2,3,4,5]

Even though clustering of polio cases was observed in rural communities in Norway and France, it was Sweden's epidemiologists/physicians who further connected polio outbreaks to ruralness and who provided the most advances in poliomyelitis in the years 1890 to 1914.[2]

Karl Oskar Medin   Many of the advances in knowledge of polio are attributed to Karl Oskar Medin. Medin is given a great deal of credit for detecting and assembling a comprehensive set of clinical features of the disease—the best effort done to this point in history. The greatest recognition of his work came when he, as a reliable, articulate, and experienced pediatrician, presented his observations to the 10th International Medical Congress in Berlin in 1890. Medin was also concerned about community care (public health aspects) of children. He was chairman of the Stockholm Board of Health from 1906–1915. He was also known for his role as an excellent teacher and had many pupils.[2]

Medin was born in 1847 in a small town near Stockholm and attended college at Uppsala, obtaining his medical licentiate at Stockholm in 1875. He was a prominent pediatrician in Sweden, a professor of pediatrics at the Karolinska Institute, and head physician at the General Orphan Sylum in Stockholm, giving him 30 years' experience in pediatric medicine in an all-child setting. Medin clarified the picture of poliomyelitis but gained for Sweden the unfortunate reputation of being the country where the worst outbreaks had occurred at the time.[2]

In 1887 Medin investigated an outbreak of 44 cases. Before that, he had stated that the cases of polio showing up at Polyclinic Hospital in Stockholm were infrequent. Attending to such an epidemic gave Medin considerable experience in dealing with polio in a great number of children.[2]

Medin divided the cases into two groups: (1) the spinal type which consisted of 27 cases of the paralytic type, and (2) those with less common signs based on unusual location of the lesions. Medin was able to establish clearly the clinical course of the disease. The site of the pathological lesion had been previously established as being in the spinal cord, but it was Medin who established that there is first a phase that affects the body's total systems, then later, a paralytic phase. He established that early minor symptoms and signs, such as fever, headache, and malaise, were symptoms of the early phase and later could (or may not) be followed by serious damage to the central nervous system. In certain areas of the spinal cord, the lesions could cause paralysis of various muscle groups or organs when the motor neurons were destroyed. Any disease involvement with the CNS always led to complications and some form of paralysis, even if it was minor. Medin followed the patients in the outbreak closely, making astute observations, documenting the early features of the disease, and observing that the disease subsided for a brief interim afebrile period, thus giving the course of the disease a biphasic pattern, with a major bout of fever experienced in both the first and last acute phases of the illness. The minor illness and its accompanying symptoms represented the first phase, and the second phase was more complicated and serious, resulting in paralysis to some parts of the body (see Figure 9.8, page 280). These observations were followed and advanced by Kling and his colleagues, including Ivar Wickman.[2]

Why the Scandinavian region experienced the first wave of the extensive polio epidemic is not clear. The epidemic of 1905 was the worst, with over 1,000 cases. It is known that polio seems to occur in rural areas as much as, if not more than, in large cities, and Scandinavia was quite rural at the time. Less exposure to a disease led to the population's having less immunity to the disease. There seemed to be higher immunity in city dwellers and lower immunity in rural populations.[2]

Ivar Wickman   Ivar Wickman, Medin's pupil, was thoroughly educated about poliomyelitis by his mentor. Wickman experienced two epidemics while working at the Medical Clinic in Stockholm—one in Stockholm and the other in Goteborg in 1903. Wickman was born in Lund in the southern tip of Sweden in 1872. He studied in Lund and Stockholm, and, later in his career, on the European continent. He passed the medical board exams in 1895, at which time he became Medin's assistant in the Stockholm Pediatric Clinic. He wrote a 300-page monograph on polio in 1905, making him one of the leading experts in the field. Wickman, a man with well-known publications and advanced training, including the advanced medical degree of "Doctor of Medicine," applied for the directorship of the now-prestigious Stockholm Pediatric Clinic, feeling sure he would be accepted for the position. He was not and consequently committed suicide in 1914 at age 42.[2]

Epidemiological Questions

Among the clinical pathological observations made by Wickman, was concern with how the agent (of which he was not sure) traveled through the community and how it entered the human host. How did it spread throughout the body, and how was it eliminated? Did it travel within the body along the nerves, in the lymph, or in the blood? From the 1905 epidemic of 1,031 cases, he wanted to know what the nature of the disease was. Was it actually contagious? How did it spread? Was it spread by direct contact with infected sick people? Did healthy people carry the agent? Was it waterborne? Foodborne? Was it spread like typhoid? (We now know the answer is yes—both are feces-borne.)[2]

Key Epidemiological Points

The number of cases was no doubt increased by Wickman's inclusion of cases of both the paralytic type and the abortive/nonparalytic type. Whether or not to include nonparalytic cases was always a subject of debate among epidemiologists and statisticians. Wickman's astute observation that the nonparalytic cases were as important to the transmission of the disease, if not more so than the paralytic cases, was a major epidemiological contribution. The abortive type, or nonparalytic cases, and paralytic cases are two ends of a continuum. Nonparalytic or abortive cases were lucky and escaped having a serious outcome from such a crippling disease, with no more than what might seem to be a bad case of the common cold. (The course of the disease ends, either because of a high immune response by the body, or because the person gets only a mild dose of the pathogen and/or a mild case of the disease, develops immunity, and is therefore, no longer susceptible.) Paralytic cases might die but most often they were crippled and devastated for life. These advanced cases suffered major or minor deformation of limbs, total loss of use of limbs, or confinement to an iron lung for the rest of their lives.

Mild cases (abortive/nonparalytic cases) were found to be just as contagious as paralytic cases and could not be ignored. A relationship between main roads and railway routes and the spread of the epidemic of 1905 was established. An association with disease spread was developed based on busy traffic centers, which allowed frequent communication between rural and urban dwellers. Wickman followed many rural outbreaks, pursuing epidemiological investigations with tireless energy.[2]

It was observed by W. Wernstedt in the 1911 epidemic that, if an outbreak visited a certain locale, in the next few years that area would be spared an epidemic. Wernstedt observed and reported that the areas hardest hit by the 1905 and 1908 epidemics had little activity during the major epidemic of 1911. He attributed this to a natural immunization process caused by past outbreaks. He also observed a reduced incidence of the disease in the following years due to this general natural immunization. Wernstedt is given credit for his observation about acquired immunity to the disease from inapparent infections.[2]

The abortive and nonparalytic cases were of major concern to public health officials and epidemiologists because of their ability to spread the disease and continue to transmit it. The paralytic phase confined a person to bed, so that the person was no longer out and about spreading the disease. To the family, and more so to the individual, the paralytic form of the disease was of major concern as it changed the lives and structure of families and in many cases ruined lives. Even though to Wickman both forms were equally infectious, the focus of the medical community seemed to be limited to the paralytic form of the disease. Attack rates of paralytic polio in rural areas was about 3.0 to 3.7 per 1,000. Wickman established that polio was not only a disease of the central nervous system, but that the disease was highly contagious, spread mainly through its subclinical infectious state, and biphasic in its course. All clinical studies done later in monkeys verified not only the clinical but the public health and epidemiological observations of Wickman.

In 1911, Kling and his team of virologists proved Wickman's observations to be correct; that is, that the mild or inapparent cases of the infection were indeed very contagious and thus of great concern in the spread of the disease. Kling and his colleagues, by isolating the pathogen in the mucous membranes, were able to show that the agent propagated itself in the mucous membranes and then penetrated them to cause the infection. The infection was spread by both the oral route and the feces route, with the feces/gastrointestinal route being more significant. Kling's virology studies confirmed the two phases of the disease, and that the abortive stage was as contagious as the paralytic phase. They also demonstrated that healthy carriers do exist during an epidemic. Studies showed that the virus persists in the throat for about two weeks in most cases, but that it could be there for as long as 180 days (6 months) and 200 days (7 months). The pathogen's ability to produce inflammation was reduced after the 14-day period, showing that the virus weakens after its acute stage.[2]

Rural Observations

Many investigations observed that rural areas often had more serious epidemics than urban areas. Wickman himself observed several times that epidemics often ravaged rural areas while sparing cities. In Sweden there was a tendency for polio to attack rural areas, especially remote villages in Sweden's sparsely settled countryside. Wickman was able to trace the movements of people during the epidemic. Ruralness seemed to contribute to the disease, due to the fact that lack of travel, remoteness of villages, and infrequent contact with outside people did not allow even a mild form of the disease to be experienced by rural folk, which would have produced immunity. Thus, outbreaks occurred often in rural areas, with the inevitable result of crippled children, partly due to a lack of immunity in infants and youth.[2]

Epidemic Curve

Wickman developed an epidemic curve of the cases. The epidemic curve for this Swedish outbreak was much like other disease outbreaks, a significant epidemiological point. For epidemic curves to occur, a population of susceptibles must be available, as well as a disease that has an identifiable course and time duration. The disease enters the population with a few cases, and as the pathogen is transmitted through the population, more and more cases occur. (See Herd Immunity in Chapter 2, Figures 2.8, 2.9.) Depending on the disease's incubation period and the usual course and duration of a case of the disease, the shorter the incubation and duration, the more pronounced the epidemic curve. What allows an epidemic to continue is the number of susceptibles in the population at risk. In a totally susceptible population, like that in the late 1800s and early 1900s in Sweden, the disease spreads like wildfire, and the epidemic curve is extreme and pronounced. What causes the epidemic to subside and diminish is the number of susceptibles left. Who is left to get the disease? The epidemic curve diminishes when susceptibles have become diseased or have died. The diseased recover and are now immune, or the still-healthy have fled and can no longer be exposed. The epidemic curve diminishes due to the recovery/immunity of the previously ill or the death of the diseased cases. Immunization/vaccination and mild cases of the disease reduce the susceptibles and stop an epidemic by herd immunity. Numbers of nonparalytic cases compared to paralytic cases vary from epidemic to epidemic. Ratio of paralytic to nonparalytic varies due to circumstances of the outbreaks.[2]

Not only did Wickman recognize that the pathogens often missed the CNS, but he realized that the abortive/nonparalytic cases actually outnumbered the paralytic cases. He learned quickly that paralysis was the dramatic side of the disease, but that if the infected cases were lucky enough to escape paralysis, they were no less contagious. Wickman observed that, in one village in the middle of the epidemic, more than half were of the nonparalytic type. He observed that the infection was spread mostly by the nonparalytic cases.[2]

Observed symptoms in nonparalytic types could be stiff neck, pain, stiffness in the back, or merely a fever. Wickman's colleagues viewed a diagnosis of infantile paralysis in the absence of paralysis as ridiculous. The skepticism would remain for many years to come.[2]

Wickman demanded that poliomyelitis be considered a highly contagious disease. Mild cases (abortive/nonparalytic cases) must also be taken seriously and considered just as contagious as paralytic cases because of their infectious nature. Wickman was as concerned with slightly ill cases and healthy carriers or inapparent cases as he was with full-blown paralytic cases. Clinical and laboratory evidence eventually proved this epidemiological observation to be true.[2]

In the summer of 1905, Wickman investigated an outbreak in a school near Tingsryd, a village of 3,000, with 18 cases occurring between August and October. The school was the primary site from which the infection spread. Twelve of the 18 attended the school, and the other 6 lived at the school. Six children from only 4 houses, who had no contact with any of the other 52 attending the school, also came down with the disease, considering both abortive and paralytic cases.[2]

Wickman held that the incubation period was 3 to 4 days to onset of the minor illness phase, with the time period to onset of fever in the paralytic phase being 8 to 10 days. Later, when studies were done with the live attenuated poliovirus vaccine, it was demonstrated that the incubation period to first onset was 3 to 4 days.[2]

Poliovirus Discovered

The poliovirus was discovered in 1908 in Vienna, by Karl Landsteiner and E. Popper.[2] In 1911, one of the worst polio epidemics of all time hit Sweden, with 3,840 cases. Scandinavia was labeled as the source and breeding ground of the polio disease, because much of the reported research occurred there; the 1911 epidemic further emphasized this negative image.[2]

The Swedish medical community, specifically the clinical virologists, were trying their best to understand and study the new findings about polio, especially because they now knew the agent was a poliovirus. In the 1911 epidemic, this presented an opportunity for a team from the State Bacteriological Institute in Stockholm to study the clinical and virological aspects of polio. The team was headed by Carl Kling.[2]

Carl Kling went to the Pasteur Institute after the 1911 epidemic subsided and became known as the world's leading authority on poliomyelitis. He was associated with the Pasteur Institute for 25 years and in 1919 was made director of the State Bacteriological Institute in Stockholm. He also made radio broadcasts about polio. He claimed that poliomyelitis was waterborne. He never married and died in 1967 at the age of 80, after 50 years of work on poliomyelitis.[2]

Kling and his team obtained tissue samples from victims who had died. Most importantly, they were able to recover poliovirus samples from various anatomical sites throughout the body, showing that the disease invaded more than just the CNS. The team also recovered samples of the poliovirus from living patients, proving that the abortive phase of the disease was just as communicable as the paralytic phase. They also were able to acquire samples of the virus in "healthy carriers."[2]

Kling and his colleagues knew the virus was a filterable virus and therefore could be separated from other material and used experimentally. They also knew that the virus caused lesions in the spinal cord and brain of monkeys and humans. The virus had been shown to be in the mucous membranes of the throat and nasal passages of monkeys as well as lymph nodes next to the small intestine (mesenteric lymph nodes). The agent was also found in the tonsils, pharyngeal mucous membranes, salivary glands of humans and monkeys, oropharynx, trachea, and, especially important, in the blood and the walls and contents of the small intestine. Fourteen fatal human cases of polio confirmed all the sites. Then 11 acutely ill patients provided specimens, and the poliovirus was recovered from basically all the same body sites in the live acute cases of the disease. Thus, monkey experiments, fatal/dead cases, and live acute cases all produced basically the same findings—that is, the pathogen was found in all the same sites throughout the body.[2]

Doubts by American researchers, physicians and scientists, and some Europeans concerning the presence of the pathogen in the gastrointestinal tract and rectum, as well as doubts concerning the virus's weakening over time, caused delays and setbacks in developing a vaccine well into the 1930s.[2]

Case Study Questions

B.1   Using the data below and a computer spreadsheet, create an epidemic curve bar graph.

Person/Disease: Cases of poliomyelitis recorded in Sweden

Place: Sweden

Time: Monthly reporting for the years of 1905, 1906, 1907; from January 1905 through July 1907

Frequency: For the y-axis of the graph: 50-case increments up to 400 cases

1905		Cases	1906		Cases	1907		Cases
Jan.	=	1	Jan.	=	48	Jan.	=	9
Feb.	=	5	Feb.	=	33	Feb.	=	9
Mar.	=	4	Mar.	=	36	Mar.	=	11
Apr.	=	4	Apr.	=	24	Apr.	=	6
May	=	8	May	=	41	May	=	5
Jun.	=	20	Jun.	=	15	Jun.	=	13
Jul.	=	138	Jul.	=	21	Jul.	=	51
Aug.	=	367	Aug.	=	32			
Sept.	=	242	Sept.	=	49			
Oct.	=	140	Oct.	=	22			
Nov.	=	69	Nov.	=	31			
Dec.	=	38	Dec.	=	24			

B.2   From the epidemic curve created in Study Question B.1 and what you have learned from this case thus far? Discuss the implications and observations of all *time* aspects of this disease. Discuss seasonal variation, cyclic trends, implication for duration of the disease, and incubation periods.

B.3   List the various names by which polio has been known.k

B.4   Discuss and explain the issues of age and its implications for the epidemiology of polio and infantile paralysis.

B.5   Why did physicians and epidemiologists have such a difficult time identifying outbreaks and the spread of polio? Explain and discuss in detail.

B.6   From your reading and study thus far, and from studying Figure 9.8, explain and discuss polio as a biphasic (two-phase) disease and the problems this two-phase process posed in investigating polio epidemics.

B.7   List the many epidemiological observations made by Wickman about infantile paralysis and its spread. Who later confirmed these observations, and how did he verify them?

B.8   What were the epidemiologist observations of Wernstedt?

B.9   Explain and discuss the terms *abortive case* and *anterior case*. What are other terms used for each of these two terms? Explain the role of these two terms in polio epidemics. What observations did Kling make about the abortive cases or phase?

B.10   When was the poliovirus discovered? Explain its characteristics and the locations in the body where it was originally discovered.

(C) FIRST MAJOR EPIDEMIC OF POLIOMYELITIS IN AMERICA: RUTLAND, VERMONT

It was in the summer of 1894 in Vermont that the first major United States poliomyelitis epidemic occurred. Charles S. Caverly, M.D., a practicing doctor, member of the state board of health and public health officer for the state of Vermont, presented a report on the epidemic. Caverly, though a very successful practicing physician, was excited about public health and epidemiology. He came from a rural area of a rural state, born in Troy, New Hampshire in 1856. He attended New Hampshire schools and Dartmouth College, graduating in 1878. He received his medical degree from the University of Vermont in 1881. He also did postgraduate work at the College of Physicians and Surgeons in New York City and was professor of hygiene and preventive medicine at the University of Vermont, from which he later received an honorary Sc.D. degree.

Caverly reported that, in Rutland county, there was an outbreak of an acute nervous disease that invariably was attended with some paralysis. The first cases occurred in Rutland and Wallingford about mid-June. The epidemic progressed through July into surrounding towns.

This first U.S. epidemic was the largest reported in the world thus far, with 132 documented cases. Six of the cases had no paralysis, but all had distinct nervous symptoms. Caverly was one of the first to recognize the abortive nonparalytic cases, even though he probably overlooked hundreds of them. This epidemic was also the first to be studied by a public health officer. From the advantage of his political position, Caverly was able to call meetings and coordinate the exchange of information.

Caverly was most diligent in his effort to identify each case. The previous summer, a small epidemic had occurred 125 miles away in Boston, making the outbreak in some nearby cities somewhat predictable. Public health officials have observed that poliomyelitis epidemics usually terminate when cold weather sets in and show up again in a neighboring city the next summer, much as they did in Scandinavia. (This makes epidemiological sense, as the new city is where susceptibles are now available. Those in the city of the recent outbreak had naturally acquired immunity yet interacted on a close personal basis for the disease to be communicated.) Caverly was able to show that the age distribution was much greater than previously reported (Dr. Mary Jacobi in 1886 had suggested that infantile paralysis was limited to children 18 months to 4 years of age.) Caverly reported cases (probably only paralytic cases) of 20 in the 9- to 12-year age range and 12 cases over age 15. The shift in age to include older age groups including adults (Franklin D. Roosevelt, the 32nd president of the United States, who served from 1933–1945, contracted poliomyelitis at age 39) was observed more frequently from this point on. Adults were not excluded from the Rutland epidemic, even though most cases occurred in children. Caverly attempted to classify cases according to sites of paralysis. The death rate from this epidemic was quite high at 13.5%. This figure held with later observations that the older the patient who contracted poliomyelitis, the greater the death rate. Caverly reported a curious observation—that the paralytic disease also affected domestic animals, with horses, dogs, and fowl dying with various types and degrees of paralysis. Dr. Charles Dana, professor of nervous diseases at Cornell University Medical College, verified that one of the fowls with paralysis of its legs had an acute poliomyelitis of the lower portion of the spinal cord. Yet Landsteiner in Vienna and Flexner could not produce cases of poliomyelitis in lower animals. Finally they turned to primates to produce experimental polio. Yet this paralytic disease has been reported throughout this era as occurring in domestic animals.

Caverly made some gross mistakes beyond the animal paralysis issue. He suggested that infantile paralysis was not contagious. He seemed to try to define the disease by the old Hippocratic theory of medicine—because heating is mentioned in 24 cases, and chilling of the body in only 4 cases, he determined that there was a general absence of infectious disease as a causative factor in the epidemic.

Despite his errors, Caverly made major contributions for his time; he was the first health officer and physician to do a major systematic study of an infantile paralysis epidemic, and he was the first to recognize and confirm the occurrence of nonparalytic cases.

Case Study Questions

C.1   What unique epidemiological observations and contributions about the epidemic of infantile paralysis were made by Dr. Caverly from his experience in rural Vermont?

C.2   What epidemiological observations did Dr Caverly make regarding age of infantile paralysis victims and polio epidemics?

C.3   What were some critical thinking and observational errors regarding epidemiology that were made by Dr. Caverly?

(D) SIMON FLEXNER, M.D. AND WADE HAMILTON FROST, M.D.: AMERICAN EPIDEMIOLOGISTS WHO INVESTIGATED POLIOMYELITIS

Flexner

When the news of Landsteiner's discovery of the poliovirus reached the United States, Simon Flexner, M.D., the new director of the Rockefeller Institute of Medical Research in New York City, took advantage of the opportunity the new discovery presented. The Rockefeller Institute was well funded, had just had much success in an attack on meningococcal meningitis, and had a well-equipped institute including facilities to handle primates, which was supported by a staff of qualified researchers.

Flexner was born in Louisville, Kentucky, in 1863. He attended local schools and received his medical degree from the University of Louisville in 1889 at age 26. He went on for postgraduate work at the newly established medical school that was the model for all medical schools in America, Johns Hopkins University School of Medicine, graduating in general and experimental pathology.

Abraham Flexner, Simon's brother and the dean of education at Johns Hopkins, concerned with the poor quality of medical education in the United States and Canada, and the lack of a standardized medical education, was also a noted figure at the time. Abraham visited and evaluated every medical school in the United States and Canada. Funded by the Carnegie Foundation, he presented his final report on the status of medical schools in 1910, which became known as the Flexner Report. From his findings, Abraham Flexner developed a model medical school curriculum based on the sciences and established Johns Hopkins University School of Medicine as the model and example for the rest of the country.

Simon Flexner was appointed associate professor of pathology and was later promoted to full professor at Johns Hopkins. He worked on several epidemics in Maryland, studying the pathology, epidemiology, and pathogenesis of various diseases. He spent time in the Philippines in 1899 studying tropical diseases in the local natives and U.S. armed forces personnel. He was responsible for identifying bacillary dysentery; the bacterium was referred to as the Flexner bacillus. He was also chairman of pathology at the University of Pennsylvania and took a directorship at the Ayer Clinical Laboratory at Pennsylvania Hospital in 1900. He served as chairman of the Federal Plague Commission to ascertain if there was an epidemic of bubonic plague in San Francisco in 1901. It was in 1903 that Simon Flexner took the post at the newly established Rockefeller Institute of Medical Research in New York.

New York had recently suffered through a poliomyelitis epidemic of about 750 to 1,200 cases in 1907. Flexner was appointed as one of 12 members of a committee appointed by the New York Neurological Society to study the polio epidemic. A report was finally produced by the committee in 1910 which included the findings of Landsteiner. Flexner also described in his work, supported by Dr. Martha Wollstein, that they had obtained samples of the pathogen from two fatal cases, one in New Jersey and one in New York in 1909. They inoculated monkeys and were able to pass the two strains from monkey to monkey in serial fashion, thus meeting Koch's second postulate (see pages 337, 389 and 390). Most of their work was on monkeys, yet they claimed that what occurred in primates was also true for humans, a statement the medical community questioned. Flexner himself noted that in different species of monkeys the poliovirus behaved differently making animal model research a bit unpredictable and making it hard to develop a protocol applicable to humans.

Simon Flexner, considered a laboratory doctor and one of the foremost experts on poliomyelitis at the time, did not have the answers for many practical questions of practicing doctors: How long was a case of poliomyelitis contagious? Why is it that poliomyelitis is contagious to some and not to others? And the key question at the time—How do you best treat poliomyelitis? The fact that the disease was known to be caused by a virus provided the general practice doctor with no cure or solution to treatment. Viruses are small, difficult to see, and mysterious. Much laboratory work was done by Flexner and his colleagues at the Rockefeller Institute and published in the *Journal of the American Medical Association* from 1909 to 1913 as news updates on poliomyelitis, again establishing Flexner as the expert on the disease.

In 1910 Flexner and his colleagues in the United States, and Landsteiner and his colleagues in Vienna, were able to demonstrate that the serum of monkeys that had recovered from experimental poliomyelitis contained antibodies (which Flexner called *germicidal substances*) that, when mixed with a small amount of active poliovirus, would actually neutralize or inactive the poliovirus and render it inert. Later, A. Netter and C. Levaditi in Paris, found the same antibodies in humans recovering from the disease. This was a landmark discovery that would benefit later vaccine research. For Flexner, this was the last major breakthrough, and his polio research started to subside, as did that of Landsteiner and his colleagues in Europe.

Stubbornly clinging to lines of thinking that are not accurate has plagued medicine from the very beginning. So it was with Flexner. He refused to accept certain clinical facts, which led him away from important discoveries, including virology as a method of clinical investigation. Flexner retired in 1935 from the Rockefeller Institute and died in 1946 before the poliovaccine was discovered and before the discovery that the poliovirus was indeed a family of viruses instead of being a single virus. Flexner was also faced with the separation at that time between practicing physicians and researchers. M.D.s were to practice medicine and not dabble in anything remotely resembling experimental research. During the 1911 epidemic in New York, Flexner worked at the Rockefeller Hospital instead of at the institute, rigidly clinging to the idea that physicians should practice their art at the bedside in the hospital, not in the laboratory. Thus, as a physician, he was not allowed to do testing in virology. Contention existed between the hospital medical director and Flexner because of the opposition to collaborative work among the physicians and the researchers. Meanwhile, the physicians wished to stretch their efforts beyond mundane medicine into the areas of research. The Rockefeller Hospital study, even though it included 200 cases, offered little insight beyond that provided by the Swedes.

Treatment offered by the Rockefeller groups was similar to that offered elsewhere: mild sedative, bed rest, and medication to control pain. From a public health perspective, cases should be treated like any other communicable disease—they should be made aware of their contagious conditions, be quarantined, and have disinfection carried out. In the wards with poliomyelitis cases, caps and long gowns were worn by those working with patients, hands were thoroughly scrubbed with soap and a nail brush, and soaked in a corrosive substance.

Two physicians, Rosenau and Brues, in 1912 set forth the theory that poliomyelitis was spread by the stable fly. W. H. Frost and a colleague (J. F. Anderson) were able to show experimentally that this was untrue. Frost relied on a clinical laboratory for his work, much as Flexner did, but also traveled the countryside, much like Wickman in Sweden, going door to door investigating poliomyelitis outbreaks. He gathered serum specimens for laboratory tests which in turn allowed statistical analysis. The use of statistics in epidemiology was greatly advanced by Frost in this era.[2]

Frost

W. H. Frost was born in 1880 in a village near the Blue Ridge Mountains of Virginia, in a family of 8 children of which he was number 7. His father was a country physician. Frost's early education was informal, as he was home-schooled by his mother. At age 15 he entered a military academy in Danville, Virginia, and later, another preparatory school. He attended the University of Virginia, graduating in 1898, went on to medical school there, and was granted his M.D. degree in 1903. He did an internship at St. Vincent's Hospital in Norfolk, Virginia. He broke family tradition and did not follow his father and grand-father to become a country doctor, but instead became a commissioned officer in the Public Health and Marine Service, as an assistant surgeon at the Marine Hospital in Baltimore. He was introduced to epidemiology when he was assigned to a yellow fever epidemic in New Orleans. From his experience in the Public Health and Marine Service, Frost learned basic public health and epidemiological skills, and insights such as observing the disease in a number of different settings.

Frost contributed much to the epidemiology of polio from 1910 to 1930. He quickly grasped the importance of knowing how polio was spread and is credited with establishing a strong foundation of statistics as a basis for epidemiological study. He was considered one of America's leading epidemiologists in the 1920s and 1930s.

In 1908 Frost was assigned to the Hygienic Laboratory. Two years later, after investigating pellagra, tetanus, typhoid, and water pollution, he was assigned to field investigations of poliomyelitis epidemics, even though he had limited knowledge of the disease. He and J. F. Anderson, the new director of the Hygienic Laboratory, learned quickly, and their involvement with this new disease led to the composition of a 50-page monograph on poliomyelitis, which they called a *précis*. This document contained subject matter not included in Wickman's 300-page monograph and not covered by the Rockefeller Institute of Medical Science. Frost would eventually become dean of the School of Hygiene and Public Health at Johns Hopkins University.[2]

Frost and Anderson addressed and recorded age of the onset of cases in various epidemics in different environmental conditions. Frost, like Wickman, observed that the disease was more contagious than medical science believed at the time, and was quick to point out that direct contact was probably one of the main means of disease transmission. Frost observed in the 1910 epidemic that the disease was transmissible from person to person, probably by direct contact, and appeared to be highly contagious under some circumstances, affecting a considerable proportion of the population of a limited area.[2]

For a short time, the stable fly and other biting insects were implicated as possible vectors of the poliovirus. Anderson and Frost in 1912–1913 tested the stable fly and showed that vectors were not generally involved in the disease's transmission. Frost had worked on poliomyelitis epidemics in Mason City, Iowa, in 1910; Cincinnati, Ohio, in 1911; and Buffalo and Batavia, New York, in 1912. He knew from experience and first-hand observation that vectors were not implicated in disease transmission but direct person-to-person contact was. Frost was able to observe the disease in different environments and settings, including large cities, small towns, and rural areas. Not since Wickman in Sweden had any other epidemiologist so painstakingly completed statistical studies on epidemics. No other epidemiologist had been afforded the opportunity to make scientific observations and draw learned conclusions on the three dimensions of investigation: close clinical observation, laboratory experiments, and statistical analysis. Frost, like Wickman, had used spot maps to mark the location of the residences of paralytic, abortive, and suspicious cases.[2]

Frost's Epidemiological Methods

Frost was able to observe increases and decreases in incidence and prevalence in rural versus city settings. He made seasonal and meteorological charts surrounding the times of epidemics. Included in his investigations were other observations of epidemics, such as sanitary conditions of individual cases, milk supply, food supply, observation of paralytic cases in humans and domestic animals, and the presence and absence of flies, mosquitoes, and other insects. His knowledge base was founded on house-to-house surveys, countless clinical observations, statistical analysis of the findings, and years of community-based experience, all confirming that poliomyelitis was spread by direct contact.[2]

Frost came to a most fundamental epidemiological conclusion: that an accurate diagnosis must be made before an investigation can proceed. In the case of poliomyelitis, the abortive case—those without paralytic symptoms—must be identified, as they are so numerous as to be of great epidemiological significance. Thus, Frost was able to use the laboratory to achieve a more accurate diagnosis of the poliomyelitis in all types of cases. He was able to collect serum samples from 9 cases in the Iowa epidemic and, with the help of Anderson, analyzed them, thus proving Flexner as well as Netter and Levaditi of France incorrect in their assumptions based on monkey experiments: that the blood of victims recovered from the disease (in monkeys at least) did not contain poliovirus. Frost showed that abortive or inapparent infections of poliomyelitis did indeed contain the antibodies.

Frost and Anderson were always extremely cautious in their claims and reports, which often weakened their position and respect. They were hesitant to make any strong affirmative stance on their discoveries for fear they would not be accepted. The investigators at the hospital of the Rockefeller Institute heard of the findings on Frost's work and themselves went on to show that human sera from recovered adults *did* have high amounts of polio antibiotics, much as paralytic patients did.

Frost was the first to use such a combination of methods and such a sophisticated arsenal against poliomyelitis, yet he was overly cautious. He observed that during epidemics the incidence of the disease was affected by susceptibility to the infection. Age was one of the key observations about poliomyelitis, with susceptibility being limited to the first half-decade of life and the risk diminishing thereafter. (Naturally acquired immunity probably accounted for this factor; either the victim had a mild case and was no longer susceptible, or had a bad case and died, or was paralyzed. Once an epidemic had passed through a community, the disease was no longer contagious until a new crop of susceptibles in the form of new children came along.) Early on, the lack of understanding of the role of the abortive, mild, or inapparent cases in a population caused Frost to conclude that widespread immunization of the population against the disease was unjustifiably radical. Frost was able to share his vast experience of poliomyelitis investigation in the 1916 epidemic.

Case Study Questions

D.1   What were the epidemiological limitations of Flexner's work on polio? List and discuss several of these limitations.

D.2   Who was Dr. Frost, and what were his contributions to epidemiological investigations of infantile paralysis/polio?

D.3   What did Dr. Frost contribute in the way of understanding modes of disease transmission in poliomyelitis?

D.4   Which specific methodologies and approaches was Dr. Frost able to use and establish as solid epidemiological methodology?

(E) POLIOMYELITIS EPIDEMIC IN LOS ANGELES, 1934

By the spring of 1934, a great deal was known about poliomyelitis. The mode of transmission was known to be person to person, the two-phase process of the disease was well understood, and mild nonparalytic infections or anterior poliomyelitis as well as paralytic infections were all understood to be major means of contagion. Animals and most insects were eliminated as vectors. It was known that some victims would die in a few days, some would have crippling paralysis, and others would recover without a sign. The poliovirus had been isolated and identified from most parts of the body—most importantly, the central nervous system; blood; saliva; gastrointestinal tract, especially the small intestine; mesenteric lymph nodes, and nasopharynx. The damage caused by the poliovirus was known to be done in the spinal cord's anterior horn of the gray matter and in brain tissue.[2]

When the poliomyelitis epidemic hit Los Angeles, many horror stories from past epidemics had been deeply implanted in the minds of medical and nursing professionals. It appears that the medical professionals at the time were well informed about the facts of poliomyelitis, yet most ignored them and, moreover, failed to inform the public. The Contagious Unit of the Los Angeles County General Hospital was responsible for most of the activities of the epidemic, and fear of the disease seemed to dominate its efforts, in spite of evidence that much of the sickness that occurred in June of 1934 was not poliomyelitis.[2]

Physicians and nurses were strained, worried, and terrified of contracting the disease themselves. By June 15, 50 cases a day were being admitted to most hospitals, yet by June 29, only 1 fatal case of poliomyelitis had occurred, producing a sample of the poliovirus. A second case produced another sample on July 4.[2]

When the Poliomyelitis Commission arrived in Los Angeles from Yale University School of Medicine, headed by Dr. Leslie T. Webster of the Rockefeller Institute of Medical Science of New York City, a public meeting was held to review the situation of the epidemic. The meeting digressed to physicians' and nurses' discussing their risk of getting poliomyelitis and whether or not they might receive disability pensions if paralyzed by the disease and disabled in the line of duty.[2]

New interns in training at the Los Angeles County Hospital were deprived of teaching and proper guidance, because the attending physicians were afraid of getting the disease and stayed away, consulting by phone instead of going to the hospital. Doctors who worked at the County Hospital in the communicable disease wards were not welcome on house calls because their patients viewed the hospital as a pest house.[2]

No one knew how much of the disease outbreak that year was really polio. Nearly all adults, especially the nurses and doctors, were afraid of getting paralytic polio. In those who got the serious form of the disease, health care providers observed much pain and weakness. But very few deaths occurred. The number of cases of paralysis was much lower than one would expect. The question was, Could it be another virus or a different strain of the virus? Dr. Webster believed that 90% of the cases were actually not poliomyelitis.[2]

Researchers had little success in searching for the poliovirus in the nasal passages of suspected victims through nasal washings. The disease could not be produced in monkeys or lab animals. Webster believed that the problem was complex and that the infantile part of infantile paralysis was missing, because most cases were in adults. The paralysis phase of the disease was also missing, as no paralysis occurred in most cases.[2]

Oral washings with ropy (an adhesive, stringy-type thread that was soaked in a special solution and swirled around in the throat in order to capture samples of mucous tissue) were done routinely. Ropy washes were able to gather even a few flakes of mucus and the debris in it. The ropy washes used a special solution that helped save samplings of potential poliovirus evidence, and preserved the specimens for months (101 days) for later study. Even after such a long time, the specimens could be spun in a centrifuge and yield the virus, so in future outbreaks, disease investigators would not need to take an army of public health workers along to gather specimens.[2]

Hysteria raged on in the main populace. Not only was the general public afraid of getting the disease, but a major part of the medical and nursing profession was also participating in the fear. Yet officials were not daring enough to tell the public that the disease was not polio. It was disclosed that half of the 1,301 suspected cases were not poliomyelitis. The actual attack rate was estimated to be from 4.4% to 10.7%.[2]

There was no doubt that Los Angeles was visited by an epidemic of poliomyelitis in the summer of 1934, but it was a mild one. Most of the people who were sick that summer were sick either from another disease (encephalitis, meningitis, or influenza) or from a mild form or a different strain of the poliovirus. Patients had atypical symptoms for polio, and the observed symptoms were rheumatoidal or influenzal with striking emotional tones of fear that they might get polio. It was observed by U.S. Public Health Service officer Dr. A. G. Gilliam, of the Los Angeles County Hospital's personnel, "Irrespective of actual mechanisms of spread and identity of the disease, this outbreak has no parallel in the history of poliomyelitis or any other CNS infections."[2]

As an unfortunate outcome of this epidemic and its resulting hysteria, patients who exhibited even a slight degree of weakness were immobilized in plaster casts. This was a common practice in the 1930s and many were subjected unnecessarily to this treatment.

Case Study Questions

E.1   By 1934 a great deal was known about poliomyelitis. Summarize all that was known about all facets of the epidemiology of polio.

E.2   How serious was the polio epidemic of 1934? What were the social, psychological, and political implications and their effects on the epidemiology of polio surrounding this case?

E.3   What were the final conclusions about the polio epidemic of 1934 in Los Angeles, and what were the implications for the future?

EPILOGUE

Polio epidemics continued across America. The last national poliomyelitis epidemic was in the early 1950s. In 1954, Dr. Jonas E. Salk began immunizing with killed (formalin-inactivated poliomyelitis viruses) vaccine, called the *poliovirus vaccine*, and later Albert B. Sabin developed the live vaccine, called the *oral poliovirus vaccine*, usually taken orally in sugar cubes. In the late 1980s, post-polio syndrome was discovered, and investigations of this late phase of poliomyelitis have continued.

REFERENCES

1. Berkow, R. (Editor). 1982. *The Merck Manual of Diagnosis and Therapy*, 14th edition. Rahway, NJ: Merck, Sharp and Dohme.
2. Paul, J.R. 1971. *A History of Poliomyelitis*. New Haven, CT: Yale University Press.
3. Millard, F.P. 1918. *Poliomyelitis (Infantile Paralysis)*. Kirksville, MO: Journal Printing Company.
4. Smith, J.S. 1990. *Patenting the Sun*. New York: William Morrow and Company.
5. Rogers, N. 1990. *Dirt and Disease*. New Brunswick, NJ: Rutgers University Press.

II

Epidemiological Associations and Societies

American College of Epidemiology (ACE)
c/o Michigan Cancer Foundation
110 E. Warren
Detroit, MI 48201
Phone: (313) 833-0710   FAX: (313) 831-8714
Founded: 1979
Publication: *Annals of Epidemiology* (quarterly)

American Epidemiological Society (AES)
c/o Dr. Phillip S. Brachman
Emory University
School of Public Health
1599 Clifton NE
Atlanta, GA 30329
Phone: (404) 727-0199
Founded: 1927
Publication: none

American Public Health Association (APHA)
Epidemiology Section
1015 15th St. NW
Washington, DC 20005
Phone: (202) 789-5600   TDD 789-5673
Founded: 1872
Publications: *American Journal of Public Health* (monthly), *Nations Health* (monthly)

American Society for Microbiology
Executive Director, Dr. Michael I. Goldberg
1325 Massachusetts Avenue, NW
Washington, DC 20005
Phone: (202) 737-3600
Founded: 1883
Publications: *Clinical Microbiology Reviews; Journal of Virology; Antimicrobial Agents and Chemotherapy; Applied and Environmental Microbiology; International Journal of*

Systematic Bacteriology; Journal of Clinical Microbiology; Microbiological Reviews; Infection and Immunity; Journal of Bacteriology; Molecular and Cellular Biology; and *Clinical and Diagnostic Laboratory Immunology*

Association for Professionals in Infection Control and Epidemiology (APIC)
P.O. Box 79502
Baltimore, MD 21279-0502
Publication: *American Journal of Infection Control*

Council of State and Territorial Epidemiologists (CSTE)
c/o Dr. McWilson Warren
20 Executive Park W., Suite 2018
Atlanta, GA 30329
Phone: (404) 982-0878
Founded: 1951
Publication: *CSTE Update* (quarterly)

International Epidemiological Association (DEA)
c/o Roger Detels, M.D.
University of California Los Angeles
School of Public Health, Rm. 71-269CHS
Department of Epidemiology
Los Angeles, CA 90024
Phone: (310) 206-2837
Founded: 1950
Publication: *International Journal of Epidemiology* (quarterly)

National Foundation for Infectious Diseases (NFID)
4733 Bethesda Avenue
Suite 750
Bethesda, Maryland 20814
Founded: 1973
E-Mail: nfid@aol.com

Society for Epidemiological Research (SER)
c/o Joseph L. Lyon, M.D.
Dept. of Family and Preventive Medicine
50 N. Medical Dr., 1C26
Salt Lake City, UT 84132
Phone: (801) 581-7234
Founded: 1967
Publication: *American Journal of Epidemiology* (bimonthly)

The Society for Healthcare Epidemiology of American (SHEA)
875 Kings Highway, Suite 200
Woodbury, NJ 08096-3172
Phone: (609) 845-1636   FAX: (609) 853-0411
Founded: 1980
Publications: *Infection Control and Hospital Epidemiology; Clinical Performance and Quality Health*

III

Epi Info and Epi Map Epidemiology Software

EPI INFO

What Is Epi Info, Version 6?

Epi Info is a series of microcomputer programs for handling epidemiologic data in questionnaire format and for organizing study designs and results into text that may form part of written reports. A questionnaire can be set up and processed in a few minutes, but Epi Info can also form the basis for a powerful disease surveillance system database with many files and record types. It includes features used by epidemiologists in statistical programs such as SAS or SPSS and database programs like dBASE. Unlike commercial programs, however, Epi Info may be freely copied and given to friends and colleagues.

There are three levels of facilities in Epi Info for processing questionnaire or other structured data. Using Epi Info on the simplest level, you can computerize a questionnaire or investigation form in a few minutes by:

- Running the main menu.
- Typing the questionnaire or form with EPED, the word processor, or another word processing program.
- Entering data in the questionnaire using the ENTER program.
- Analyzing the data using the ANALYSIS program to produce lists, frequencies, crosstabulations, means, graphs, and accompanying statistics.

As your knowledge of the program grows, you will use additional features to shape data entry and analysis to your needs. You will probably want to:

- Insert error checking, skip patterns, and automatic coding in the questionnaire using the CHECK program.
- Select records, create new variables, recode data, manipulate dates, and carry out conditional operations with IF statements during ANALYSIS.
- Incorporate these operations into program files so that they can be performed repeatedly or by other persons unfamiliar with programming.

- Import and export files from other systems like SAS, SPSS, dBASE, and Lotus 1-2-3.
- Change the names of variables in the data file using the CHECK program.

The third level of features is important if you are setting up a permanent database system, a large study, or want to customize Epi Info's operations to suit special 12 needs. For such purposes, you can:

- Program the data entry process to include mathematical operations, logical checks, color changes, pop-up boxes, and custom routines, written in other languages.
- Specify the format of reports from ANALYSIS to produce customized tables.
- Enter data into more than one file during the same session, moving automatically among several questionnaires within ENTER.
- Link several different types of files together in ANALYSIS so that questions can be answered that require data from more than one file.
- Compare duplicate files entered by different operators to detect data entry errors.

EPED, the editor included with Version 6, contains a programming system for text, called EPIAID, which parallels Epi Info's facilities for structured data. Programs are included to guide you through the creation of questionnaires and the design of an epidemic investigation. The text produced can be used as part of an investigation report. EPIAID programs can be written to assist in letter writing or production of reports for other purposes.

Version 6 of Epi Info contains many new features, such as a configurable pull-down menu system, new commands for programming data entry and analysis, the capacity to sort and relate very large files, a program to analyze data from complex sample surveys, a new epidemiologic calculator, and a batch processing program for nutritional anthropometry. Files created by previous versions of Epi Info can be used in Version 6. With a few revisions, programs written for Version 5 can be run in Version 6.

EPI INFO can be obtained free of charge and downloaded from the home page of the Centers for Disease Control and Prevention's Epidemiology Program Office's home page (see Appendix IV).

EPI MAP

What Is Epi Map 2?

Version 1.0 released:	April 1993
Version 1.01 released:	June 1994
Version 2.0 released:	December 1995
Version 2.01 released:	January 1997

Epi Map is a program for IBM-compatible microcomputers that displays data using geographic or other maps. Data values may be entered from the keyboard or supplied in Epi Info or dBASE files. The data may be counts, rates, or other numeric values. In Color/Pattern maps, the values are represented as shading or color patterns for each geographic entity. In Dot Density maps, randomly placed dots proportional in number to the values are placed in each entity. Epi Map also produces Cartograms, in which the value for each geographic entity is allowed to control the size of the entity.

Outline maps are supplied with Epi Map, and others can be created or edited within Epi Map. A complete map can be traced from a transparency in less than an hour in many cases—with less trouble than locating a suitably digitized "ready-made" map.

The text of the Epi Map Manual is contained in the help file accessible from Help (<F1>) on the main menu. Copies may be printed in plain text format or with illustrations and better typography, from a Microsoft Word (Version 6) file available via the Internet (see below).

Epi Map is designed to work independently or as a companion to Epi Info, a system of computer programs produced by CDC and the World Health Organization, providing public-domain software for word processing, database, and statistics work in public health.

EPI MAP can be obtained free of charge and downloaded from the home page of the Centers for Disease Control and Prevention's Epidemiology Program Office's home page (see Appendix IV).

APPENDIX

IV

Internet Sites

(All Internet addresses are preceded with http://)

Census Bureau
www.census.gov/

Centers for Disease Control and Prevention Search—CDC Search
www.cdc.gov/search.htm

Communicable Disease Surveillance Centre, United Kingdom
www.open.gov.uk/cdsc/cdschome.htm

Emerging Infectious Diseases (Journal—CDC)
www.cdc.gov/ncidod

Emerging Infectious Diseases and the Law
www.cdc.gov./ncidod/eid/vol12no4/fidler.htm

Emory University School of Public Health plus links
www.gen.emory.edu/MEDWEB/medweb.html

Epidemiology Links and Information, University of California San Francisco
www.epibiostat.ucsf.edu/epidem/epidem.html

Epidemiology Naval Research Studies
mac088.nhrc.navy.mil.default.htm

Epidemiology Program Office, Centers for Disease Control and Prevention
www.cdc.gov/epo/index.htm

FEDSTATS—70 agencies that produce statistics
www.fedstats.gov/regional.html

HCFA (Health Care Financing Administration) home page
www.hcfa.gov/

HCFA (Health Care Financing Administration) Stats and Data
www.hcfa.gov/stats/stats.htm

Infection Control Association
www.medscape.com/shea

Morbidity and Mortality Weekly Report
www.gen.gov/epo/mmwr/mmwr.html

National Center for Chronic Disease Prevention and Health Promotion (CDC)
www.cdc.gov/nccdphp/nccdhome.htm

National Center for Environmental Health (CDC)
www.cdc.gov.nceh/ncehhome.htm

National Center for Health Statistics
www.cdc.gov/nchs.www/nchshome.htm

National Center for Injury Prevention and Control (CDC)
www.cdc.gov/ncipc/ncipchm.htm

National Institute for Occupational Safety and Health (NIOSH) (CDC)
www.cdc.gov/niosh/home page.html

National Institutes of Health
www.nih.gov/

National Library of Medicine
www.hm.hlm.nih.gov/

Scientific data, surveillance, health statistics, and laboratory information
www.cdc.gov/scientific.htm

Social Statistical Briefing Room—Health Statistics—White House
www.whitehouse.gov/fsbr/health.html

Statistical agencies
www.fedstats.gov/index20.html

Statistics and epidemiological information from the World Health Organization
www.who.ch/whosis/whosis.htm

Tuberculosis reference from the Department of Informatics of Columbia University and
the New York City Bureau of Tuberculosis Control
www.cmpc.columbia,edu/tbcpp/

Vital Statistics of the United States
www.cdc.gov/nchswww/products/pubs/pubd/vsus/1985/1985.htm

Weekly Epidemiological Record
www.who.ch/wer/wer_home.htm

World Health Organization
www.who.ch/welcome.html

Yale University Biomedicine: History of Science, Technology and Medicine
http:info.med.yale.edu/library/resources/history/

Yale University Epidemiology and Public Health Library
www.library.yale.edu/eph.html

Index